Clinical Problems, Injuries and Complications of Gynecologic and Obstetric Surgery

Third Edition

"Chance favors only the prepared mind."

Louis Pasteur, 1854

Clinical Problems, Injuries and Complications of Gynecologic and Obstetric Surgery

Third Edition

Edited by

David H. Nichols, M.D.

*Visiting Professor of Obstetrics, Gynecology,
and Reproductive Biology
Harvard Medical School
Chief of Pelvic Surgery
The Women's Care Division of the
Massachusetts General Hospital
Boston, Massachusetts*

John O. L. DeLancey, M.D.

*Associate Professor of Obstetrics and Gynecology
University of Michigan School of Medicine
Director, Division of Gynecology
Department of Obstetrics and Gynecology
University of Michigan Medical Center
Ann Arbor, Michigan*

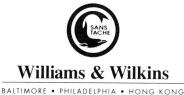

Williams & Wilkins

BALTIMORE • PHILADELPHIA • HONG KONG
LONDON • MUNICH • SYDNEY • TOKYO

A WAVERLY COMPANY

Editor: Charles W. Mitchell
Project Manager: Victoria M. Vaughn
Copy Editor: Susan Zorn
Designer: Wilma E. Rosenberger
Illustration Planner: Lorraine Wrzosek

Copyright © 1995
Williams & Wilkins
428 East Preston Street
Baltimore, Maryland 21202, USA

Accurate indications, adverse reactions, and dosage schedules for drugs are provided in this book, but it is possible that they may change. The reader is urged to review the package information data of the manufacturers of the medications mentioned.

Printed in the United States of America

First Edition 1983
Second Edition 1988

Library of Congress Cataloging-In-Publication Data

Clinical problems, injuries and complications of gynecologic and obstetric surgery / edited by David
H. Nichols, John O. L. DeLancey—3rd ed.
       p. cm.
  Rev ed. of: Clinical problems, injuries, and complications of gynecologic surgery, 2nd ed. c1988.
  Includes bibliographical references and index.
  ISBN 0-683-06497-5
  1. Generative organs, Female—Surgery—Complications—Case studies. 2. Obstetrics—Surgery—
Complications—Surgery. I. Nichols, David H., 1925– . II. DeLancey, John O. L. III. Clinical problems,
injuries, and complications of gynecologic surgery.
  [DNLM: 1. Genitalia, Female—surgery. 2. Genital Diseases, Female—surgery. 3. Surgery, Opera-
tive—adverse effects. 4. Wounds and Injuries. 5. Postoperative Complications. WP 660 C641 1995]
RG104.2.C55 1995
618' .0459—dc20
DNLM/DLC   94-44911
for Library of Congress   CIP

                                        94 95 96 97 98
                                 1 2 3 4 5 6 7 8 9 10

This book is dedicated to Raymond A. Lee, M.D., George W. Morley, M.D., and John D. Thompson, M.D.—three most exemplary models as effective teachers of gynecologic surgery throughout the world. Each has shown that there is no better task than to strive for perfection both in decision making and technical skills, which go hand-in-hand in the operating room.

PREFACE

During the seven years since publication of the second edition of this book, much new surgery has appeared in the armamentarium of the gynecologic surgeon. Operative laparoscopy and aspects of laser therapy have become more widely embraced. Surgeons need to be comfortable with transvaginal, transabdominal, and translaparoscopic surgical solutions to frequent problems so that they may choose the best alternatives from a wide range of choices, responding to the specific needs of the patient rather than limiting choices to specific procedures with which they are familiar.

Cost-effectiveness is essential in surgical practice today. We must reduce when possible the length of hospital stay by preventing surgical complications or, failing that, recognizing them promptly so that appropriate treatment is instituted without delay.

The original intent of *Clinical Problems, Injuries and Complications of Gynecologic and Obstetric Surgery* remains the same: to stimulate resourceful thinking in the surgically inclined reader, who will develop solutions to all problems and choose from them those that best fit the needs of each particular patient. To these ends, chapters have been added, others updated, and a few chapters deleted. A number of new and respected authors are included in this new edition.

The editors again acknowledge that many surgical problems have several alternate and effective solutions, but each author was asked for his or her reasoning for a particular solution. The reader is urged to study the chapter abstract and mentally prepare a response to the problem, then read the remainder of the chapter to understand the author's conclusion, recommendation, and reasoning. These problems and their solutions are without provincial boundaries, and are truly international. Former collaborator Dr. George W. Anderson, a dedicated and thoughtful teacher, has retired from professional duties, and the senior author welcomes a respected colleague, John O. L. DeLancey, as coeditor. Our work together on this edition has been both pleasant and productive, and we look forward to its continuation in future editions.

David H. Nichols, M.D.
John O. L. DeLancey, M.D.

ACKNOWLEDGMENTS

Respectful and friendly appreciation is expressed to the publisher's senior editor Charles W. Mitchell for his enthusiasm and encouragement, to project manager Vicki Vaughn for her patient and effective persistence in keeping the project moving always in a forward direction, and to artist Lori Vaskalis for her prompt response to our needs.

CONTRIBUTORS

Barrie Anderson, M.D., *Professor and Director of Fellowship Program, Gynecologic Oncology, Department of Obstetrics and Gynecology, University of Iowa Hospitals and Clinics, Iowa City, Iowa*

Michael Aronson, M.D., *Assistant Professor of Obstetrics and Gynecology, Tufts University School of Medicine; Director, Division of Urogynecology/Pelvic Reconstructive Surgery, New England Medical Center, Boston, Massachusetts*

Ricardo M. Azziz, M.D., *Associate Professor of Obstetrics and Gynecology, Department of Obstetrics and Gynecology, The University of Alabama at Birmingham, Birmingham, Alabama*

Jerome L. Belinson, M.D., *Chairman, Department of Gynecology, Cleveland Clinic Foundation, Cleveland, Ohio*

James L. Breen, M.D., *Chairman, Department of Obstetrics and Gynecology, Saint Barnabas Medical Center, Livingston, New Jersey*

Douglas Brown, Ph.D., *Ethics Curriculum Consultant, Department of Obstetrics and Gynecology, Louisiana State University, New Orleans, Louisiana*

Sheila E. Buchbinder, M.D., *Senior Attending, Department of Obstetrics and Gynecology, Overlook Hospital, Summit, New Jersey*

R. Clay Burchell, M.D., *Retired Chair, Department of Obstetrics and Gynecology, Lovelace Medical Center; Clinical Professor, Department of Obstetrics and Gynecology, University of New Mexico School of Medicine, Albuquerque, New Mexico*

John W. Caldwell, J.D., *Special Assistant U.S. Attorney, Department of Justice, El Paso, Texas*

Denis Cavanagh, M.D., *Professor and Director, Division of Gynecologic Oncology, Department of Obstetrics and Gynecology, University of South Florida College of Medicine, Tampa, Florida*

William A. Cliby, M.D., *Assistant Professor, Department of Obstetrics and Gynecology, Division of Gynecologic Surgery, Mayo Clinic, Rochester, Minnesota*

John T. Comerci, Jr., M.D., *Instructor, Department of Obstetrics and Gynecology, Division of Gynecologic Oncology, Albert Einstein College of Medicine, Bronx, New York*

William T. Creasman, M.D., *Sims Hestor Professor and Chairman, Department of Obstetrics and Gynecology, Medical University of South Carolina, Charleston, South Carolina*

William E. Crisp, M.D., *Professor, Cancer Research Institute, Arizona State University, Phoenix, Arizona*

Alan H. DeCherney, M.D., *Professor and Chairman, Department of Obstetrics and Gynecology, Tufts University School of Medicine, Boston, Massachusetts*

John O. L. DeLancey, M.D., *Associate Professor, Chief, Division of Gynecology, Department of Obstetrics and Gynecology, University of Michigan Medical Center, Ann Arbor, Michigan*

Julian E. De Lia, M.D., *Associate Professor, Department of Obstetrics and Gynecology, Medical College of Wisconsin, Milwaukee, Wisconsin*

Philip J. DiSaia, M.D., *The Dorothy Marsh Chair in Reproductive Biology, Professor, Department of Obstetrics and Gynecology, University of California, Irvine, Orange, California*

Bruce H. Drukker, M.D., *Professor and Chairperson, Department of Obstetrics, Gynecology and Reproductive Biology, Michigan State University, East Lansing, Michigan*

Thomas E. Elkins, M.D., *Abe Mickal Professor and Head, Department of Obstetrics and Gynecology, Louisiana State University School of Medicine in New Orleans, New Orleans, Louisiana*

Tommy N. Evans, M.D., *Professor Emeritus, Department of Obstetrics and Gynecology, Good Samaritan Regional Medical Center, Phoenix, Arizona*

Augusto G. Ferrari, M.D., *Professor of Clinical Obstetrics and Gynecology, Chairman, Department of Obstetrics and Gynecology, Instituto Scientifico H.S. Raffaele, University of Milan, Milan, Italy*

Charles E. Flowers, Jr., M.D., *Distinguished Professor and Chairman Emeritus, Department of Obstetrics and Gynecology, University of Alabama, Birmingham, Alabama*

Luigi Frigerio, M.D., *Clinical Associate in Obstetrics and Gynecology, Instituto Scientifico H.S. Raffaele, University of Milan, Milan, Italy*

Arlan B. Fuller, Jr., M.D., *Assistant Professor of Obstetrics and Gynecology, Harvard Medical School; Director, Gynecologic Oncology Service, Department of Gynecology, Massachusetts General Hospital, Boston, Massachusetts*

Phillip C. Galle, M.D., *Reproductive Endocrinology, Springfield, Illinois*

Donald G. Gallup, M.D., *Professor, Department of Obstetrics and Gynecology, Section of Gynecologic Oncology, Medical College of Georgia, Augusta, Georgia*

Celso-Ramón García, M.D., *The William Shippen, Jr. Emeritus Professor of Obstetrics and Gynecology, Department of Obstetrics and Gynecology, University of Pennsylvania Medical Center, Philadelphia, Pennsylvania*

Ray V. Haning, Jr., M.D., *Associate Professor of Obstetrics and Gynecology, Brown University Program in Medicine; Director, Gynecologic Endocrinology, Women's and Infants Hospital, Providence, Rhode Island*

Michael P. Hopkins, M.D., *Professor, Department of Obstetrics and Gynecology, Northeastern Ohio Universities College of Medicine; Chairman, Department of Obstetrics and Gynecology, Akron General Medical Center, Akron, Ohio*

William J. Hoskins, M.D., *Chief, Gynecology Service, Avon Chair of Gynecologic Oncology Research, Department of Surgery, Memorial Sloan-Kettering Cancer Center, New York, New York*

William W. Hurd, M.D., *Associate Professor, Obstetrics and Gynecology, University of Michigan, Ann Arbor, Michigan*

W. Glenn Hurt, M.D., *Professor, Department of Obstetrics and Gynecology, Medical College of Virginia, Virginia Commonwealth University, Richmond, Virginia*

John H. Isaacs, M.D., *Professor Emeritus, Department of Obstetrics and Gynecology, Loyola University of Chicago, Maywood, Illinois*

Howard W. Jones, Jr., M.D., *Professor, Department of Obstetrics and Gynecology, Eastern Virginia Medical School, Norfolk, Virginia*

John C. Lathrop, M.D., *Clinical Associate Professor, Department of Obstetrics and Gynecology, Brown University, Providence, Rhode Island*

Raymond A. Lee, M.D., *Professor, Department of Obstetrics and Gynecology, Division of Gynecologic Surgery, Mayo Clinic, Rochester, Minnesota*

Lewis Russell Malinak, M.D., *Professor, Vice Chairman of Clinical Affairs, Department of Obstetrics and Gynecology, Baylor College of Medicine, Houston, Texas*

Donald E. Marsden, M.D., *Professor of Obstetrics and Gynecology, Hobart University School of Medicine, Hobart, Tazmania, Australia*

Kathleen Martin, M.D., *Department of Obstetrics and Gynecology, Rochester General Hospital, Rochester, New York*

Fred M. Massey, M.D., *Clinical Professor, Department of Obstetrics and Gynecology, The University of Texas Health Science Center at San Antonio, San Antonio, Texas*

Byron J. Masterson, M.D., *J. Wayne Reitz Professor and Chairman, Department of Obstetrics and Gynecology, University of Florida College of Medicine, Gainesville, Florida*

Henry C. McDuff, M.D., *Clinical Professor of Gynecology, Emeritus, Brown University Medical School, Providence, Rhode Island*

Edward J. McGuire, M.D., *Director, Division of Urology, University of Texas, Houston, Texas*

Abe Mickal, M.D., *Emeritus Professor and Chairman, Department of Obstetrics and Gynecology, Louisiana State University, New Orleans, Louisiana*

John J. Mikuta, M.D., *Franklin Payne Professor, Gynecologic Oncology, Department of Obstetrics and Gynecology, University of Pennsylvania School of Medicine, Philadelphia, Pennsylvania*

George W. Mitchell, Jr., M.D., *Clinical Professor, Department of Obstetrics and Gynecology, University of Texas Health Science Center at San Antonio, San Antonio, Texas*

Fred S. Miyazaki, M.D., *Head, Section of Gynecologic Urology, Department of Obstetrics and Gynecology, Kaiser Permanente Medical Group, Los Angeles, California*

J. George Moore, M.D., *Professor, Department of Obstetrics and Gynecology, UCLA School of Medicine, Center for the Health Sciences, Los Angeles, California*

George W. Morley, M.D., *Norman F. Miller Professor, Department of Obstetrics and Gynecology, University of Michigan Medical Center, Ann Arbor, Michigan*

David Muram, M.D., *Professor and Chief, Section of Pediatric and Adolescent Gynecology, Director, Division of Gynecology, University of Tennessee, Memphis, Memphis, Tennessee*

David H. Nichols, M.D., *Visiting Professor of Obstetrics, Gynecology, and Reproductive Biology, Harvard Medical School; Chief of Pelvic Surgery, Vincent Memorial Obstetrics and Gynecology Service, Massachusetts General Hospital, Boston, Massachusetts*

David Landel Nichols, B.A., M.A., J.D., *Assistant United States Attorney, Department of Justice, El Paso, Texas*

Leslie W. Ottinger, M.D., *Visiting Surgeon, Massachusetts General Hospital; Associate Professor of Surgery, Harvard Medical School, Boston, Massachusetts*

Lisa M. Peacock, M.D., *Associate Professor, Section of Obstetrics and Gynecology, Emory University Hospital, Atlanta, Georgia*

Karl C. Podratz, M.D., Ph.D., *Professor and Chairman, Department of Obstetrics and Gynecology, Mayo Medical Center, Rochester, Minnesota*

Robert F. Porges, M.D., *Professor and Acting Chairman, Department of Obstetrics and Gynecology, New York University School of Medicine, New York, New York*

Joseph H. Pratt, M.D., *Emeritus Professor of Gynecologic Surgery, Mayo Clinic, Rochester, Minnesota*

John F. Randolph, Jr., M.D., *Associate Professor, Department of Obstetrics and Gynecology, University of Michigan Medical Center, Ann Arbor, Michigan*

Harry Reich, M.D., *Advanced Laparoscopic Surgery Consultant, Wyoming Valley Health Care Systems, Wilkes-Barre, Pennsylvania; New York Center for Gynecologic Laparoscopic Surgery, New Rochelle, New York*

James A. Roberts, M.D., *Professor, Department of Obstetrics and Gynecology, University of Michigan Medical Center, Ann Arbor, Michigan*

John A. Rock, M.D., *James Robert McCord Professor and Chairman, Department of Gynecology and Obstetrics, Emory University School of Medicine, Atlanta, Georgia*

Robert E. Rogers, M.D., *Professor, Obstetrics and Gynecology, Chief, Gynecology Section, Indiana University School of Medicine, Indianapolis, Indiana*

Susan I. Salzberg, M.D., *Resident Physician, Department of Obstetrics and Gynecology, University of Michigan Medical Center, Ann Arbor, Michigan*

William D. Schlaff, M.D., *Associate Professor, Vice Chairman/Chief, Department of Obstetrics and Gynecology/Reproductive Endocrinology, University of Colorado Health Sciences Center, Denver, Colorado*

Richard H. Schwarz, M.D., *Professor of Obstetrics and Gynecology, State University of New York Health Science Center, Brooklyn, New York*

Bobby L. Shull, M.D., *Professor of Obstetrics and Gynecology, Department of Obstetrics and Gynecology, Texas A&M University Health Science Center, Scott and Chite Clinic and Hospital, Temple, Texas*

Greg Simolke, B.S., *Department of Obstetrics and Gynecology, Baylor College of Medicine, Houston, Texas*

Andrew E. Slaby, M.D., Ph.D., M.P.H., *Clinical Professor of Psychiatry, New York University Medical School, New York, New York*

Richard E. Symmonds, M.D., *Emeritus Professor and Chair, Division of Gynecologic Surgery, Mayo Clinic, Rochester, Minnesota*

M. Leon Tancer, M.D., *Emeritus Professor of Clinical Obstetrics and Gynecology, Department of Obstetrics and Gynecology, Columbia-Presbyterian Medical Center, New York, New York*

John D. Thompson, M.D., *Professor, Department of Gynecology and Obstetrics, Emory University School of Medicine, Atlanta, Georgia*

James M. Wheeler, M.D., M.P.H., *Clinical Assistant Professor, Department of Obstetrics and Gynecology, Baylor College of Medicine, Houston, Texas*

Clifford R. Wheeless, Jr., M.D., *Associate Professor, Department of Obstetrics and Gynecology, The Johns Hopkins University School of Medicine, Baltimore, Maryland*

Winfred L. Wiser, M.D., *Professor and Chairman, Department of Obstetrics and Gynecology, University of Mississippi School of Medicine, Jackson, Mississippi*

Anne K. Wiskind, M.D., *Active Staff, Department of Obstetrics and Gynecology, Piedmont Hospital, Atlanta, Georgia*

Stephen Bernard Young, M.D., *Director, Division of Urogynecology and Pelvic Reconstructive Surgery, Department of Obstetrics and Gynecology, University of Massachusetts Medical Center, Worcester, Massachusetts*

CONTENTS

SECTION I. LAPAROTOMY

SECTION II. ADNEXAL SURGERY

SECTION III. LAPAROSCOPIC AND FERTILITY SURGERY

SECTION IV. ENDOSCOPIC SURGERY

SECTION V. VAGINAL SURGERY

SECTION VII. INTESTINAL PROBLEMS AND INJURIES

SECTION VIII. PELVIC CANCER SURGERY

SECTION IX.   PROBLEMS OF MINOR GYNECOLOGIC SURGERY

SECTION X.   OBSTETRIC SURGERY

Section XI. Medical, Endocrine, and Miscellaneous Problems

SECTION I

LAPAROTOMY

1

Managing Unexpected Findings at Myomectomy: Adenomyosis and Multiple Small Leiomyomas

John O. L. DeLancey

Case Abstract 1

A 36-year-old nulligravid patient complained of hypermenorrhea, dysmenorrhea, and pelvic pressure. On pelvic examination, she was found to have a uterus enlarged to the size of a uterus at 12 weeks gestation. Sonographic examination indicated the presence of uterine leiomyomas and normal ovaries. A hysterosalpingogram demonstrated a generally enlarged uterine cavity and bilateral tubal patency. With the patient's consent, a myomectomy was planned. A generally enlarged and somewhat irregular uterus was found when the abdomen was opened. No specific myomas were detectable. Incision into the masses revealed a whorled pattern of dense fibrous tissue with some slight discoloration but nothing to suggest malignancy. No cleavage was plane present and the surgeon was faced with the problem of what to do.

DISCUSSION

The most common reason for the uterus to be enlarged and irregular in size is the presence of leiomyomas arising from the uterine wall. However, this is not the only reason for this enlargement. Endometrial carcinoma, sarcomas, and other pelvic malignancies are familiar well-recognized reasons for the uterus to be enlarged, and this must be kept in mind when scheduling a patient for surgery because of presumed leiomyomas. In these situations, hysterectomy is indicated, and, apart from performing a preoperative dilatation and curettage to detect malignancy, there is no intraoperative dilemma about the course of action to be followed. Although diagnostic imaging has increased our ability to visualize the pelvic organs, the resolution of these tests will probably not always be able to discriminate between adenomyomas and leiomyomas. When the enlarged uterus fails to contain well-circumscribed lesions that can be shelled out, the surgeon is faced with two possibilities. The abdominal incision may be closed and the patient may be informed of the findings, or an operation may be carried out to reduce the size of the uterus. The decision between these options must be based on the surgeon's detailed knowledge of the patient's symptoms and also on her desire to avoid hysterectomy. In an individual who

Figure 1.1. Both encapsulated intramural ade- nomyoma and diffuse adenomyosis are illustrated. (Reprinted with permission from Thompson JD, Rock JA (eds): *Te Linde's Operative Gynecology,* ed. 7. Philadelphia, JB Lippincott, 1992, p. 464.)

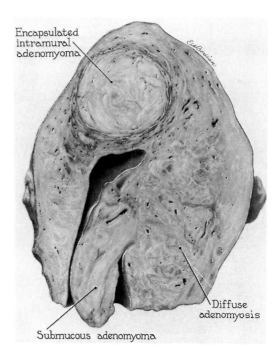

Encapsulated intramural adenomyoma

Diffuse adenomyosis

Submucous adenomyoma

wishes to retain the ability to bear children, removing a uterus that does not contain cancer would be unjustified unless the patient has requested this to relieve her symptoms.

The possibility that the operative findings may differ from what the surgeon thought preoperatively should be anticipated. One needs to discuss the possibility that ovarian malignancy might be present, and also consider other causes for uterine enlarge- ment; adenomyosis and adenomyoma should be kept in mind. Localized adenomyosis may occur in conjunction with diffuse adenomyosis (Fig. 1.1) or as a more global process (Fig. 1.2).

The irregular contour of the uterus in these instances indicates that reduction of the uterine size will often still be possible despite the absence of a cleavage plane surrounding the hyperplastic uterine wall (3). When specific nodular, enlarged areas are localized within the myometrium, these can be directly resected to reduce the size of the uterus and to remove the glandular elements (Fig. 1.3). This is important because it is these glandular elements that are probably causing the pain with menstru- ation. Care should be exercised to avoid damage to the fallopian tubes during this part of the operation. Adequate hemostasis is needed so that the walls of the uterus may be anatomically approximated if the cavity is entered. One or several areas may need to be resected to achieve adequate reduction in size. Palpation of the uterine wall will be the best guide to the location of the various areas of enlargement, and opening the cavity to permit full exploration of the uterus is usually advisable. Examination of a frozen section to exclude the possibility of malignancy is probably prudent even though the characteristic appearance of adenomyosis and adenomyomas is different from that of the uterine sarcomas.

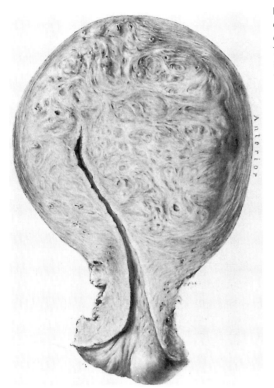

Figure 1.2. Diffuse adenomyosis involving most of the uterus, yet normal myometrium can still be discerned. (Reprinted with permission from Thompson JD, Rock JA (eds): *Te Linde's Operative Gynecology*, ed. 7. Philadelphia, JB Lippincott, 1992, p. 464.)

Instances will also arise in which the uterus is generally enlarged without any specific area of nodularity. When this occurs, resection of specific areas of disease is not feasible. The surgeon must be guided by the patient's wishes. Some women may wish to have the uterus preserved if this is feasible but readily accept the possibility that it may need to be removed. In this situation, hysterectomy is the best course to follow. On the other hand, other women feel strongly that loss of the uterus will pose a significant psychologic or physiologic trauma to their body. Although the physician may not agree with the patient about the sequelae of hysterectomy, a woman who firmly believes that removal of the uterus will result in sexual dysfunction will probably have significant problems adjusting to having lost her uterus. In this setting, sexual dysfunction is to be expected. When faced with a situation where myomectomy is not possible in a woman who wants to retain her uterus, a hysterectomy should not be performed unless ureteral obstruction is present, significant anemia has occurred, or other problems that put the patient at significant risk are present and no possibility of retaining the uterus exists. The possibility of stopping the operation at the end of the exploratory laparotomy portion and not performing the hysterectomy should be considered.

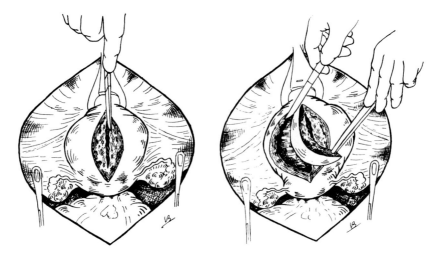

Figure 1.3.   Excision of localized adenomyosis. *A.* Incision through thickened area into the uterine cavity. *B.* Excision of thickened wall to be followed by closure of the uterine wound. (Reprinted from Bonney V: Adenomyomectomy. In: *The Technical Minutiae of Extended Myomectomy and Ovarian Cystectomy.* New York, Paul B. Hoeber, 1946, pp. 239–258.)

Case Abstract 2

A 35-year-old nulliparous woman with hypermenorrhea leading to anemia (Hb = 9 g %) was found to have an irregular enlarged uterus, enlarged to the size at 14 weeks gestation. Endometrial biopsy revealed secretory endometrium, and the cavity sounded to 8.5 cm. An ultrasound examination revealed normal ovaries and a uterus of mixed echogenicity consistent with leiomyomas. After suppression with a GnRH analog to restore the patient's hematocrit, a myomectomy was planned. After the abdomen was opened, the uterus was found to contain innumerable small (1 to 2 cm) myomas.

DISCUSSION

Myomectomy is easiest when a single myoma is present. The number of myomas that may occur, however, is almost limitless. The great British gynecologist Victor Bonney once removed over 200 myomas from a single uterus. In most clinical situations, a balance must be struck between the time spent removing myomas and the impact of the operation on the patient's problem. In a patient who wishes to retain fertility, myomectomy offers an acceptable approach to treatment of the enlarged, symptomatic uterus despite the presence of multiple myomas (10,11). Pregnancy rates after surgery are high enough to justify the attitude that preserving the uterus will result in successful pregnancy in approximately 40% of women (1).

In the situation described in the case summary, where many small myomas were found, the primary indication for surgery was anemia. Therapy should therefore focus on the bleeding problem as much as on the size of the uterus. Myomas are most likely to cause increased menstrual flow when they are submucosal or intracavitary. A hysteroscopy, a dilatation and curettage, or even a hysterosalpingogram would have allowed the surgeon to know preoperatively whether this type of myoma was present. Furthermore, for unknown reasons the dilatation and curettage is often therapeutic and might have avoided major surgery altogether.

If a submucous myoma or myomas had been found, transvaginal removal of pedunculated myoma (2) or hysteroscopic resection of sessile myoma might have been all that was necessary to alleviate the bleeding. Among 92 women undergoing resectascopic myomectomy, 24 of 28 that had dysmenorrhea had resolution of their pain, and 65 of 80 experienced resolution of their dysmenorrhea (5). Therefore, when the size of the uterus, impingement on the ureter, or uncertainty about the presence of ovarian cancer is not the primary problem, evaluation of the uterine cavity prior to myomectomy seems prudent in a woman who feels strongly about retaining her uterus. Although resectascopic excision would have left the patient with an enlarged uterus, it would have had a good chance of alleviating her symptoms without eliminating her fertility. This would have avoided the laparotomy, which placed the surgeon in the unenviable position of deciding between extensive myomectomy and hysterectomy in a woman who wished to preserve her uterus.

Should myomectomy be carried out in the presence of large numbers of myomas? The chance of myomas recurring after myomectomy is lowest when only a few myomas are found, yet, even though larger numbers of myomas have a greater risk of needing subsequent removal, there may be adequate time for reproduction before recurrence occurs. Myomectomy is easiest, and the risk of recurrence is lowest, when one or a few myomas are present (4). At the other end of the spectrum, myomas may be so numerous that myomectomy is not possible (9). Between these two extremes a decision must be made about how many myomas it is reasonable to resect. This will depend on the surgeon's skill and resourcefulness in performing myomectomy.

When large numbers of small tumors are encountered, several surgical techniques will simplify the operation. First, hemostasis will be important, since removing large numbers of myomas may be time-consuming. A firm rubber catheter (16 French red rubber Robinson) may be placed through holes placed in the broad ligament over the uterine arteries and tied tightly enough so as to occlude not only the uterine arteries, but also the blood flow that might come up through the uterus from the cervical connection between the uterine artery and vaginal artery. Rubber-shod Bainbridge vascular clamps may be placed between the adnexal structures and the uterus with the tube passing atraumatically through the hole in the clamp, or atraumatic clamps may be placed on the ovarian vessels (6). This permits absolute hemostasis so that blood loss is kept to a minimum and the surgeon can see the operative field. Although there is some decrease in bleeding with pretreatment using GnRH analogs (8), there is also some indication that they may make the small myomas smaller. In one study, 6 months after myomectomy 63% of women who had preoperative suppression had sonographically detectable myomas, and 13% of those who had not been pretreated had detectable myomas (7). Since the clinical course of these groups in the short term was the same, the importance of these findings remains to be determined. We have found that surgical hemostasis using a tourniquet and clamps is superior to pharmacologic techniques, allowing for even the most extensive myomectomy to be performed safely.

Once hemostasis has been obtained, dissection of the myomas may be carried out expeditiously but carefully. When clusters of myomas exist together with little intervening myometrium, the group may sometimes be excised all together, but usually the techniques used to dissect myomas from their surrounding tissues are employed. It is imperative to proceed quickly because there will be a large number of tumors to remove.

When many myomas are present, the surgeon must decide whether complete removal of all myomas is feasible. In this situation, since the patient's primary problem is hypermenorrhea, a submucous myoma should be sought. If many of the superficial myomas are removed but the one causing the excess bleeding is missed, the patient will continue to bleed to the point of anemia. Many surgeons will obtain a hysterosalpingo-gram preoperatively to assure themselves of tubal patency, and this will also indicate the presence of myomas that impinge on the cavity. If this is not done, then the cavity should be sought and the presence or absence of intracavitary myomas should be determined. The surgeon should not hesitate to attempt removal of all of the myomas, but if this is not possible, the maximum feasible without putting the patient at undue risk should be accomplished.

Conservative surgery for the enlarged uterus requires surgical improvisation, resourcefulness, skill, and judgment. With careful preparation, the patient's as well as the surgeon's goals may be met. Simply performing a hysterectomy because myomectomy might be challenging may leave a patient unsatisfied with her situation.

REFERENCES

1. Babaknia A, Rock JA, Jones HW Jr: Pregnancy success following abdominal myomectomy for infertility. *Fertil Steril* 30:644–647, 1978.
2. Ben-Baruch G, Schiff E, Menashe Y, Menczer J: Immediate and late outcome of vaginal myomectomy for prolapsed pedunculated submucous myoma. *Obstet Gynecol* 72:858–861, 1988.
3. Bonney V: Adenomyomectomy. In *The Technical Minutiae of Extended Myomectomy and Ovarian Cystectomy*. New York, Paul B. Hoeber, 1946, pp. 239–258.
4. Candiani GB, Fedele L, Parazzini F, Villa L: Risk of recurrence after myomectomy. *Br J Obstet Gynaecol* 98:385–389, 1991.
5. Corson SL, Brooks PG: Resectoscopic myomectomy. *Fertil Steril* 55:1041–1044, 1991.
6. DeLancey JOL: A modified technique for hemostasis during myomectomy. *Surg Gynecol Obstet* 174:153–154, 1992.
7. Fedele L, Vercellini P, Bianchi S, Brioschi D, Dorta M: Treatment with GnRH agonists before myomectomy and the risk of short-term myoma recurrence. *Br J Obstet Gynaecol* 97:393–396, 1990.
8. Friedman AJ, Rein MS, Harrison-Atlas D, Garfield JM, Doubilet PM: A randomized, placebo-controlled, double-blind study evaluating leuprolide acetate depot treatment before myomectomy. *Fertil Steril* 52:728–733, 1989.
9. Lapan B, Solomon L: Diffuse leiomyomatosis of the uterus precluding myomectomy. *Obstet Gynecol* 53:82S–84S, 1979.
10. Smith DC, Uhlir JK: Myomectomy as a reproductive procedure. *Am J Obstet Gynecol* 162:1476–1479, 1990.
11. Verkauf BS: Myomectomy for fertility enhancement and preservation. *Fertil Steril* 58:1–15, 1992.

2

Huge Cervical Myomata

Celso-Ramón García

Case Abstract

A 36-year-old nulligravida complained of constant, left lower quadrant pelvic and abdominal pain that increased prior to menstruation. Although the menstruation was reported to be regular, lasting the normal 3 to 5 days, she described the flow as becoming very heavy over the past several years. She reported dyspareunia that limited her sexual activity to only six occasions. Abdominal examination only disclosed a suggestion of a palpable mass just above the symphysis pubis. Ultrasound disclosed a myomatous uterus with several myomas, the largest being 12 cm and located low in the pelvis as a cervical myoma. She pressed for a myomectomy after laparoscopy confirmed the myomatous uterus with this largest cervical myoma occupying the entire lesser pelvis and displacing a short partially effaced stubby cervix anteriorly. Chromopertubation, accomplished with difficulty, disclosed fill and spill of the right tube, but a left anterior small myoma compressed the lateral fundal area with no fill or spill noted on that side. The bladder was located above the symphysis, with the body of the uterus being retroflexed, disclosing many small myomas. Hysterectomy was discussed as a possible option. Control of bleeding was assessed in preparation for myomectomy as well as hysterectomy. Concerns were also expressed over the dissection of the uterine vessels since the cervical myoma caused an anteflexion as well as a retrocession of the uterus deep into the lesser pelvis.

DISCUSSION

Uterine fibroleiomyomas are very frequently encountered benign tumors that are clinically more apparent after the age of 30 or 35 and rarely prior to age 19. Uterine myomas can occur in all locations of the uterus, and their growth direction is believed to create the varied locations and distortions that they produce. Most commonly they are present in the uterine body or project from the body as a pedunculated myoma. The cervix is a collagenous structure that contains smaller amounts of smooth muscle than the uterine body but more elastic tissue. This can, and often does, permit submucous myomas to protrude from within the uterine cavity through the endocervix following softening, effacement, and dilatation of the cervix with extrusion or prolapse of the myoma, often on a long stalk. On rare occasions inversion of the uterus can occur during this gradual expulsion of a submucous myoma. Determining the extent and type of pathology, as well as the surgical management, can be very problematical. Fortunately, the cervix appears to have considerable retentive "memory," since following the avulsion or the excision of these myomas, the cervix regresses to normal within 4 to 5 weeks.

Myomas that arise from the isthmic-cervical tissue are much less common than those arising in the uterine body. Moreover, the frequent histologic demonstration of continuity between capillary muscular walls and the fibers of the smooth muscle tumors is believed to explain the source of this benign neoplastic growth. Although the etiology of myomas is not clear, the sparse smooth muscle elements in the cervix may perhaps relate to the infrequency with which they occur within this structure. Myomas in the cervical location have been stated to occur at a frequency of 1.2% to 8%. When thay are located in the cervix, the slow rate and particularly the direction of growth play an important role, not only in the variation and the accommodation of the patient to her symptoms, but also in the specific clinical and surgical management.

Although uterine body myomas may be present in the submucosal, intramural, and subserosal loci, they also project from the uterine surface or into its cavity as pedunculated structures. Their size can vary from barely detectable to enormous size. Cervical myomas have special features. These tumors may grow in various directions. As they continue to enlarge there may be a counterresistance to the adjacent pelvic structures as well as the bony pelvis itself. Their infrequency and few early signs and symptoms, as well as their slow rate of growth, tend to make the patient less aware of their presence, and they may be missed early on or in the absence of periodic pelvic examinations.

The cervical myoma presents different clinical features. When the direction of growth is anterior, the myoma bulges and dissects the vesicouterine space, dislodging the bladder and directing the uterus posteriorly. A posterior cervical myoma grows by dissecting the subperitoneal space in the pouch of Douglas, obliterating the cul-de-sac and growing between the surface of the rectum and the sacrum as well as into rectovaginal space. The lateral myoma grows into the broad ligament and on rare occasions will not only displace the ureter but may also involve the rectum and sigmoid. An even more difficult cervical myoma is the central one that may develop in an encircling manner surrounding the endocervix, expanding laterally with the uterus body sitting on top, looking dwarfed by comparison. Alternatively, the direction of growth may be within the endocervical canal with a lateral expansion of a pedunculated myoma dilating the endocervix. These may be more difficult to detect early and more formidable to manage.

The secondary effects of the compression of expanding myomas may produce pain or cause indirect effects on other body systems, such as on the ureters with possible hydronephrosis, or on the rectum with constipation, hemorrhoids, or pain, as well as general pelvic vascular stasis, which may lead to peripheral leg edema or even varices over time. Compression of the bladder and urethra have also produced difficulty or inability to void. The woman may present with a supple abdomen without ascites and a pelvic mass that can best be appreciated on rectal examination but that can offer varying degrees of vaginal cavity compromise. The cervix is very often inaccessible by speculum examination. The mass may be firm or it may be soft, suggesting a degeneration of the myoma.

Myomas are noted for the numerous variations in their size, number, and location, and the many variations in pathologies with which they may be associated or present. Thus, the better the preoperative assessment, the more accurately the woman can be counseled. When the extant pathology is documented in this manner, the woman has a better opportunity to accept and support the physician's judgment than if she submits to a proposed approach based on a less firm assessment that relies more on clinical judgment or intuition. Moreover, the more specific the possible approaches that can be planned preoperatively based on the detailed preoperative assessment, the better the chances of a successful procedure with the least amount of blood loss.

Although fibroids prolapsing through the cervix should be removed from below, the extirpation of a huge cervical myoma from below can be a very vexing experience fraught with many difficulties. Rochet and associates from France detail an exploration and morcellation of a huge cervical myoma by dissecting through the transverse perineal body, since the very low cervical myoma had dissected down through the planes of the rectovaginal septum with bulging of the perineal body. Such oddities depict the ingenuity and thorough understanding of the pelvic anatomy that is needed to address the various complexities that the huge cervical myoma can present. Although a hysterectomy might be viewed as a preferable option, a myomectomy often may be needed as a requisite to gaining access to the appropriate dissection of the vessels of the pelvic dissections because of the distortions produced by the myomas.

There can be considerable variability in the findings of the palpable surface and consistency of the myoma. The softer myomas more often reflect degeneration or necrobiotic changes. Limitation of mobility can be related to adhesion as well as constraint or impingement of the myoma to the bony pelvis. The presence of endometriosis is another complexity often associated with myomas. Moreover, pelvic inflammatory disease, ovarian cysts, and other neoplasms can also be confounding.

Clinical assessment might call upon less invasive approaches such as ultrasound, CT scan, or MRI to help define the extent of the problem and the relationships to the other structures. Hysterography may be very difficult when the cervix is severely displaced. Yet it is very helpful to define the cervical and uterine cavities and their contents. An excretory urogram will outline the ureteral deviations from normal, both in dilatation and in location. In this case, the excretory urogram confirmed the lack of ureteral involvement. Cystourethroscopy may also be an aid when feasible. Finally, laparoscopy is an indispensable aid in assessing the extent of the possible pathology that may coexist with that of the myomas. It helps define, before the laparotomy, the status of the adnexa and bowel, whether there are several adnexal compromises, adhesions, and so on.

Perioperative adjuvants include those agents aimed at improving the preoperative status, the intraoperative status, and the postoperative course of the women. These include the use of meticulous hemostasis, starting with the abdominal incision and extending through the operative procedure as well as in the closure of the abdominal incision. The controversy regarding the use of a midline versus a transverse incision is beyond the scope of this chapter. The approach that will give the greatest exposure for the specific surgeon's experience and judgment is the appropriate one. Ensuring excellent exposure is paramount. The Shaw ™ Scalpel with the heated blade, microelectrocoagulation, and the Coherent ™ CO_2-Ultra-Pulse Laser can be used. The last mentioned not only contributes to reducing blood loss but also improves the speed with which the procedure is performed. The use of vasoconstrictors, such as diluted Pitressin (20 units/40 to 50 ml), injected into the myometrium blanches the uterine mass.

Much controversy surrounds the preoperative use of the GnRH analogs in the preoperative management of myomas. Although the reduction in volume of most myomas has been documented in most studies, the reduction in diameter is less dramatic. Many support preoperative GnRH use for such a person as the woman in this case presentation. I have not been convinced that the diameter reductions in these large myomas are dramatic enough to justify exposing women to the unpleasant side effects of GnRH analogs, such as the menopausal changes, the histamine reactions, the arthralgia, and so on that they may tolerate, perhaps with dutiful tolerant indignation, while offering a desire to please. It is hard to demonstrate an improved, facile, more hemostatic surgery attributable to this therapy, despite the claims to the contrary. The undesirable side effects of GnRH analogs, although believed to be transient, are severe enough in some women that they discontinue its use. Moreover, since the reduction in diameter size is greater in the smaller myomas, the recurrence rate is greater with its use. This medical approach for the management of myomas has yet to receive the approval from the Food and Drug Administration. The occurrence of allergic reactions can be, has been, and should be of considerable concern. This is particularly the case with the long-acting injectable approach. Therefore, despite the widespread use of these agents in the man-agement of myomas, I believe they should be applied as a clinical experiment and as such used with oversight to record the actual frequency of the side effects and complications in view of their perceived theoretical value. This is particularly so in view of the continuing, albeit rare, histamine reactions that have plagued the agonist analogs and even more so the antagonists since their earliest appraisals. Hemostasis is best ensured by placing a rubber tubing tourniquet around the entire uterus, tubes, and ovaries; this will reduce the amount of blood loss when one is dissecting out the myomas. This technique has not caused ischemia to the ovaries and uterus in hundreds of women carefully followed long-term. The ischemia is well tolerated and probably limited to under 5 hours (4 to 5 hours). Animal data support that ischemia of over 12 hours is needed to observe atrophy of the uterus.

Manual dislodgment of the pelvic mass with attempts to elevate the organ were futile. The patient's strong expression of the desire to retain her reproductive potential was a significant contributing factor. A tourniquet application presented diffi-culties because of the constraints of the cervical myoma and the lesser pelvis. A dilute Pitressin solution was injected into the myometrium prior to the placement of a traction suture, applied as low in the midline of the cervical myoma as was technically feasible. Using steady traction upwardly out of the pelvis permitted the placement of a second traction suture inferiorly to the first, and with a traction rocking motion this delivered the cervical uterine mass out of the pelvis. This then permitted the application of a rubber tourniquet around the entire mass, ensuring hemostasis to permit the enucleation of the cervical myoma through a posterior midline elliptical incision placed around the traction sutures over the thinnest area of myometrium covering the myoma. This midline incision over the central part of the myoma extended laterally for a centimeter on either side of the traction sutures, which further facilitated the dissection of the myoma through the cap-sule down to the base; the pedicle at the base was clamped and ligated. The closure of the defect(s) was accomplished with the use of a continuous no. 3–0 Vicryl ™ Suture applied as a radial stitch with a concentric pattern, occluding or obliterating the void of the bed of the enucleated fibroid. Several other myomas (20 in number) were also excised and the defects repaired. Total operative time was under 3 hours. Postoperative follow-up reveals normal size and shape of the uterus. The patient has had normal menses and coital activity is satisfactory. It is hoped that pregnancy is forthcoming.

In this case, the assessment of the uterine-cervical fibroid by laparoscopy also gave one the opportunity to judge the status of the adnexa as well as the uterus itself. One could be better assured that the myoma was deliverable from the lesser pelvis with pressure from below. Despite the presence of other uterine myomas, this enormous cervical myoma could be seen arising from below the uterosacral ligaments, filling the lesser pelvis and accounting for the inability to perform a speculum examination during the initial office pelvic examination. Even under anesthesia there was difficulty in viewing the well-covered pinpoint cervical os because of its inherent marked displacement. Nonetheless, it was feasible to perform a hysteroscopy, which revealed the presence of submucous myomas in the left anterior fundal area, explaining the inability to demonstrate patency of that left oviduct by hysterosalpingography. After the fundal myomectomy, patency of the left oviduct was demonstrated.

Although the ingenuity of the human is infinite, it is with the huge cervical myoma that all of our resources are needed to carry out the corrective surgery, whether by hysterectomy or by myomectomy. In this case the mobilization of the entrapped cervical myoma facilitated its removal and thus preserved reproductive function.

SELECTED READINGS

Ferenczy A: Benign lesions of the cervix. In: Blaustein A: *Pathology of the Female Genital Tract*, ed. 3. New York, Springer-Verlag, 1987.

Fluhman CF: *The Cervix Uteri and Its Diseases*, ed. 1. Philadelphia, WB Saunders, 1961.

García C-R, Pfeifer S: Myomectomy. In: Nichols DH (ed): *Gynecologic and Obstetric Surgery*. St. Louis, Mosby-Yearbook 36:606–623, 1993.

González Calzada GJ: Isthmico-cervical myomatosis as a surgical problem. *Ginec Obstet Mex* 54:176–180, 1986.

Rochet et al: Voluminous cervical fibroid. *Bull Fed Soc Gynecol Obstet Lang Fr* (France) 23:616–617, 1971.

Saleh MT et al: Myomatosis isthmicocervical. *Ginec Obstet Mex* 59:246–248, 1991.

3

Intraoperative Hemorrhage

Bryon J. Masterson

Case Abstract 1: Insecurely Tied Infundibulopelvic Ligament

During a total abdominal hysterectomy and bilateral salpingo–oophorectomy performed through a Pfannenstiel incision to relieve a 35-year-old patient of a symptomatic fibroid uterus, it was evident that there was some unexpected ovarian endometriosis present. As an initial step in the operation, it was decided to perform a simultaneous bilateral salpingo–oophorectomy. The infundibulopelvic ligament on each side was clamped and ligated, and the hysterectomy was commenced. Exposure was a problem, and several packs were inserted to push the bowel away from the operative field. When the removal of the uterus had been completed, pelvic peritonealization considered, and the lower packs removed, it was evident that the tie holding the right infundibulopelvic ligament had partially slipped. A 5- to 7-cm hematoma was already evident in the stump of the right infundibulopelvic ligament. The tie was removed and dissection initiated to find the source of bleeding. The hematoma rapidly increased in size and bleeding increased, but the specific source of bleeding became more elusive.

DISCUSSION

Identification of the Problem

The patient has had an ovarian artery or vein retract from the original tie and is now bleeding into the retroperitoneal space. The operator should always aggressively identify this type of bleeder at the time of surgery. Retroperitoneal accumulation of blood, with associated protracted ileus, abdominal discomfort, and on occasion retroperitoneal abscess formation, can produce significant morbidity.

Prevention of the Problem

The term *infundibulopelvic ligament ligation* should be abandoned, since the process involved is really the ligation of the ovarian artery and veins. The use of large crushing clamps across the venous plexus is hazardous. The most secure method is to pass a suture around the vessels after they have been dissected free and the ureters have been identified. This should be followed with a suture ligature placed distally with the needle placed to the central portion of the venous plexus and tied in front and behind. Ovarian vein hematomas will almost never occur if the veins are handled this way. If, however, the crushing clamps are placed, particularly if the less desirable double-clamp technique is used, hematomas are not uncommon.

14

Management of This Problem

The operator is now faced with the difficulty of identifying a vessel in a somewhat edematous and engorged space. The operator should grasp the lower end of the veins with a small clamp, identify the ureter, and dissect sharply upward in the retroperitoneal space, constantly observing the ureter. Additional exposure can be attained by incising up either gutter and reflecting the colon, or medially and reflecting the peritoneum.

As soon as one has reached the top of the hematoma as identified by resumption of the veins into a more normal caliber, one should place a right-angled clamp about them. One then passes a tie around the veins at this point, again carefully identifying the ureter. One may perform suture ligature, noted above, or occasionally a large clip may be placed below the vein. The hematoma, thus isolated, should be removed. Any small venous contributors to this hematoma should be clipped with small clips, or electrocautery may be used. The distal ends of the veins near the hysterectomy site should again be inspected to make sure that they are not contributing to the hematoma formation. A dry pack should be placed with some pressure over the site where the hematoma has been removed. One rarely encounters difficulty in controlling such bleeding if sharp dissection and precise vessel ligation are performed. The operator should avoid the tendency to place large clamps and sutures in and around this hematoma because this will only injure adjacent structures and will almost never accomplish the desired results of precise ligation of the contributing vessels and removal of the trapped hematoma. If necessary, the ovarian artery of either side may be ligated near its origin from the aorta just below that of the renal arteries, proximal to the hematoma.

Case Abstract 2: Damage to Internal Iliac Vein

During ligation of the left internal iliac artery for control of persistent angle bleeding following hysterectomy, the wall of the internal iliac vein was lacerated. Hemorrhage was temporarily controlled by direct pressure to the vein. A call for a vascular surgeon was fruitless.

DISCUSSION

Injury to adjacent structures in pelvic surgery is almost always due to poor exposure. Exposure may be limited by too small an incision, inadequate assistance, poor instruments, pelvic masses such as a cervical fibroid obscuring the area, blood obscuring the visualization, inappropriate anesthesia, or poor operative lights. The injury has occurred in this particular case at the time of ligation of the internal iliac artery for control of bleeding at the vaginal angle. The author would disagree with the surgeon that unilateral ligation of an internal iliac artery is of much value in the control of pelvic bleeding from the vaginal angle. One need only look at the intense arterial anastomosis around the vaginal tube to realize that such a maneuver offers little chance of producing hemostasis. A much more appropriate maneuver would be to isolate the artery in question with appropriate exposure and to ligate it at its source. Secondly, bleeding as described in this case, at the vaginal angle, is often venous in origin and not influenced by isolating and ligating the internal iliac artery. One can demonstrate this by ligating the internal iliac artery during the course of a radical hysterectomy and then producing an operative injury in an area that will subsequently be excised. Bleeding will be brisk and not affected by unilateral internal iliac artery ligation. One can further demonstrate this by placing a vascular clamp across the entire arterial tree and dividing an artery or vein below the site of ligation. One will be unable to detect the difference in bleeding volume whether the vessel is clamped or not, because of the intense pelvic anastomosis so well demonstrated with pelvic arteriography. In managing the defect produced, the operator is faced with the control of bleeding in a structure that frequently cannot be mobilized. The exiting branches of the internal iliac vein are fixed and fragile, and may produce almost uncontrollable hemorrhage if injured. Great care must be exercised in manipulating this venous tree. The initial response to such bleeding should be prompt pressure directly applied upon the defect against the pelvic wall. The surgeon should then advise the anesthesiologist to secure an additional 4 units of blood for transfusion, immediately secure additional lighting, both overhead and the flexible intraoperative type, and get an additional suction and any additional assistance needed. Where extensive blood loss is anticipated, the Cell Saver may be a worthwhile choice to reduce blood consumption. The Cell Saver recovers and provides washed, relatively plasma-free blood for reinfusion into the patient.

Complications from reinfusion must be kept in mind. Washing the blood cells with sterile saline solution does not ensure that there is no contamination. However, Schweiger noted no correlation with clinical infection and positive blood cultures.

When transfusion volumes exceed 20 red blood cell units of any kind, significant thrombocytopenia will result. In addition, following transfusion reaching 12 units of plasma-free red blood cells, significant prothrombin time and partial thromboplastin time prolongations consistently occur. Delicate thumb forceps, needle holders, building clamps, and other vascular instruments should be brought to the operative site, and hopefully such instruments are in the operator's usual instrument set. Kocher and Heaney clamps and other nonvascular instruments are hazardous in the extreme in handling delicate branches of the internal iliac vein. Delicate swaged-on vascular suture of no. 5–0 size, monofilament type is most useful, and hemostatic clips of both small and large size with long appliers should be immediately at hand.

The operator should direct an assistant to maintain pressure on the vein by pressing it gently against the pelvic wall. The vein can then be exposed by lifting the left round ligament strongly upward. One should place a medium Deaver retractor above the femoral artery and dissect upward to the bifurcation of the common iliac artery. Then one identifies the ureter and directs the scissors downward along its medial leaf. The operator should enter the pararectal and paravesical spaces and identify the obliterated hypogastric artery and the obturator nerve. The entire internal iliac venous tree may be ligated with impunity, as may any of its branches, so one need not preserve the integrity of this vein to continue vascular function of the pelvis. One places two suction tips in the wound, places a flexible fiberoptic light source over the pelvic wall, and gently removes the sponge stick pressed against the venous defect. The surgeon may be delighted to find that the bleeding has ceased. Less fortunately, he or she may be amazed by the volume of blood escaping from a relatively small defect in the vein. The surgeon must not attempt to operate on this venous defect with Kocher, Heaney, or other large crushing toothed clamps. By doing so one may convert a small defect, which can be easily managed with a single clip, to a laceration involving two or three venous trunks, which may only be controlled by a complex procedure requiring numerous blood transfusions.

As soon as the operator has clearly identified the defect and its size, he or she replaces the sponge stick and puts a sucker directly near the defect. If the defect is small, a small clip or two will quickly close the hole in the vein and control bleeding. The presence of a clip on the defect makes its suture infinitely more difficult, since the clip will be incorporated in the suture and the defect will not close. Therefore, one should avoid using clips with large lacerations when suture is contemplated. If the defect is large, one may divide the vein by placing large clips on each end of the defect. One must remember that the vein in this area is not a simple tube but a branching system that may have veins entering its lateral surface that cannot be seen by the operator. In this case, one may place a running vascular suture in the vein and control bleeding. If, however, the laceration is large and several venous trees have been torn where several perforators enter, a truly hazardous circumstance exists. When concerted effort does not produce control of the bleeding and hemorrhage is life-threatening, two maneuvers remain: (a) sew over the entire area with a 0 chromic suture in a continuous fashion; (b) realize that some of the pelvic plexus of nerves may sustain some injury during this maneuver, and inform the family at the conclusion of the procedure.

As a last resort, one can tightly pack the pelvis with a large breast roll gauze and layer the gauze into the pelvis in such a way that its removal will not produce knots, causing difficulty in its extraction from the wound. Before placement, one soaks the upper portion of the roll with Betadine and brings it out to the edge of the abdominal wound. One then closes the wound with retention sutures and leaves a 4- to 5-cm defect for pack removal untied. The patient should be sent to the intensive care unit and observed carefully. If bleeding is controlled, the patient should be brought back to the operating room in 48 hours. The operator should then administer a light anesthetic, remove the pack, and irrigate the wound gently to remove any superficial hematoma. He or she should tie the retention sutures, being careful not to manipulate the area of the old venous injury and to not use any sutures in the skin. Although hernias are increased when packs are used through the incision, little other morbidity is usually noted. Other methods to be considered are arterial catherization and selective Gelfoam embolization. Pitressin infusion may also be useful.

The operator must avoid injury to the internal iliac venous system by carefully exposing the area before any manipulations are performed, and must also avoid the double-clamp system of pelvic surgery. One will rarely be faced with a lacerated internal iliac vein if this advice is followed.

SELECTED READINGS

Bergan JJ, Dean RH, Yao JT: Vascular injuries in pelvic cancer surgery. *Am J Obstet Gynecol* 124:562, 1976.

Boldt J, Kling D, Zickmann B, et al: Acute preoperative plasmapheresis and established blood conservation techniques. *Ann Thorac Surg* 50:62–68, 1990.

Leslie SD, Toy PT: Laboratory hemostatic abnormalities in massively transfused patients given red blood cells and crystalloid. *Am J Clin Pathol* 96:770–773, 1991.

Magrina JF, Moffat RE, Masterson BJ, et al: Selective arterial infusion of Pitressin for the control of puerperal hemorrhage after hypogastric artery ligation. *Obstet Gynecol* 58:646, 1981.

Masterson BJ: *Manual of Gynecologic Surgery*, ed. 2. New York, Springer-Verlag, 1986.

Schweiger IM, Gallagher CJ, Finlayson DC, et al: Incidence of Cell-Saver contamination during cardiopulmonary bypass. *Ann Thorac Surg* 48:51–53, 1989.

4

Transabdominal Myomectomy — Broken Needle

L. Russell Malinak
James M. Wheeler
Greg Simolke

Case Abstract

Myomectomy was planned for a 28-year-old nulligravida with hypermenorrhea and an enlarged, irregular uterus. Following enucleation of the fibroid tumors from the uterus, the myometrium was being closed in layers. As the deeper stitches were being placed, an audible "clack" was heard. When the needle holder was withdrawn, it was evident that the tip of the needle had been broken. The location of the broken tip was unknown; the surgeon suspected it was retained by the myometrium.

DISCUSSION

Exposure is often a problem when operating in the depths of the female pelvis. Manipulation of instruments in restricted spaces with restricted visualization is occasionally associated with a surgical complication—a broken needle. This event invariably occurs in the deepest, most inaccessible layer of a closure, as in the myomectomy described above. A broken needle implies an imbalance of forces—excessive resistance offered by the tissue, the use of an inappropriate needle, or the application of undue force by the surgeon.

To minimize the likelihood of this complication, it is necessary to select the proper needle. The characteristics of the specific needle are mandated by the type of tissue to be sutured. Tissue tensile strength, shear strength, weave, penetrability, density, elasticity, and thickness are mechanical factors that should be considered (7). Clinical situations may further affect these mechanical factors. For example, fibrosis in the myometrium adjacent to a myoma or lack of a discrete capsule, as with an adenomyoma, may complicate closure.

One basic assumption must be made when considering the ideal needle for a given application: the tissue being sutured should be altered as little as possible by the needle, since the only purpose of the needle is to introduce the suture into the tissue. The needle should be constructed of suitably strong material and designed so as to minimize needle damage, breakage, or alteration of its physical characteristics (7).

Breakage of surgical needles can be avoided by proper use of needle holders. There are two important considerations in grasping the needle: location and angle. The needle may be grasped near the swaged eye so that the point protrudes after inserting the stitch, making it easier to retrieve the needle from the tissue. This maneuver is suitable for soft tissues such as subcutaneous fat. For greatest driving force in tough tissue, the needle is grasped between midpoint and tip. As the needle is advanced, the holder is repositioned nearer the midpoint, and the needle is further thrust through the tissue—the so-called "ratchet" technique. In dense tissue, the needle should not be grasped near the eye.

The angle of the needle to the needle holder may be perpendicular, obtuse, or acute. A perpendicular angle is preferred, since the needle can be driven through tissue by rotating the needle holder on its long axis. This results in more controlled delivery of the needle through tissue. In situations where perpendicular application is not practical, the least acute or obtuse angle of application is preferable.

The importance of the surgeon's grip on the needle holder is related to the strength with which needles may be thrust into tissue. The pencil grip, used in gynecologic microsurgery, is the most delicate grip, and is unlikely to provide the force necessary to break a needle. The thenar and thumb-ring finger grips are intermediate in strength to the palmed grip. The palmed grip, therefore, is most likely associated with broken needles, since surgeons adopt this grip only when they expect significant tissue resistance (1).

In the interest of saving operating time, it is common during closure after myomectomy to attempt to force the needle through both sides of the myometrial defect. It is usually prudent, however, to pass the needle through one side of the myometrium, bring it completely out at the deepest point, and then enter the myometrium of the other side.

Needles bend before they break. If a surgeon feels a needle bending, this is a signal that excessive force is being applied. Perhaps a thicker, more stout needle should be selected. All needles that are bent should be discarded, never to be straightened and reused. In the ideal situation, the surgeon should inspect each needle for its integrity prior to placing it into the patient.

To summarize thus far, proper selection of suture materials and use of surgical technique are of paramount importance in preventing breakage of needles in tissue. The surgeon must do the following:

1. Appreciate the nature of the tissue about to be sutured.
2. Know the needle characteristics and their practical application to various tissues.
3. Use the proper needle location and angle in grasping with the needle holder.
4. Use a grip on the needle holder that will not transmit excessive force.
5. Discard bent needles; it is wiser to have wasted a bent needle than to risk breakage.

In gynecologic surgery, needle breakage is most common in difficult settings where exposure is poor and the surgeon is in some way compromising good technique.

What techniques can the surgeon use to identify and remove the broken needle tip from the patient?

Perhaps the initial question is, "Does the needle tip need to be removed?" Although patients live normally with a variety of foreign bodies in their tissues, there are specific reasons why broken needles should be removed (5). The needle could migrate to a position in which adjacent anatomic structures might be compromised (3). The needle can also move to a surgically less accessible position (2). Long-term medical complications of retained broken needles include infection and nerve irritation (8). Psychologically, many patients will manifest anxiety regarding a retained needle in their genital tracts, including fears of damage to their sexual partner or their fetus. Medicolegally, plaintiffs with retained foreign bodies have been awarded compensation even if no demonstrable harm has occurred, simply on the principle that a surgical instrument—especially one that breaks—is ipso facto negligence.

Although in other subspecialties (e.g., neurosurgery) it may be of greater risk to attempt removal of a broken needle than to leave it behind, in most situations in gynecologic surgery, attempted removal of the needle is indicated.

Immediately on hearing the telltale "clack" of a broken needle, the surgeon should not withdraw the needle holder, nor avert his or her gaze from the surgical field. All available light should be directed onto the field. Good retraction and assistance are mandatory. A radiopaque marker, such as a surgical hemostatic clip, should be placed at the entry point of the needle (4). A different-sized clip can mark the expected exit site of the needle as if it had continued to arc through the tissue. Once the field is marked, the surgeon can gently probe the wound so as not to advance the broken tip any deeper into the tissue. It may be difficult to appreciate the "feel" of the needle fragment when it is small or the surrounding tissue is particularly firm. Often a small incision made perpendicular to the expected course of the needle will reveal the retained part. Use of a sterile strong magnet has been described to retrieve metallic foreign bodies. Small hand-held electronic instruments (Roper-Hall electro-acoustic metal foreign body locator) that are used in ophthalmologic surgery for localization of metallic foreign objects may be useful. If multiple attempts at probing the wound fail, then an imaging technique is indicated to help localize the retained needle (6).

The most available technique to help demonstrate a retained metallic object is radiography. An x-ray will confirm the presence of the fragment. This is the first priority if incision or probing fails to reveal the needle. A minimum of two views—anterior-posterior and lateral—with the use of markers (e.g., 18- to 20-gauge needles) inserted perpendicularly to the expected path of the broken needle may aid in localization. However, we question the utility of this method for localization. Recent experimental attempts at radiographic localization of a broken needle in an extirpated uterus have been very difficult. Intraoperative fluoroscopy via a c-arm device is the preferred radiographic technique. Needles can be advanced in one or several planes under fluoroscopic control until their tips lie in close proximity to the buried metal object; an incision can then be made down the shaft of the needle to retrieve the foreign body.

Ultrasonographic localization of retained metallic fragments is increasingly available. Modern ultrasound units found in obstetric departments often have sector-scanning capability; linear array units are unlikely to have the resolution necessary to retrieve needle tips. Currently, small transducers for sector scanners are available to perform transvaginal pelvic ultrasonography. These transducers are 1 cm square and would be small enough to help in needle localization in abdominal or vaginal cases. Ideally, if probing the wound fails to retrieve the needle tip, an ultrasonographer should be consulted. A 7.5- or 10-MHz in-line transducer is placed within a sterile probe cover (a surgical glove will do); sterile sonographic gel is placed in contact with the transducer inside the probe cover—it is not smeared on the uterus. With serial scanning and use of one or several probes, most needle fragments will be localized. When the retained needle is found, it should be grasped with a needle holder, then "backed out" or advanced along the tract of prior anticipated passage. In most cases, it should not be pulled straight up from its imbedded site. This maneuver would be acceptable only if an incision large enough to expose the entire needle had been made, an unlikely situation in myomectomy closure. A needle holder with a finer point than that in use when the needle broke may be useful.

Although computerized tomography (CT) and nuclear magnetic resonance (NMR) imaging have superior resolution in identifying metallic objects, their bulk makes them highly unlikely to be of any use in the intraoperative location of a broken needle. These advanced instruments may have their greatest utility in carefully following migration of retained foreign bodies toward vital structures.

REFERENCES

1. Anderson RM, Romfh RF: *Technique in the Use of Surgical Tools.* New York, Appleton-Century-Crofts, 1980, pp. 41–48.
2. Crouse VL: Migration of a broken anesthetic needle: Report of a case. *SC Dent J* 18:16–19, 1970.
3. Fraser-Moodie W: Recovery of broken needles. *Br Dent J* 105:79–85, 1958.
4. Leidelmeyer R: The embedded broken off needle. *JACEP* 5:362–363, 1976.
5. Orr D: The broken needle: Report of a case. *J Am Dent Assoc* 107:603, 1983.
6. Roper-Hall MJ (ed): *Stallard's Eye Surgery*, ed. 7. Philadelphia, JB Lippincott, 1980, pp. 773–801.
7. Trier WC: Considerations in the choice of surgical needles. *Surg Gynecol Obstet* 149:84, 1979.
8. Wigant FT: Otalgia caused by a broken needle in the pterygomandibular space: Report of a case. *J Oral Surg* 18:77–78, 1960.

5

A Small Transverse Pfannenstiel Incision and a Large Pelvic Tumor

William E. Crisp

Case Abstract

A 46-year-old patient had known for years of some fibroid tumors, but in the year preceding admission the tumors had slowly and progressively enlarged. Menses were regular, and no menopausal symptoms were evident. The uterus now extended to the patient's umbilicus. Total abdominal hysterectomy was recommended.

The abdomen was opened through a small Pfannenstiel incision and the pelvis was explored. The presence of multiple fibroids within the uterus was confirmed; the ovaries and tubes seemed grossly normal. There were so many large nodularities in the uterus that it could not be delivered "in one piece" through the incision.

DISCUSSION

Selecting the appropriate incision for abdominal gynecologic surgery is the primary step in ensuring a successful operation. Adequate exposure is essential.

The abdomen was opened via a small suprapubic Pfannenstiel incision and suspected pathology was confirmed, but the surgeon could not deliver the uterus through the incision. The problem was that the surgeon had compromised his proposed operation by an inappropriate incision. How could this predicament be avoided?

The problem the surgeon now faces with an inappropriate incision could have been avoided by the usual workup of a large pelvic mass, thought to be a myomatous uterus but could represent adnexal pathology or retroperitoneal pathology (lymphoma, etc.) or even a pelvic kidney, any of which could accentuate uterine size. Evaluation of the pelvic tumor by ultrasound or CAT scan or even MRI is now a routine procedure for any large pelvic mass.

Examination under anesthesia with or without a uterine sound is also essential in evaluating a pelvic mass before deciding which incision is appropriate.

SOLUTION

The operative findings confirmed the presence of a uterus irregularly enlarged with multiple fibroids. The solution to the problem is to either modify the Pfannenstiel incision to get more room or decrease the size of the uterus by myomectomy.

In this particular patient, both adnexa were normal and there were multiple leiomyomas, so the risk of sarcoma was minimal because a sarcoma will usually present as a single uterine enlargement. The menses had been regular and the patient was only 46 years old, so the risk of an endometrial cancer was also minimal. The patient, therefore, was a good candidate for myomectomy.

The technique of myomectomy depends on the location of the fibroids in the uterus. Ideally, it is best if you can ligate as much of the blood supply of the uterus as possible before removing the fibroids. If technically possible, both infundibulopelvic ligaments should be ligated and cut. The bladder flap should then be taken down so that the uterine vessels can be easily ligated. The peritoneal surface over the greater curvature of the fibroid is then incised and the fibroid can usually be bluntly dissected from the uterine base. If the uterine blood supply cannot be safely ligated, a uterine tourniquet can be placed around the uterus or the uterus can be debulked in a similar manner and bleeding controlled with figure-of-eight sutures. The Bonney clamp, which was designed for myomectomy, has not proven useful with a large uterus in our hands.

If the fibroids are intraligamentary, the broad ligament should be opened and the course of the uterer identified, as well as any distortions of vascular anatomy, before the fibroid is removed.

If it is the surgeon's choice to modify the incision, he or she has several options. If the Pfannenstiel incision is immediately suprapubic, it can be converted to a Cherney incision by cutting the tendinous insertion of the rectus and pyramidalis muscles and then extending the incision in a curvilinear manner toward the anterior superior spine of the ileum.

In closing the Cherney incision, it is important to identify the full thickness of the cut ends of the tendon and reattach it to the undersurface of the rectus sheath below the incision. Permanent sutures such as 0 Prolene, with parallel mattress sutures that are tied all at the same time, are appropriate. This is because the tendon of the rectus muscle retracts with potential hernia formation if it is not securely reattached.

If the original incision was placed more cephalad over the body of the rectus muscle, a muscle-cutting incision (Maylard) could be made and then extended in a curvilinear manner toward the anterior superior spine of the ileum. The rectus muscles are divided completely in a transverse fashion. The inferior epigastric vessels are always encountered and must be identified and ligated. The segmental innervation of the rectus muscle from the lateral edges of the muscle allows it to heal automatically with a new inscription, obviating the need to approximate the cut ends of the rectus.

If the patient's anatomy or the pelvic pathology limits the advantages of the extended transverse incision, the surgeon should not hesitate to convert the Pfannenstiel incision to a midline incision, giving the patient a T-shaped scar. Appearance is a secondary consideration to adequate exposure.

SELECTED READINGS

Thompson JD, Rock JA (eds): *Te Linde's Operative Gynecology*, ed. 7. Philadelphia, JB Lippincott, 1992.
Wheeless Cr Jr: *Atlas of Pelvic Surgery*. Philadelphia, Lea & Febiger, 1981.

6

Panniculectomy as Incidental Procedure

Joseph H. Pratt

Case Abstract

A chronically obese 42-year-old patient with a symptomatic myomatous uterus was advised to have an abdominal hysterectomy. She agreed to this recommendation and expressed the wish that her surgeon remove her abdominal panniculus at the same time.

DISCUSSION

Panniculectomy is the removal of excess fatty tissue and skin to provide access to the abdomen or to leave the female patient with an improved appearance. Unfortunately, gynecologic surgeons have almost completely overlooked this very obvious part of the total patient care of a surgical patient. Plastic surgeons, however, have most adequately filled the void, and their literature abounds in variations of techniques for the removal of excess adipose tissues and the reconstruction of the body's surface (4, 6).

The first panniculectomies were done for relatively enormous aprons and folds of skin and fat. Kelly (1) wrote in 1910 that these masses should be removed, if only for cosmetic effect to the patient. As much as a 78-lb (35–40 kg) panniculus has been reported (3), but 19 lb (18.6 kg) is the largest I have excised (5). A panniculectomy per se, utilizing large compressing stay sutures, will result in a relatively small loss of blood. A panniculectomy as a part of a surgical procedure to aid in removal of the uterus must be done in a manner that leaves the lower abdominal wall exposed for a laparotomy incision, and for this reason, 200 to 400 ml of blood may be lost during the panniculectomy.

There are two indications for a panniculectomy in association with an abdominal hysterectomy. Most women have some excess fat in the lower abdominal wall, and in some the fat may be 6 to 9 cm in thickness. There also may be large hanging aprons of tissues that actually rest against the front of the thighs. The skin beneath these folds is often chronically excoriated, inflamed, thickened, and pigmented. The most effective way to sterilize such an area is to remove it in toto, along with the thickened adipose tissues. Thus, one indication for a panniculectomy is to excise chronically infected areas and facilitate the exposure of the lower abdominal wall. This method requires transverse elliptical incisions that excise a large "watermelon" section of tissue (2). The lower abdominal wall thus exposed is only 1 to 2 cm in thickness from external rectus fascia to peritoneum, and any further incisions give excellent exposure to the pelvis.

The second indication for a hysterectomy–panniculectomy is appearance. There may not be enough adiposity to make the hysterectomy more difficult, yet by the addition of a modified panniculectomy, the surgeon can remove with almost no risk the majority of unsightly "stretch" marks, tighten-up excess flabby abdominal skin, and re-move enough lower abdominal wall and fat to give the patient a more stylish figure. Of course, along with removal of such excess unsightly tissues, hernias should be repaired if they are present. A diastasis recti, or even relaxed rectus fascia, can be imbricated to aid in the reconstructed appearance of the lower abdomen. Not only is there no increased risk of a resulting ventral or umbilical hernia, but, because of attention to technique, imbri-cation of fascia, and removal of excess loose skin, the abdominal wall is better supported than it was preoperatively.

In the first instance, the approach to the pelvis is facilitated, and in both instances the patient's general appearance is improved. There are drawbacks such as "dog ears" at the end of large transverse incisions when a large quantity of tissue is removed. Hematomas or seromas may require drainage, and some decreased sensation is always present from the extensive undermining of skin that is often necessary.

The umbilicus poses a problem. If considerable skin must be removed, the umbilicus will be displaced downward. In such cases, the best technique is to leave the umbilicus attached by a pedicle to the fascia, excise what tissues are necessary, and then bring the umbilicus out through a small circular midline incision that does not displace the umbilicus from its physical relationship to costal margins, symphysis, and iliac crests. Four to six skin sutures are all that are required to reattach the umbilicus to the skin.

For excision of a moderate or large panniculus in association with or as preparation for primary pelvic surgery, a transverse elliptical incision should be used. The fascia is widely exposed, and access to the abdomen is facilitated. The transverse diameter may be of any size, and often is between 30 to 70 cm. A vertical V of tissue may be excised in the midline to shorten the incision, and very often a V incision is necessary at the lateral ends to reduce the quantities of tissue there. Drainage is always necessary because of the extensive raw surfaces. Large vertical figure-of-eight sutures will help tack the skin flaps to the fascia, obliterate cavities, and hold the skin in apposition. These transverse inci-sions of the lower abdomen are large, the suture scars show, and the incisions are not cosmetically pleasing (Fig. 6.1).

When a panniculectomy or a "tummy tuck" is basically for cosmetic purposes, not as a specific aid to the pelvic procedure, then a different approach is indicated. A review of some of the articles in the plastic surgery journals is most helpful. These surgeons have spent much time and thought on the problem. In an effort to remove stretch marks, excise unsightly flabby skin, and so forth, undermining may be carried up to the costal margins. The lines of the incision should be marked preoperatively to be certain of symmetry. Depending on the tissue to be removed, the umbilicus may be transplanted through the upper skin flap. The final transverse skin incision should be at or below the hairline and be compatible with the wearing of a bikini bathing suit. Since the upper skin flap almost always is longer than the lower, some modification of a W incision in the lower skin flap is a helpful technique (Fig. 6.2).

Postoperatively, one watches for evidence of seromas or hematomas. All extensive incisions require drainage for at least 2 days. When tension on the suture line is

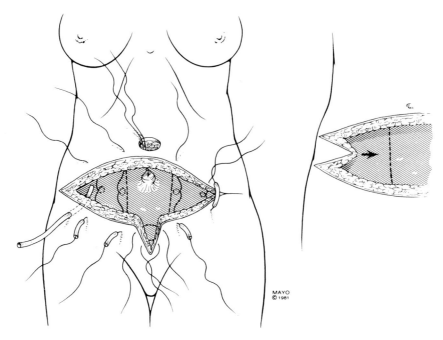

Figure 6.1. "Watermelon" incision with lower flap V; transplantation of umbilicus. At right is representation of incision closure to prevent "dog ears."

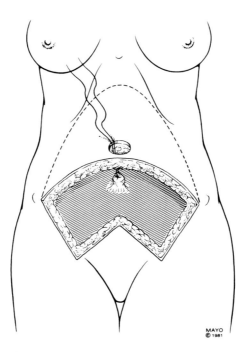

Figure 6.2. W incision.

considerable, and some tension is necessary to make the skin flap adhere to the fascia, then a modified "jackknife" position in bed is helpful for the first 48 hours. When snug compression dressings are utilized postoperatively to compress the skin to the fascia, the patient must be observed for evidence of respiratory difficulties.

As a general statement, patients are very happy to have this added attention, since this is the only part of an operation they can really see postoperatively. It behooves the gynecologic surgeon to be acquainted with techniques, to be cognizant of possible complications yet ready to advise the patient first of possible improvements in appearance, and to vary his or her normal operative approach as seems indicated.

REFERENCES

1. Kelly HA: Excision of the fat of the abdominal wal—lipectomy. *Surg Gynecol Obstet* 10:229, 1910.
2. Masson JK: Lipectomy: The surgical removal of excess fat. *Postgrad Med* 32:481, 1962.
3. Meyerowitz BR, Gruber RP, Lamb DR: Massive abdominal panniculectomy. *JAMA* 225:408, 1973.
4. Pitanguy V: Abdominal lipectomy: An approach to it through an analysis of 300 consecutive cases. *Plast Reconstr Surg* 40:384, 1967.
5. Pratt JH, Irons GB: Panniculectomy and abdominoplasty. *Am J Obstet Gynecol* 132:165, 1978.
6. Regnault P: Abdominoplasty by the W technique. *Plast Reconstr Surg* 55:265, 1975.

7

Symptomatic Genital Prolapse in a Patient Desiring More Children

David H. Nichols

Case Abstract

A 33-year-old primipara had been troubled by progressive and disabling feelings of pelvic discomfort, backache, and a bearing-down sensation when on her feet since the birth of her first child 6 months previously. The patient was a gestational diabetic, and labor was electively induced at the 36th week of gestation after amniocentesis study confirmed fetal lung maturity. A 12-hour induced labor with a prolonged first stage accompanied by much bearing down prior to full dilation of the cervix brought forth by spontaneous delivery without episiotomy a healthy 7-lb, 9-oz male infant. A second-degree perineal laceration was noted and repaired.

From that event to date the uterine cervix had protruded from the vagina, and the daytime protrusion was gradually increasing. A ring pessary was worn but briefly, the patient finding it uncomfortable and difficult to retain. Because the patient had expressed an intense desire for more children, she requested gynecologic help, but had no interest in hysterectomy at that time. There was no coincident urinary incontinence or gastrointestinal symptoms. There was no relevant past or family history, but the patient had taken oral contraceptives for 3 years prior to conception.

Pelvic examination confirmed the presence of a third-degree uterine prolapse with descent of the vaginal vault, minimal cervical elongation, a displacement upper vaginal cystocele, and a low rectocele. The uterus was not enlarged and was freely movable. No adnexal pathology was palpated. Voluntary contractions of her pubococcygei were of poor intensity. The pelvis was of gynecoid configuration. Laboratory blood studies and urinalysis and cervical cytology were within normal limits.

DISCUSSION

A progressive and symptomatic uterovaginal prolapse in a patient who wishes more children is a problem best solved, temporarily, by wearing a properly fitted ring pessary. This will permit coitus and conception, and will provide comfort to the patient until about the fifth month of gestation, at which time the pessary can be removed, and the size of the uterus usually will be large enough to retain the pregnancy and its container within the abdomen until after delivery, when the pessary can be reintroduced and the process repeated until childbearing has been completed and the patient can plan definitive surgery by vaginal hysterectomy and repair. Retention of a suitable pessary requires strong pubococcygei, permitting the pessary to rest on top of a strong levator plate.

When the pessary cannot be retained, as in the patient described, and conservation of the uterus is required, there are three primary surgical choices from which a proper operation may be selected that will relieve the patient's symptoms and yet preserve her fertility.

A transvaginal Manchester-type operation can be useful. An elongated cervix should be amputated at a point just below the internal cervical os, and the shortened cardinal ligaments sewn together in front of the remaining cervix, raising it within the pelvis and pushing it backward into the hollow of the sacrum. Coincident appropriate colporrhaphy can be accomplished. The risks concerning future pregnancy following a Manchester-type operation are four:

1. Postoperative cervical stenosis may develop that may make conception difficult. This can be prevented by periodic cervical dilatation and postoperative sounding of the cervical canal.
2. The residual cervix could be mechanically incompetent and dilate and efface prematurely during preganancy. If diagnosed in a timely fashion, a vaginal or abdominal cerclage could be performed.
3. Premature rupture of the membranes might occur near the beginning of fetal viability, and a very premature infant delivered at high risk for survival.
4. Fibrosis of the scarred residual cervix might produce a soft tissue dystocia and all of its problems during subsequent labor.

Transabdominal construction of a retroperitoneal sacrocervical ligament using fascia lata or a synthetic bridge such as Mersilene mesh would bring the cervix back into the hollow of the sacrum and would not interfere with subsequent labor and delivery (1).

A third option would be for transvaginal sacrospinous cervicopexy, possibly bilateral, in which the uterosacral ligaments at the site of junction to the cervix would be sewn to the coccygeus muscle–sacrospinous ligament complex, preferably using a buried permanent monofilament suture. This too should be followed by an anticipated normal labor and delivery. Coincident colporrhaphy would not be encouraged, lest the resultant surgically small vagina would not dilate sufficiently to permit safe vaginal delivery.

For the patient described, and who is without demonstrable cervical elongation, the author's choice would be for the second option—a transabdominal construction of a sacrocervical ligament—and the author would anticipate a normal future labor and delivery. Colporrhaphy to relieve symptoms might be required at some *future* date after completion of the childbearing process.

REFERENCE

1. Nichols DH: Fertility retention in the patient with genital prolapse. *Am J Obstet Gynecol* 164:1155–1158, 1991.

8

Ruptured Tubo-Ovarian Abscess

Richard H. Schwarz

Case Abstract

A ruptured right tubo-ovarian abscess was discovered at laparotomy for suspected appendicitis in a 30-year-old infertility patient. The abscess was on the patient's right side, but the appendix was not involved in the process. The tube and ovary of the left side of the pelvis were grossly normal, although now bathed in the purulent exudate from the ruptured right tubo-ovarian abscess. A 4-cm leiomyoma was palpable in the uterine fundus.

DISCUSSION

The critical problem presented by this case is to strike a balance between a desire to preserve the potential of childbearing in this relatively young infertile woman and the risk that surgical conservatism may not resolve the life-threatening problem. This decision would be far less difficult if the patient were multiparous or perimenopausal, or even if the opposite tube and ovary were grossly diseased, suggesting a poor prognosis for any future reconstructive surgery. In such circumstances, total abdominal hysterectomy with bilateral salpingo-oophorectomy would be the approach of choice and would offer the most certain chance of cure. Unilateral adnexal removal, however, is the better option for this patient.

Although it is not common to have totally unilateral involvement with pelvic inflammatory disease, it is certainly more common than previously thought, or taught, to have markedly disparate involvement of the two sides. Up to 40% of tubo-ovarian abscesses are unilateral, a finding first brought to the attention of clinicians in dealing with infections associated with intrauterine contraceptive devices. This information does permit the surgeon to consider a conservative approach. The worst-case outcome for the patient, if this approach is used, would be the need for a second operation. This might arise if the less obvious disease in the residual tube progressed despite perioperative antibiotics or a secondary pelvic operative site (pelvic) abscess formed. The latter could, of course, occur even if hysterectomy and bilateral salpingo-oophorectomy were done.

The surgical procedure in this patient should be a simple salpingo–oophorectomy on the side of the abscess. The myoma described should not be removed since an incision into the uterus would provide a focus for secondary infection. Surgical steps should include obtaining aerobic and anaerobic cultures (best done from the pus in the abscess or even a piece of the abscess wall); exploration of the abdomen to locate and break up any loculations of pus; and thorough lavage with copious amounts of warm saline solution. Although some would suggest irrigation with antibiotic solutions, the author believes there is some risk of absorption of excess quantities of antibiotics from inflamed serosal surfaces. In general, the author believes antibiotics are most effectively delivered in such patients by the intravenous route.

There are always questions concerning surgical drainage in these cases. Should there be drainage? Of what area? Through what portal? The author believes this patient should have drainage, and there are two reasonable options for the route. If the cul-de-sac is free, a drain can be placed through that area into the vagina. A T-tube or a mushroom catheter is appropriate, and placement can be facilitated by an assistant exerting upward pressure with an open-ring forceps or long hemostat placed in the posterior vaginal fornix. This same instrument can then be used to pull the drain down into the vagina after a stab wound in the cul-de-sac has been made. This route has the advantage of gravity. An alternate is placement of a drain through a lateral stab wound (drains should not be brought out through the primary incision). The tip of the drain may be placed in the cul-de-sac or at the site of the abscess. Finally, in such a patient, the wound should be dealt with by delayed primary closure of the subcutaneous tissue and skin.

With the approach outlined it is important to keep in mind that with the increased use of sophisticated imaging technology and laparoscopy, it is more likely now that the diagnosis of a tubo-ovarian abscess would have been made, or at least suspected, prior to laparotomy and hopefully before rupture had occurred. This would then have afforded options not applicable in this case, including intensive antibiotic therapy. Recent studies indicate that 75% of tubo-ovarian abscesses diagnosed by sonography can be successfully managed conservatively with broad-spectrum antibiotic treatment. Unruptured abscesses have also been successfully managed by percutaneous or transvaginal aspiration and drainage guided by sonography or other imaging techniques. This may be a consideration when the response to antibiotics is incomplete, before proceeding to laparotomy, provided the patient is under close supervision and there is no evidence of rupture. The long-term outcome with this approach and even with intensive antibiotic therapy has not been well studied, particularly as to the need for later surgical treatment. Nonetheless, the occurrence of a ruptured abscess demands surgical intervention.

SELECTED READINGS

Brown SE, Allen HH, Robins RN: The use of delayed primary wound closure in preventing wound infection. *Am J Obstet Gynecol* 127:713, 1977.

Casola G, van Sonnenberg E, Dagostino HB, Harker CP, Varney RR, Smith D: Percutaneous drainage of tubo-ovarian abscesses. *Radiology* 182(2):399–402, 1992.

Franklin EW, Hevron JE, Thompson JD: Management of pelvic abscesses. *Clin Obstet Gynecol* 16:66, 1973.

Mead PB, Beecham JB, Maeck S Jr: Incidence of infections associated with intrauterine contraceptive devices in an isolated community. *Am J Obstet Gynecol* 125:79, 1976.

Reed SD, Landers DV, Sweet RL: Antibiotic treatment of tubo-ovarian abscess: Comparison of broad-spectrum beta-lactam agents versus clindamycin-containing regimens. *Am J Obstet Gynecol* 164:1556–1561, 1991.

Shulman A, Maymon R, Shapiro A, Bahary C: Percutaneous catheter drainage of tubo-ovarian abscesses. *Obstet Gynecol* 80:555–557, 1992.

Soper DE: Surgical considerations in the diagnosis and treatment of pelvic inflammatory disease. *Surgical Clinics of North America* 71:947–962, 1991.

Teisala K, Heinonen PK, Punnonen R: Transvaginal ultrasound in the diagnosis and treatment of tubo-ovarian abscess. *Br J Obstet Gynaecol* 97:178–180, 1990.

9

Ovarian Remnant Syndrome

Raymond A. Lee

Case Abstract

The patient, a 35-year-old gravida I, para I weighing 173 pounds, presented with pelvic pain. Her past history was significant in that her first operation was an abdominal exploration in 1983, at which time an endometrioma was removed from the right ovary. She subsequently underwent five additional laparoscopic procedures from 1979 to early 1991, at which time endometriosis was cauterized, but no tissue was ever obtained at any of these procedures. Her second major abdominal operation was in 1991, at which time a total abdominal hysterectomy and bilateral salpingo–oophorectomy were done for persistent pain from endometriosis. Her third abdominal operation was done in 1992, at which time her local surgeon removed an ovarian remnant along the left side of the pelvis, which was flush with the left ureter. Following this operation, she received pelvic radiation in five separate treatments with a total dose of 1500 cgy. Following all of this treatment, the patient was unable to have sexual relations because of pelvic pain but did experience normal bowel and bladder function.

On the author's initial examination, the patient could not permit an accurate pelvic examination because of pelvic discomfort. Under anesthesia, one was able to palpate a thickened, firm mass along the left pelvic sidewall at approximately the area where the left ureter would enter the bladder. The right pelvis felt normal.

DISCUSSION

The ovarian remnant syndrome is an unusual complication of bilateral oophorectomy, usually when combined with hysterectomy. The patient often presents with pain, with or without a definable pelvic mass.

Predisposing Factors

Conditions associated with dense adhesions, diffuse inflammatory reaction, or distortion of pelvic anatomy leading to a difficult dissection may result in retention of a fragment of ovarian tissue. The most frequent predisposing conditions are endometriosis, pelvic inflammatory disease, diverticulitis, and previous operations with the resultant adhesions. There is an apparent increase in the frequency of the ovarian remnant syndrome. This probably results from more widespread use of ultrasonography or computed tomography scanning in evaluating the patient with recurrent or persistent pain after bilateral oophorectomy.

Symptoms

Usually, the condition occurs within 5 years after bilateral salpingo–oophorectomy. The most frequent presenting symptom or sign is pelvic pain with a mass. Occasionally, the patient may have pelvic pain without a discernible mass or may have a symptomatic mass. The pain may vary from a sensation of pelvic pressure to a dull ache or a sharp stabbing pain. Occasionally, there may be dyspareunia, and gastrointestinal or urinary symptoms may be a part of the clinical pattern. The patient may experience temporary hot flashes immediately after the operation only to have them spontaneously disappear, suggesting the resurgence of estrogen production. It is possible that older patients undergoing oophorectomy under similar conditions may retain portions of the ovary yet remain asymptomatic because of the lack of ovarian activity.

Diagnosis

Knowledge of the clinical history of this entity is critical in making the diagnosis. A palpable mass or thickening is identifiable in most patients. Because of the frequent extraperitoneal location of the remnant or presence of extensive adhesions, laparoscopic examination is rarely beneficial or helpful in making the diagnosis. Ultrasound examination and computerized tomography scans are helpful in further delineating the size and the location of a mass. Preoperative pyelography may also define the status of the ureter, demonstrating effects of a previous operation or a current ovarian problem, which may foretell surgical obstacles. The FSH value lends support to the diagnosis. The presence of premenopausal levels of FSH in the absence of exogenous hormone confirms that residual ovarian tissue is present. However, we have seen patients with histologically normal ovarian tissue who had postmenopausal gonadotropin levels suggesting that the remaining ovarian tissue was not active enough to suppress these hormones. The surgeon should be prepared to dissect the ureter throughout its pelvic course because it always will have some involvement.

Treatment

Through a lower midline incision, exploration of the upper abdomen was entirely normal. The doctors had placed, preoperatively, ureteral stents up both ureters. Beginning above the pelvic brim on the left side, we dissected the ureter throughout its course and carried out an en bloc resection of the distal ureter with a thickened, scarred mass involving the branches of the internal iliac artery and vein. They also dissected the right ureter, removing a thickened, scarred area and its medial surface just superior to the dome of the bladder. The pathology report read:

> Specimen reveals a 5 × 4 × 1.6 cm mass in the left side and a 7 × 4.5 × 1 cm mass on the right side. The right pelvic mass reveals luteinized ovarian stroma. The left pelvic sidewall reveals a portion of luteinized ovarian tissue identified. Complete cross section of the segments shows ureter present. Back of bladder shows fibrosis with no ovarian tissue identified. Sections from the back of the bladder and pelvic sidewall show endometriosis.

Postoperatively, the patient did well, and her left ureteral stent was removed 3 months following this procedure, after which an IVP revealed normal renal function.

The author favors operative excision of the mass with identification of the ureter in an extraperitoneal position, beginning above the level of the previous operation. After the perirectal and perivesical spaces are developed, the anterior division of the internal iliac vessels is usually ligated in preparation for further ureteral dissection. Staying close to the ureter, one applies tension to the mass to provide the necessary countertraction for sharp dissection (Fig. 9.1). Rather than concentrating on excision of the mass, attention is directed to complete dissection of the ureter throughout its pelvic course (Fig. 9.2). After this is accomplished, the surgeons completely excise the ovarian remnant with its contiguous peritoneum and surrounding tissues. Some have advocated the use of radiotherapy (as was done in this patient) to produce a castrating level of radiation. The author has had no firsthand experience with the use of radiation; however, secondhand experience would suggest that this is not very successful. In the multioperated patient, the presence of a ureteral catheter may aid in the identification of the ureter and facilitate the dissection of the ovarian remnant. Usually, a ureteral catheter is unnecessary and not routinely placed because its unyielding nature may add to the potential of ureteral injury. Excellent exposure with appropriate traction and countertraction and perfect hemostasis will facilitate the dissection of contiguous structures (bowel, bladder, vessels, and nerve routes) to ensure safe, complete removal of the ovarian remnant (Fig. 9.3). In most patients, and in all of those undergoing repeated operations, Hemovac catheter drainage is carried out in an extraperitoneal fashion to prevent hematoma or lymphocyst formation. Successful excision of the mass is associated with prompt relief of symptoms and few complications.

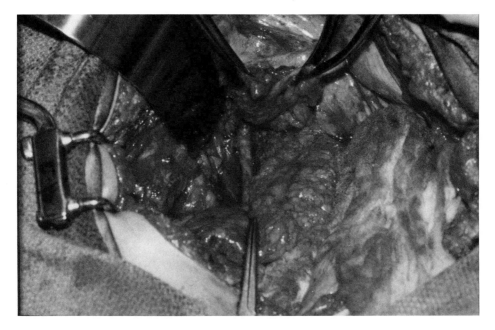

Figure 9.1. Tension is applied medially on the mass with the major vessels of the leg held laterally, exposing the partially dissected left ureter.

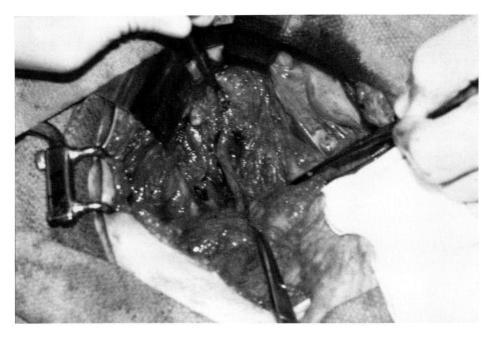

Figure 9.2.   With the major vessels retracted laterally, the completely dissected left ureter is exposed from the brim of the pelvis to its entrance into the bladder.

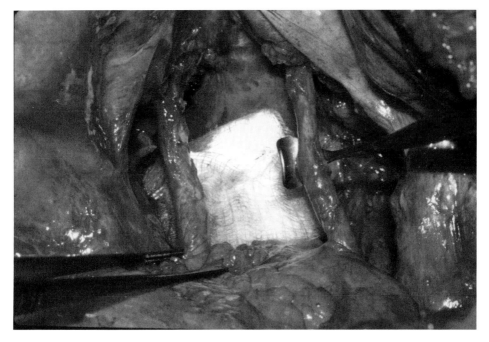

Figure 9.3.   Bilateral dissection of the pelvic sidewalls results in both ureters being free from the level of the sacrum to their entrance into the bladder.

10

Coexisting Genital Procidentia and Rectal Prolapse

M. Leon Tancer

Case Abstract

A 76-year-old multipara complaining of a mass between her thighs, anal incontinence, and the frequent inability to initiate micturition was found to have coexisting massive genital and rectal prolapse (Fig. 10.1). Upon replacing the genital prolapse, urinary incontinence was demonstrated during a Valsalva maneuver.

DISCUSSION

Some degree of genital prolapse is a common finding in gynecologic practice, and total genital prolapse, procidentia, is not unusual. What is unusual is the coexistence of procidentia with massive rectal prolapse. Not surprisingly, colorectal surgeons report some degree of genital prolapse in up to 70% of female patients with rectal prolapse, probably because most such patients are elderly. However, they too find the coexistence of rectal prolapse and procidentia to be highly unusual.

The coexistence of genital procidentia and massive rectal prolapse places one on the horns of a therapeutic dilemma. Should the two prolapsed organs be treated at different times and by different surgeons? If so, which should be treated first, and what procedure or procedures should each surgeon perform? Or is there a rational approach to their simultaneous surgical management?

It is well recognized that the failure to correct all existing anatomic defects when managing genital prolapse often leads to an unsatisfactory therapeutic result and the expectation of the need for future surgery. Therefore, multiple procedures are commonly performed using either a suprapubic or transvaginal approach. Defects should be determined preoperatively and may exist in any combination. Surgery, therefore, may involve any combination of the following procedures: removal of the prolapsing uterus; correction of midline, anterior, and posterior vaginal wall defects; prevention or excision of an enterocele sac; shortening of the cardinal ligament complex; replacement of the vesical neck to its retropubic site; repair of a paravaginal defect; and, of major significance, attachment of an incompetently supported vaginal apex to a fixed pelvic structure.

The anatomic defect present in rectal prolapse is the loss of the normal position of the rectum in the hollow of the sacrum where intra-abdominal pressure compresses the rectum against the supporting levator ani. It is the contraction of the

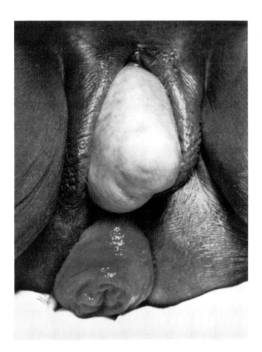

Figure 10.1.   Actual procidentia uteri and rectal prolapse at time of surgery.

levator ani that then angulates the rectum to help maintain fecal continence. A congenitally long sigmoid mesentery allows the rectosigmoid to migrate from its normal position in the sacral hollow to adopt a longitudinal attitude overlying the anal orifice, through which the rectum intussuscepts. As a result, the anal sphincter becomes dilated excessively and loses tone, and the rectum evades angulation by the contracting levator. Hence, fecal incontinence is a common complaint.

A transabdominal procedure, sacral rectopexy, repositions the rectum in the sacral hollow. Subsequently anal sphincter tone returns to normal and the rectum again becomes susceptible to angulation by the contracting levator ani. Fecal incontinence as well as rectal prolapse disappears.

As previously stated, a major defect in genital procidentia is the lack of effective support for the vaginal apex. This defect has been successfully managed by sacral–colpopexy. It would appear rational to accomplish both sacral suspensions simultaneously. Since most of the multiple defects associated with procidentia can be corrected transabdominally, the necessary procedures to do so can be carried out through the same incision. Only the repair of a rectocele or reconstruction of a defective perineal body would require the addition of a vaginal approach.

The technique of combined rectal and vaginal sacropexy as depicted in Figures 10.2 through 10.5 begins after the bowel is packed out of the field and the rectosigmoid is held to the left. The posterior parietal peritoneum is incised in the midline, from the level of the sacral promontory down to the junction of the rectum and sigmoid. The right ureter is identified. The retrorectal space is developed by gentle blunt and sharp dissection to the level of the coccyx. The prolapsed rectum is grasped and drawn into the pelvis. A trapezoidal piece of Teflon mesh measuring 12 cm in length, 7 cm at its distal end, and 3 cm at its proximal end is sutured to the posterior rectal wall with no. 00 silk so

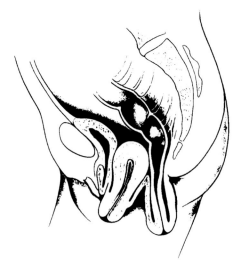

Figure 10.2. Sagittal view of procidentia uteri and rectal prolapse.

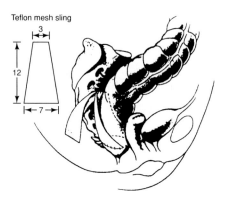

Figure 10.3. Mesh attached to S2–S3 interspace. Rectum drawn into hollow of sacrum.

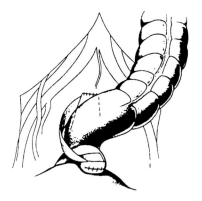

Figure 10.4. Free mesh attached to apex of vagina.

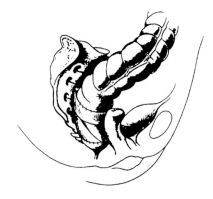

Figure 10.5. Vagina and rectum in parallel lying in hollow of sacrum.

that the wide edge is at the rectal ampulla and the graft covers the posterior rectal wall. The proximal end of the graft is free and is drawn to the level of the S2–S3 interspace, causing the rectum to lie well in the hollow of the sacrum (Fig. 10.3). An oblong piece of mesh measuring 3 × 12 cm is then cut. One 3-inch end and the free end of the mesh previously attached to the posterior rectum are sewn simultaneously to the S2–S3 inter-vertebral ligament with interrupted no. 00 silk sutures. This fixes the rectum in the hollow of the sacrum and leaves a free end of the oblong mesh for further use. The free mesh (Fig. 10.4) is brought around the right side of the fixed rectum, cut to the appropriate length, and sutured to the posterior wall of the upper vagina so that the vagina will lie in the hollow of the sacrum directly anterior to the fixed rectum. The medial edge of the second mesh is attached to the lateral rectum and curved around it to the posterior vagina to close any potential space (Fig. 10.5). The cut edges of the posterior parietal peritoneum are approximated, and the abdomen closed.

Although simultaneous prolapse of the uterus and rectum is uncommon, this technique of repair addresses this most distressing condition satisfactorily.

Surgical management consisted of a supravaginal hysterectomy with inverted cervical conization, bilateral salpingo–oophorectomy, simultaneous sacral colporec-topexy and Burch retropubic colpopexy carried out through a Maylard incision, followed by a posterior colpoperineorrhaphy with high anterior levator plication.

Selected Readings

Amico JC, Marino AW: Prolapse of the vagina in association with rectal procidentia. *Dis Colon Rectum* 11:115, 1968.

Azpuru CE: Total rectal prolapse and total genital prolapse. *Dis Colon Rectum* 17:528, 1974.

Kupfer CA, Goligher JC: One hundred consecutive cases of complete prolapse of the rectum treated by operation. *Br J Surg* 57:481, 1970.

Parks AG: Anorectal incontinence. *Proc R Soc Med* 68:681, 1975.

Ripstein CB: Surgical care of massive rectal prolapse. *Dis Colon Rectum* 8:34, 1965.

Tancer ML, Fleischer M, Berkowitz BJ: Simultaneous colpo-recto-sacropexy. *Obstet Gynecol* 70:951, 1987.

Zhioua F, Ferchiou JM, Pira A, Jedoui A, Meriah S: La promonto-fixation uterine et l'intervention d'Orr-Loygue dans l'association prolapsus genital et prolapsus rectal. Rev fr. *Gynecol Obstet* 88: 277, 1993.

The Missing Sponge

Charles E. Flowers, Jr.

Case Abstract

Following completion of a vaginal hysterectomy and repair, a final sponge count was reportedly short by one. A recount was unrewarding.

DISCUSSION

It is important that the surgeon believe the sponge count: there is a missing sponge until every possibility of error is eliminated. Today, it is rare for operating personnel to make mistakes in the sponge count. In the majority of hospitals, laparotomy pads are placed in five units in each pack, and sponges are placed in ten units of each pack. When a pack is broken on the operating table, the scrub nurse and the circulating nurse both count the sponges. If there is an error, that group of sponges is removed from the operating theater. After sponges are used they are placed back in a container, five in the laparotomy sponge container and ten in each sponge container. At the conclusion of the procedure, it is only necessary to count the remaining sponges to be sure that all are present.

If a sponge is missing, the pathology specimen is first checked, then the space around the operating table and the shoe soles of the personnel in the operating theater. A recount is made. If the sponge is still missing, an x-ray of the abdomen is mandatory.

The operator must assume responsibility for every sponge he or she uses in a procedure. Appropriate surgical technique dictates that no free sponges be used in the abdomen and that all laparotomy pads be marked with a ring or instrument. If it is necessary to place a free sponge deep within the pelvis or the recesses of an anterior or posterior repair, it is preferable to put a suture through the sponge and clamp it with an instrument so that it can be easily retrieved. If a fairly large sponge is necessary, a laparotomy pad may be cut in half or thirds and appropriately marked.

During the time that the flat plate of the abdomen is being ordered and taken, a recheck of the count should be made. However, one should not yet take down the anterior or posterior repair or open the peritoneum. One should wait until the flat plate of the abdomen is available and can be examined in the operating room. When the sponge is located, it is retrieved by the simplest method possible. Remember that a blood-soaked sponge or pad more or less assumes the color of its operative environment, making it more difficult to spot.

The old adage "an ounce of prevention is worth a pound of cure" is also true in surgery. The surgeon should refrain from using free sponges, mark the sponges he or she does use, and work very closely with the operating room personnel.

In this litiginous society, one must be thoughtful about what is told to a patient. If the sponge is found before the peritoneal cavity is closed, simple operative maneuvers can be made to retrieve the sponge: it is unnecessary to inform the patient concerning the event. However, if an x-ray of the abdomen is taken to locate a sponge it is important to indicate to the patient what was done.

An obstetrician and gynecologist can usually see the opaque string of the sponge. However, consultation with a radiologist is extremely important if there are problems of interpretation. Occasionally, it may be necessary in the obese patient to make a second film of greater intensity.

12

Pending Evisceration After Laparotomy

Byron J. Masterson

Case Abstract

A large amount of pink stained serous fluid was exuding spontaneously from the center of a healing laparotomy incision on the third postoperative day. The patient was a 40-year-old diabetic.

DISCUSSION

This patient had impending evisceration. The fluid frequently seen preceding evisceration is peritoneal fluid. When found, a differential diagnosis of seroma, fat necrosis, infection, fistula, or urine from a severed patent urachus should be made. Peritoneal fluid is generally clear or pink in appearance, nonpurulent, and profuse, and its discharge is painless to the patient.

The major problem here is a proper diagnosis. Before the surgeon can treat the problem, he or she must carefully investigate the wound. If the wound has a significant separation, use of a sterile powder-free glove is an efficient way to probe the wound. It should be remembered that the skin, although it seals in 24 hours, is relatively loosely affixed and may be easily separated if necessary. Should the entire fascial wound be separated, immediate reoperation is necessary.

In such patients, the fascial suture will almost invariably be found to be intact but tied too tightly, with necrosis occurring in the suture loops. Often the suture is placed too near the margins of the wound. Active collagenolysis is present in normal incisions. The area of collagenolysis will extend further laterally if there is infection, promoting dehiscence by weakening the fascia.

Management, therefore, requires full assessment of the wound. If the patient has a fascial dehiscence, she should be taken back to the operating room. There the devitalized tissue should be removed with a sharp scalpel and the wound closed with a delayed absorbable suture of adequate gauge. The use of no. 0 or no. 1 PDS (polydiaxanone) or Maxon, placed 2 to 4 cm lateral to the edge of the wound and loosely approximated, will produce an excellent wound closure. Intraoperative antibiotic coverage is useful but need not be continued after the procedure.

If the patient exudes only a minimal amount of clear fluid, the diagnosis may be fat necrosis and skin may be reapproximated. Where purulent drainage is involved, infection is present. Early antibiotics, excision of dead tissue, and secondary closure have been very successful. Such closure can be performed under local anesthesia with 1%

Xylocaine and 10 mg intramuscular morphine. The skin is prepared and the wound is closed with interrupted closure of the skin. A number of large series have been closed using this procedure with a minimum of complications. However, it is critical that the operator make certain that the fascia is intact and the problem is only a subcutaneous one before this closure is attempted.

SELECTED READINGS

Bergan JJ, Dean RH, Yao JT: Vascular injuries in pelvic cancer surgery. *Am J Obstet Gynecol* 124:562, 1976.

Daly JW: Dehiscence, evisceration and other complications. In: Masterson BJ (ed): *Clinical Obstetrics and Gynecology* 31(3). Philadelphia, JB Lippincott, 1988.

Dodson MK, Magann EF, Meeks GR: A randomized comparison of secondary closure and secondary intention in patients with superficial wound dehiscence. *Obstet Gynecol* 80(3–1):321–324, 1992.

Magrina JF, Moffat RE, Masterson BJ, et al: Selective arterial infusion of Pitressin for the control of puerperal hemorrhage after hypogastric artery ligation. *Obstet Gynecol* 58:646, 1981.

Masterson BJ: *Manual of Gynecologic Surgery*, ed. 2. New York, Springer-Verlag, 1986.

13

Postoperative Septic Pelvic Thrombophlebitis

James L. Breen
Brian Casey

Case Abstract

A 36-year-old multipara had undergone total abdominal hysterectomy and bilateral salpingo–oophorectomy because of chronic, recurrent pyosalpinx. She had had four episodes of clinical flare-up with chills, fever, pain, and menorrhagia during the year preceding surgery. These episodes had become more frequent, with the most recent one 7 weeks prior to the surgery.

Surgery was complicated by many old and new pelvic adhesions. A right tubo-ovarian abscess spilled into the abdominal wound during the course of surgery. The pelvis was irrigated with 2 quarts of sterile saline and the vaginal vault closed.

There was considerable postoperative pain and a sustained fever varying between 102° F and 104° F beginning the first postoperative day. Intravenous penicillin and chloramphenicol were administered. By the third postoperative day the fever was spiking in character, with a tachycardia sustained even when the temperature was at its nadir. Temperature spikes up to 104° F were preceded by a shaking chill followed by profuse sweating. Examination at this time revealed minimum pelvic tenderness with no palpable masses.

DISCUSSION

The patient described in the case presentation fulfills the classic description of the "pelvic cripple." Despite treatment of the initial episodes of pelvic inflammatory disease, the patient continued to have flare-ups with fever, pain, menorrhagia, and pelvic masses. The initial episode may have been a postpartum or postabortal infection, pelvic inflammatory disease from a sexually transmitted pathogen, or a complication of previous pelvic surgery. In most instances, regardless of age, a problem of this degree is usually resolved with surgical intervention by performing a total abdominal hysterectomy and bilateral salpingo–oophorectomy.

Based on the history, findings at surgery, the amount of surgical dissection necessary, and the rupture or "leak" of the abscess, a stormy postoperative course should have been anticipated. Now, 3 days after surgery, the clinician is faced with a patient who is febrile, very ill, and unresponsive to the usual therapeutic measures. In light of this, several preoperative, intraoperative, and postoperative phophylactic measures must be considered.

In order to manage gynecologic patients with postoperative febrile morbidity, the clinician must understand the microorganisms involved; the techniques of identifying them; their spectum of activity; the toxicity of proposed antibiotics; and the role of surgery in draining collections of purulent material. There are no uniformly satisfactory methods to culture specimens from deep-seated infections such as parametritis, pelvic cellulitis, and septic pelvic thrombophlebitis. We can overcome this handicap, however, by understanding those organisms that cause pelvic infections, the majority of which are caused by endogenous organisms normally found in the vaginal flora. These organisms become opportunistic pathogens in tissues damaged by trauma or exogenous pathogens such as *Neisseria gonorrhoeae*. The organisms most often involved in postoperative infections in pelvic surgery are listed in Table 13.1. The cause of pelvic infections after pelvic surgical procedures usually involves both aerobic and anaerobic bacteria. In addition to well-recognized pathogens such as Beta-hemolytic streptococci, *Escherichia coli*, *Neisseria gonorrhoeae*, *Chlamydia trachomatis*, and coagulase-negative staphylococci, anaerobic bacteria are commonly recovered in patients with postoperative pelvic infections. The most common anaerobic organisms isolated include peptostreptococci, peptococci, *Bacteroides bivius*, *B. digiens, B. fragilis*, and *Fusobacterium* species (9).

Differential Diagnosis

The differential diagnosis of conditions potentially responsible for this patient's fever are outlined in Table 13.2. Pelvic surgery in the presence of chronic pelvic inflammatory disease places the patient at an increased risk for any or all of the complications listed. Descriptions of these conditions generally list chronic pelvic inflammatory disease as a prime etiologic risk factor, yet all etiologies must be considered while the site, or sites, of infection are sought. An immediate threat to life would come from gram-negative sepsis with endotoxic shock, clostridial sepsis, necrotizing fasciitis, and septic pelvic thrombophlebitis with septic embolization.

Febrile morbidity, or temperature elevation in an otherwise asymptomatic patient, is not part of the differential diagnosis in this particular patient; however, it is still

Table 13.1   Organisms Recovered from Pelvic Infections

Aerobic bacteria	*Streptococcus*	Anaerobic bacteria	*Peptostreptococcus*
Gram-positive	*Staphylococcus*	Gram-positive cocci	*Peptococcus*
Gram-positive rods	*Diphtheroids*	Gram-positive rods	*Clostridium* species
	Listeria monocytogenes		
Gram-negative rods	*Escherichia coli*	Gram-negative rods	*Bacteroides* species
	Klebsiella		*Fusobacterium* species
	Pseudomonas		
	Proteus		
	Enterobacter		
	Serratia		

Table 13.2   Differential Diagnosis in Septic Postoperative Patients

Febrile morbidity
Atelectasis and pneumonia
Urinary tract damage or infection
Infected pelvic hematoma
Vaginal cuff cellulitis
Wound infection (clostridial or necrotizing fasciitis)
Bacterial resistance to appropriate or inappropriate antibiotic therapy
Generalized peritonitis
Endotoxic shock
Pelvic cellulitis
Pelvic or intra-abdominal abscess
Septic pelvic thrombophlebitis

an important consideration during the initial evaluation of postoperative patients. Temperature elevation is but one sign of infection, and is relied upon too heavily as an indicator of postoperative pelvic infection. Recurrent temperature elevations are commonly observed after pelvic surgery. The tendency to initiate antimicrobial therapy for the diagnosis of "presumptive pelvic infection" should be avoided in the absence of other signs and symptoms of infection. Transitory febrile morbidity occurring within 48 hours of surgery usually disappears without therapy (3).

An additional and common cause of early postoperative fever and tachycardia is pulmonary atelectasis, which, if untreated, leads to pneumonitis. It occurs to some degree in every patient, and undoubtedly contributes to febrile morbidity after pelvic surgery. Atelectasis is more frequently observed after abdominal than after vaginal surgery. The tenderness of abdominal incisions promotes abdominal stinting, which leads to hypoventilation and nonclearance of secretions and is the basis for atelectasis (3). The patient described here had a prolonged operation followed by considerable pain and probable abdominal distention, all of which are contributing factors. Physical findings may be absent but basilar rales are usually heard on auscultation. Roentgenographic findings may also be equally unrevealing but may detect extensive atelectasis.

Urinary tract infections and injuries are a significant source of postoperative infection, with recent studies suggesting an incidence of 10% to 35% in gynecologic patients (6). Extravasation of urine from injuries of the ureter into the peritoneal cavity or retroperitoneal space will result in high spiking fevers and chills in the very early postoperative period. Pyuria and flank pain may be present but are more commonly seen in conventional urinary tract infections.

Hematoma formation or intra-abdominal bleeding, in the face of active infection, can also cause fever. A falling hematocrit or an expanding mass on examination or by imaging techniques would suggest this, and immediate reoperation may be necessary. Eventually, if unresolved, this could lead to pelvic and/or abdominal abscess formation.

Cuff cellulitis is a very mild form of pelvic infection that develops at the vaginal surgical margin after hysterectomy. The vaginal cuff becomes hyperemic and indurated for several days. Additionally, a purulent vaginal discharge may be noted with tenderness at the vaginal margin. Though most women develop subclinical cuff cellulitis after hysterectomy, few require antimicrobial therapy. However, cuff cellulitis may progress, causing lower abdominal or pelvic pain with marked tenderness at the vaginal cuff. Coupled with a low-grade temperature, these findings are indicative of an infectious process requiring antibiotics. Response to broad-spectrum parenteral antibacterial therapy is usually prompt. Mild cases may be successfully treated with oral antimicrobials.

Wound infections are a frequent occurrence when surgery is performed in the presence of active pelvic infections. Bacterial contamination, blood and foreign material left in the wound, the inappropriate use or placement of drains, delayed closures, and inappropriate prophylactic antibiotic selection determine whether a wound infection will develop. Although clinical recognition of wound infections occurs 5 to 6 days after surgery, there are two exceptions: clostridial infections and necrotizing fasciitis. Members of the *Clostridium* species are endogenous to women, particularly to the gastrointestinal tract, and can also be found in the genital tract of asymptomatic women. The diagnosis of clostridial infection should be based on clinical findings with early gram staining and microbiologic workup serving as an adjunct. Clostridial anaerobic myonecrosis (clostridial gas gangrene) is dramatic in its sudden onset, with rapid involvement of skin and subcutaneous tissue. *Clostridium perfringens* is responsible in 60% to 80% of cases, and clinical signs occur between 12 and 72 hours postoperatively. The resultant effects are due to exotoxins produced by the *Clostridium* species (5). *C. perfringens* alone produces at least 12 different toxins that differentially cause local hemolysis and soft tissue necrosis. These toxins are also responsible for systemic reactions, including intravascular hemolysis and renal failure. Septic shock and hypofibrinogenemia may occur, with hepatorenal failure occurring in the terminal stages of the disease.

The early clinical signs of clostridial infection are similar to those of necrotizing fasciitis. In necrotizing fasciitis the wound is excruciatingly painful and is characterized by dark vesicles, dusky discoloration, and widespread ecchymosis in the surrounding skin. Crepitation occurs occasionally. Progression to anesthesia of the affected area with subcutaneous and fascial necrosis results in extensive undermining of the skin. Hemolytic *Streptococcus*, hemolytic *Staphylococcus*, and a variety of virulent gram-negative bacteria are responsible. The characteristic cutaneous manifestations and the initial systemic signs of a clostridial infection should alert the physician to a diagnosis of necrotizing fasciitis. Tachycardia out of proportion to the degree of fever is consistently found. The early differential diagnosis of the two conditions can be made on a Gram's stain of the wound exudate.

The choice of an initial antibiotic regimen is not difficult when one considers the potential pathogenic organisms and their antimicrobial susceptibility. With the recognition that postoperative pelvic infections are frequently polymicrobial in nature, newer treatment strategies include regimens with activity against aerobic and anaerobic pathogens. Although the treatment of these polymicrobial infections has traditionally been with a combination of chloramphenicol and penicillin, as in this patient, or an aminoglycoside plus clindamycin, single broad-spectrum antibiotics are also effective. Monotherapy helps avoid side effects (such as aplastic anemia, from chloramphenicol) as well as the increased indirect cost of administration amd monitoring.

The more contemporary regimes include cephalosporins, extended-spectrum penicillins, monobactams, carbapenems and fluoroquinolones. Although these antibiotics are effective alternatives to the aminoglycosides, several lack adequate anaerobic coverage and require the addition of metronidazole or clindamycin. The development of cephalosporins with a broader spectrum and a longer half-life provides the clinician with several excellent first-line antibiotics in treating postoperative pelvic infections. Cefoxitin has been demonstrated in numerous studies to be an effective single agent in treating postoperative pelvic infections. Newer cephalosporins such as ceftizoxime, cefotaxime, and cefotetan provide adequate cost-effective alternatives, though a potential drawback is the increased rate of resistance against anaerobic bacteria (9).

Of the newer broad-spectrum antimicrobials introduced, the single antibiotic regimes may prove to be the most useful for the empiric treatment of polymicrobial infections. The extended-spectrum penicillins are always active against anaerobes and have been shown to be as effective as cefoxitin or combination therapy in treating pelvic infections. Because these regimes are more effective with fewer treatment failures and are more costly to administer, they should be reserved for resistant cases. Finally, since oral antibiotics are commonly used to complete therapy for postoperative pelvic infections, amoxicillin clavulanate or fluoroquinolones plus metronidazole should be considered as an effective oral regimen (9).

One final concern in antibiotic failure is the observation that the antibiotic susceptibility patterns of bacteria, especially the gram-negative enteric bacilli, vary from hospital to hospital. Clinicians should be updated to sensitivity patterns of clinical isolates from their microbiology laboratories to aid in direct antibiotic therapy.

Generalized peritonitis and endotoxic shock are common complications of the spontaneous rupture of tubo-ovarian abscesses. Although a tubo-ovarian abscess was ruptured in the case presented, appropriate measures were taken. It is the delayed operation, in the face of rupture, that causes the high mortality associated with this condition. When signs and symptoms of septicemia are manifest, careful observation for signs of shock is indicated. The organisms most often associated with endotoxic shock are sensitive to second- and third-generation cephalosporin, as well as chloramphenicol. The greatest number of these organisms will also respond to an aminoglycoside. The addition of an aminoglycoside without discontinuing the penicillin, chloramphenicol, cephalosporin, or clindamycin will provide coverage of most pathogens in sepsis.

Infections at the operative site are the most common cause of fever following hysterectomy. There is a reported febrile response of 20% to 30% for abdominal hysterectomy and of 30% to 40% for vaginal hysterectomy (3). These infections range from minimal pelvic cellulitis to pelvic abscess formation to septic pelvic thrombophlebitis. Serious infection manifested by early-onset sepsis or late-onset abscess formation can occur after surgery, especially if the operative field was contaminated. Prolonged operating time, raw surfaces, poor hemostasis, and the absence of preoperative antibiotic prophylaxis are associated with a higher likelihood of infection at the operative site.

These infections are caused by a mixed aerobic and anaerobic bacteria found in the flora of the lower genital tract and bowel. The infection, as recently demonstrated in the animal model, occurs in two phases (12). In animal studies, the first phase, manifested by peritonitis and sepsis, was due to gram-negative facultative aerobic bacteria, especially *Escherichia coli*. The second phase, characterized by the formation of abscesses, was caused by anaerobic bacteria, in particular *B. fragilis*. The biphasic disease process occurs in those pelvic infections that the obstetrician-gynecologist encounters, that is, postpartum infections.

The diagnosis of pelvic cellulitis is suggested by fever occurring 2 to 4 days after surgery. When host defense mechanisms cannot confine the inflammatory response to the vaginal surgical margin, infection extends into the contiguous pelvic soft tissues of the parametrium. The symptoms are usually more severe than in cuff cellulitis and will include complaints of back or leg pain in addition to the abdominal or pelvic pain. Temperatures are usually more elevated and the patient's complaints are commonly localized to one side (3). Although some induration may be noted, no masses are palpable, and, infrequently, a small amount of drainage may be encountered on probing the vaginal cuff.

A vaginal cuff or pelvic abscess typically presents 3 to 6 days after surgery and is accompanied by a fever with pelvic or rectal pressure and a palpable pelvic mass at the vaginal apex. In the absence of hematoma formation, pelvic abscess is an extremely uncommon infection in patients undergoing abdominal or vaginal hysterectomy. An ultrasound scan aids in locating intra-abdominal abscesses and demonstrates its progression or regression. Combination antimicrobial therapy is the treatment of choice, and regression usually occurs. The signs and symptoms of sepsis will persist in the presence of an abscess despite adequate antibiotics until drainage is established spontaneously, surgically, or by CT-scan-directed aspiration.

The case presented depicts a patient with septic pelvic thrombophlebitis. Septic pelvic thrombophlebitis has been described as "enigmatic fever," that is, persistent in spite of proper antibiotic therapy. High spiking fevers ($> 102°$ F) with disparate tachycardia, chills, and minimal pelvic findings are the rule. Pelvic infection initiates the phlebitic response in the pelvic veins. There is intimal disruption with fibrin deposition at the site. This process is invaded by *E. coli*, hemolytic streptococci, *Bacteroides* species, and *Peptostreptococcus* species. Liquefaction and fragmentation may then occur with embolization (3).

Clinically, pelvic vein thrombophlebitis has two distinct presentations. The first is as described above. The "enigmatic fever" persists despite appropriate antibiotic regimes and in spite of subjective clinical improvement. Patients with this presentation generally do not appear critically ill, and therefore the disease process may be easily confused with drug fever, pelvic abscess, or a collagen disease. More commonly there is acute thrombosis of one or both ovarian veins. This most often involves the right side and can be misdiagnosed as appendicitis. Patients with *right ovarian vein syndrome* may not be febrile but do suffer acute lower abdominal pain that is progressive and that may radiate to the groin, upper abdomen, or flank. Nausea, vomiting, and abdominal distention may also accompany this entity (2).

The diagnosis of septic pelvic thrombophlebitis depends upon which of the two clinical syndromes the patient presents with. Patients with *right ovarian vein syndrome* may have a palpable abdominal mass on exam and an IVP that reveals notching of the proximal ureter resulting from dilated collateral vessels. Recent studies have reported successful diagnosis of ovarian vein thrombosis with ultrasound, but a normal sonogram does not exclude the diagnosis of septic pelvic thrombophlebitis (7). CT scan and MRI are the two most meaningful noninvasive tests in diagnosing thrombosis of the larger pelvic veins. More invasive tests such as venography may be more definitive but may be dangerous in the critically ill patient.

In patients with enigmatic fever and thrombosis of the smaller veins of the pelvis, CT and MRI are likely to be negative. The use of heparin at this point would be both therapeutic and diagnostic, since the response is usually dramatic. Consequently, it would be reasonable to allow 24 to 48 hours for a therapeutic trial with heparin before going to the next step, which would likely be a laparotomy. Heparin will not mask other types of infection. Anaerobic bacteria have a propensity for causing phlebitis, and *Bacteroides fragilis* produces a heparinase that facilitates septic phlebitis. It is unknown, at this time, why the appropriate antibiotics do not resolve the condition without the addition of heparin. Therefore, if a response is noted, the diagnosis is assured, and therapy should be continued for 7 to 10 days. The intravenous route by continuous infusion is preferred, with a goal of maintaining appropriate clotting tests one and one-half to two times the control value. The antibiotics should also be continued. Long-term anticoagulation with Coumadin or subcutaneous heparin should only be considered in patients with documented pulmonary embolism.

Conclusion

When performing surgery for residual pelvic inflammatory disease, postoperative morbidity should be anticipated and prophylactic measures taken. These measures may include (a) proper timing of surgery, (b) preoperative antibiotics, (c) careful dissection and hemostasis, and (d) proper use of drainage.

The optimal time to perform surgery for chronic pelvic inflammatory disease is between flare-ups rather than when the patient is acutely ill. At least 4 to 6 weeks from the last attack would be ideal. However, an acute inflammation not responding to medical therapy is also an indication for operative intervention. In a series where more aggressive approaches were taken during the active phases, significant intraoperative and postoperative complications occurred (5).

The surgeon has the most important role in preventing infection. Failure to adhere to good surgical principles often results in postoperative complications. Handling tissues gently, maintaining meticulous hemostasis, eliminating dead space, avoiding bowel and urinary tract damage, and avoiding the spread of purulent material with liberal use of lavage are of utmost importance in these cases.

The use of antibiotics for prophylaxis should serve only as an adjunct to the surgeon's abilities. Antibiotics given before obstetric or gynecologic surgery have been found to significantly reduce febrile morbidity and shorten hospital stay. The ideal prophylactic antibiotic should be nontoxic, effective in treating most organisms found in the endogenous flora, long-acting, and inexpensive. Cefotetan or cefazolin provides the necessary spectrum of coverage, and because of their extended half-lives these antibiotics have been found to be appropriate for single-dose prophylaxis (8). Recent studies have indicated that short-term prophylaxis is as effective as long-term prophylaxis, and that the acute decrease in the load of pathogenic microorganisms during the immediate perioperative period by short-term prophylaxis makes extended prophylaxis superfluous (8,9).

The final consideration in this case is drainage. There were three areas where drainage may have been indicated. In light of the bacterial contamination of the wound, a subcutaneous drain (Penrose), brought out lateral to the skin incision, was indicated. In severe infections, however, it is sometimes better to leave the wound open and perform secondary closure at a later date (1). The use of intra-abdominal drainage will depend on factors such as the extent of raw surfaces and the inability to excise the abscess cavity completely. In this case the Penrose drain could have been brought out through the vaginal vault. It has been shown that even in an uncomplicated hysterectomy a considerable amount of serosanguineous fluid collects in the retroperitoneal space (10). Postoperatively, morbidity is reduced if this fluid is evacuated. Alternatively, a closed suction sump drain may be placed retroperitoneally and brought out through the flank if the vaginal vault is closed. Lastly, nasogastric suction should be employed to avoid an ileus that is almost certain to occur if significant bowel manipulation and contamination occur. Two of the most commonly associated findings in wound dehiscence are bacterial contamination of the wound and mechanical factors such as abdominal distention. In addition, if a midline incision is necessary, a Smead-Jones wound closure should be considered (11). With a mortality of 10% to 20%, dehiscence is a complication to be avoided.

REFERENCES

1. Brown SE, Allen HH, Robins RH: The use of delayed primary wound infections. *Am J Obstet Gynecol* 127:713, 1977.
2. Gibbs RS: Severe infections in pregnancy. *Medical Clinics of North America* 73:3, 1989.
3. Hemsell DL: Infections after gynecologic surgery. *Obstet Gynecol Clinics of North America* 16:2, 1989.
4. Henderson WH: Synergistic bacterial gangrene following abdominal hysterectomy. *Obstet Gynecol* 49:245, 1977.
5. Kaplan AL, Jacobs MM, Ehresman JR: Aggressive management of pelvic abscess. *Am J Obstet Gynecol* 98:982, 1975.
6. Kingdom JC, Kitchener HC, MacLean AB: Postoperative urinary tract infection in gynecology: Implications for an antibiotic prophylaxis policy. *Obstet Gynecol* 76:4, 1990.
7. Rudoff JM, Astrauskas LJ, et al: Ultrasonographic diagnosis of septic pelvic thrombophlebitis. *J Ultrasound Med* 7:287, 1988.
8. Sevin BU, Ramos R, Gerhardt RT, et al: Comparative efficacy of short-term versus long-term cefoxitin prophylaxis against postoperative infection after radical hysterectomy: A prospective study. *Obstet Gynecol* 77:5, 1991.
9. Stein GE: Patient costs for prophylaxis and treatment of obstetric and gynecologic surgical infections. *Am J Obstet Gynecol* 164:2, 1991.
10. Swartz WH, Tanaree P: Suction drainage as an alternative to prophylactic antibiotics for hysterectomy. *Obstet Gynecol* 45:305, 1975.
11. Wallace D, Hernandez W, Schlaerth JB, et al: Prevention of abdominal wound disruption utilizing the Smead-Jones closure technique. *Obstet Gynecol* 56:226, 1980.
12. Weinstein WM, Onderdonk AB, Bartlett JG, et al: Experimental intra-abdominal abscesses in rats: Development of an experimental model. *Infect Immunol* 10:1250, 1974.

14

Postoperative Necrotizing Fasciitis

Raymond A. Lee

Case Abstract

A 65-year-old diabetic patient with a 3-cm grossly malignant-appearing lesion on the left labia majora underwent confirmatory biopsy, radical vulvectomy, bilateral lymphadenectomy, and sartorius transplant. The following is a copy of the pathology report: "Grade 2 invasive squamous cell carcinoma, 3.5 × 3.1 cm with 14 negative nodes."

Twenty-four hours after surgery, her temperature was 39.4°C and there was evidence of necrosis of the skin edges with purulent discharge between the suture lines. A culture was obtained, and she was placed on triple antibiotics. Her temperature elevation continued 3 days later.

DISCUSSION

Necrotizing fasciitis is a severe, synergistic bacterial infection that results in necrosis of the superficial and deep fasciae. This patient had an unusually high fever and necrosis of the wound edges very early after the operation, alerting the physician that the wound infection might be more than trivial.

Predisposing Factors

Predisposing factors include advancing age, atherosclerosis, obesity, malnutrition, diabetes mellitus, and previous radiation and operative trauma. The condition is most commonly found in the lower extremities, perineum, groin, back, or buttocks. Perineal and vulvar involvement are frequently seen in the obese diabetic patient. Minor infections may trigger the event in the compromised patient. The disease may smoulder initially and then progress rapidly, with subcutaneous necrosis of fat and fascia secondary to bacterial toxins and with thrombosis of vessels leading to gangrene and bullae in the skin. The mortality rate is from 30% to 60%. Necrotizing fasciitis is a synergistic infection usually combined with gram-positive cocci and gram-negative rods. Often the offending anaerobic bacteria are *Peptococcus*, *Peptostreptococcus*, or *Bacteroides* species. Beta-hemolytic streptococci may be cultured in about 50% of the cases, with many other organisms probably acting as secondary contaminants.

Clinical Presentation

Necrotizing fasciitis may be fulminant or slowly progressive. The patient usually has a fever and may experience prostration due to rapid changes in fluids and electrolytes. Toxicity and leukocytosis can be striking and out of proportion to the apparent extent of the condition. Given sufficient time, the infection travels in a centrifugal direction, and the skin becomes tense and brawny and may have a purple discoloration, with vesicular formation progressing to gangrene (Fig. 14.1). The skin becomes anesthetic because the subcutaneous nerves die as a result of thrombosis of the underlying nutrient vessels within the necrotic fasciae. The clinical clues are (1) cellulitis that fails to respond promptly to antibiotic treatment; (2) development of blisters over an area of cellulitis; (3) development of ecchymosis over an area of cellulitis; and (4) presence of gas in the incision, as detected by palpation.

Treatment

Survival depends on early recognition and immediate surgical debridement to healthy tissue margins (Fig. 14.2). All indurated, edematous tissue that is crepitant or does not bleed easily when incised should be removed. After the initial debridement, persistent or progressive necrotizing fasciitis is suggested by the presence of continued leukocytosis, fever, or seropurulent discharge from the wound margins. Multiple debridements may be necessary (Fig. 14.3). Cleansing of the wound is facilitated by whirlpool baths and frequent changes of wound dressings (Fig. 14.4). The wound should be dressed open while the patient is in strict isolation, with plans for a split-thickness skin graft later to cover the wound areas (Fig. 14.5). Broad-spectrum antibiotics are useful adjuncts to assist in the control of infection after the operation and may shorten the hospital stay, but

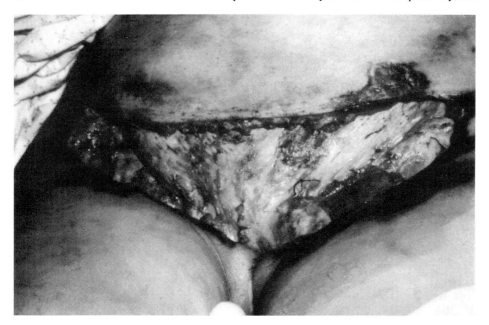

Figure 14.1.   Necrosis of operative site of radical vulvectomy.

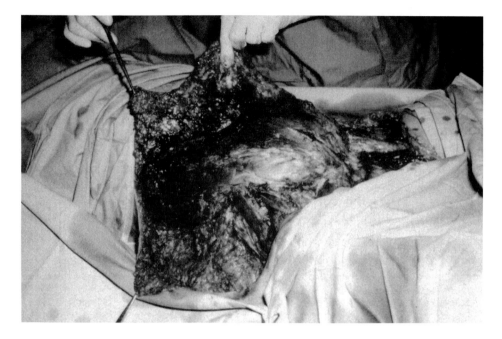

Figure 14.2.   Initial radical debridement.

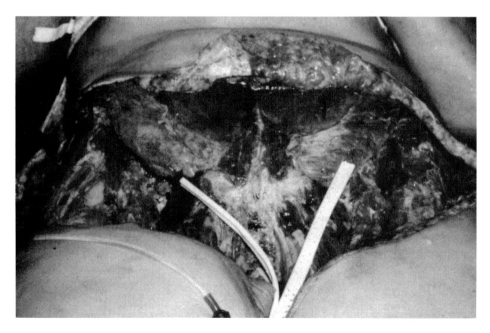

Figure 14.3.   Surgical site after fourth debridement.

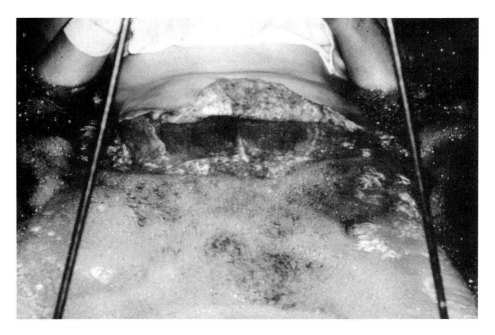

Figure 14.4.   Patient in a whirlpool bath.

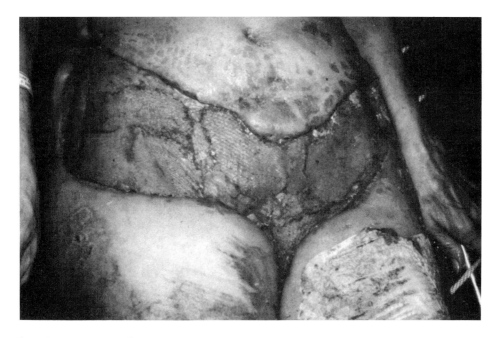

Figure 14.5.   Three days after skin graft.

they remain secondary to definitive operative intervention. Initial treatment consists of penicillin, clindamycin, an aminoglycoside, intravenously administered fluids, and blood transfusion as necessary, with supplemental calcium and general patient support. Death from necrotizing fasciitis is most commonly due to overwhelming sepsis or a combination of diabetes and vascular insufficiency. Early recognition and immediate surgical debridement are the hallmarks of successful management.

SELECTED READINGS

Addison WA, Livengood CH III, Hill GB, et al: Necrotizing fasciitis of vulvar origin in diabetic patients. *Obstet Gynecol* 63:473–479, 1984.

Defore WW Jr, Mattox KL, Dang MH, et al: Necrotizing fasciitis: A persistent surgical problem. *JACEP* 6:62–65, 1977.

Roberts DB, Hester LL Jr: Progressive synergistic bacterial gangrene arising from abscesses of the vulva and Bartholin's gland duct. *Am J Obstet Gynecol* 114:285–289, 1972.

Stone HH, Martin JD Jr: Synergistic necrotizing cellulitis. *Ann Surg* 175:702–710, 1972.

15

Dyspareunia After Radical Hysterectomy

Abe Mickal

Case Abstract

A Wertheim radical hysterectomy with bilateral salpingo-oophorectomy and pelvic lymphadenectomy had been performed upon a 44-year-old multipara. One year after surgery, there was no evidence of malignant disease in the pelvis, but the patient and her husband complained of the vagina now being too short for marital comfort. This observation was confirmed on pelvic examination, when a depth of but 3 inches was determined. There was a thick ligneous scar occupying the vault of the vagina.

DISCUSSION

The Patient, Cancer, and Quality of Life

The main thrust of therapy for cervical cancer as well as for all gynecologic malignancies is for a high cure rate and/or a respectable survival rate. In the past, emphasis on cure took precedence over the well-being of the patient with regards to the emotional, sexual, and psychologic aspects of her life. Fortunately, these views are being constantly modified as doctors learn to better relate with the patient and treat the cancer patient as a total being and not just focus on the disease process itself.

Vasicka and associates (11) have called attention to this problem. They state that

> . . . although the cure of the disease is the primary objective in the therapy of cervical cancer, preservation of function of organs adjacent to the diseased area, namely the bladder, vagina, and rectum, seems to be of no less importance. Each, however, has functions which are difficult to replace. . . . the vagina is not functionally comparable to the urinary bladder or rectum, and, therefore, it has been much more frequently neglected during the application of therapeutic measures for cancer of the cervix. . . . Even though the mutilation, shortening, or complete occlusion of the vagina does not kill the patient, it may produce serious psychosomatic implications which may make adequate social and marital post-treatment adjustment impossible.

They further state that the doctor's objective is not only to save life but to make that life worth living, and especially this is true with patients suffering from cervical carcinoma.

Siebel et al. (9, 10) compared sexual enjoyment in patients with carcinoma of the cervix who had been irradiated versus those who had been surgically managed: 45%

of the irradiated patients reported decreased enjoyment as compared to 25% of the surgically treated patients. Sexual enjoyment was the same or improved in 28% of the irradiated patients as compared to 70% of those managed surgically.

Abitbol and Davenport (1) similarly reported shortening of the vagina and interference with sexual functions in 22 of 28 patients irradiated for cervical cancer as compared to only 2 of 32 surgical patients. Decker and Schwartzman (3) reported similar findings.

The foregoing reports illustrate that sexual function is definitely affected in the treatment of invasive cervical cancer, with irradiation therapy being the more serious offender. One must be very careful in evaluating such subjective data, since no two women have similar sexual behavior nor do they have the same degree of malignancy or anatomic configurations. The emotional and psychic impact of cancer on a particular patient, her mate, and their relationship is also difficult to assess. There are no other areas in gynecology where more individualization is required in the overall management of patients than with cervical cancer and its impact on the anatomic, psychosomatic, and sexual aspects of a patient's life.

Preservation of ovarian function at the time of surgery for cervical carcinoma results in less degenerative changes of the vagina. Sexual function is improved by making coitus less painful and more enjoyable. Other causes or factors in dyspareunia besides the postsurgical pain with intercourse are post-trauma infections, lack of communication between couples, poor or incomplete knowledge of the sex act (psychosexual), and fear and pain.

Prevention of Complications

The patient presented for discussion was 44 years of age, and certainly removal of the ovaries was warranted. The ligneous scar at the vault was most likely caused by a postoperative infection. It was assumed that the cervical cancer had been cured to date and the problem at hand related to a shortened, scarred vagina with dyspareunia.

One was concerned that the complaints of the couple occurred 1 year after surgery, since this should have been the year of most frequent observation and evaluation. Much of the problem presented may have been averted if preventive measures and counselling had been instituted earlier during this first post-therapy year.

There appears to be no contraindication to the use of estrogens in cases of carcinoma of the cervix. In younger patients with this disease process, the ovaries are left in situ with no apparent complications. The late Dr. Milton McCall (6) of Louisiana State University Gynecologic Service had a large series of patients with early malignant lesions of the cervix for whom a Schauta-Amreich vaginal hysterectomy was done with the ovaries left in situ. These patients were followed for many years, and their prognosis was not noticeably affected, nor were there any serious consequences to the ovaries being left in place. There was minimal shortening of the vagina in these patients, and the vast majority reported no serious compromise of their sexual activity.

The Author's Approach to This Problem

The procedures used in helping this couple to regain a satisfactory sexual life would be as follows:

1. Frank discussion of the problem with husband and wife. This would involve complete disclosure of their sexual attitudes, including the positive

as well as the negative aspects. Encouragement to both partners, regarding free discussion with each other of the good and painful aspects of their relationship. They need to freely advise and help each other in seeking solutions for a more pleasant experience. The attitude, concern, and compassion of the physician will do much to breach the barriers of a troublesome sex life. Many couples' frustrations are benefited by good dialogue with an understanding physician. The feeling of help on the horizon is often a very effective medication.

2. Oral use of low-dose estrogen, 0.3 mg Premarin or similar preparation, on a daily basis until desired results are achieved, then on a cyclic basis—3 weeks on, 1 week off, or one tablet every other day indefinitely as long as results are satisfactory.

3. The use of a vaginal lubricant at times of coitus (K–Y jelly, an estrogen cream, or a short burst of a vaginal foam principally directed at the introitus). If penetration can be easily facilitated, then the rest of the performance may be enhanced.

4. Vaginal evaluation and dilation at 7- to 10-day intervals in the office after 10 to 14 days on estrogen therapy may induce elasticity of the vaginal canal. This, coupled with an active sex life at home, may reap the desired results.

5. The author would not recommend surgery as long as progress is being made. If after 4 to 6 months there is no noticeable improvement, he then would contemplate the following surgical approach: (a) Multiple linear transverse incisions of the stenosed or ligneous scarred vault. The incisions must be through the total thickness of the vaginal wall. (b) Suture ligation of active bleeding areas only. (c) Tight packing of vagina after estrogen cream application to the vault for 36 to 48 hours. (d) Excision of any of the ligneous scar (8) should be limited to only the thick, dense areas. One should not sacrifice any more vaginal wall than is absolutely necessary, since we are dealing with a restricted vagina.

6. If after a sufficient period of concentrated efforts, including the incision of the scarred vault, no satisfactory progress has been achieved, then one must consider additional surgical procedures. The time frame of events would be 10 to 12 months from the beginning or 6 to 8 months after the initial surgical approach to the vault. It is expected or hoped that, with estrogen therapy, dilation, and incising of the vault scar that the patient's problem would be minimized. The patient had a 3-inch vagina to begin with, and hopefully these efforts increased the depth by .5 to 1 inch.

The two surgical procedures most often used to increase the vaginal depth are the Williams (12) and the McIndoe (7) operations. Which of these two procedures will produce the best results in this case would depend on the following:

1. Complete evaluation of the couple's problems as of this time and an assessment of their needs for satisfactory sexual relations. This must be done individually and collectively to understand their individual as well as their combined problems.

2. Explanation of surgical procedures available with the positive as well as negative aspects, including operative risk and postoperative care.

3. The author's choice would be a modified Williams operation, since only about an inch or so is needed to achieve a 5-inch vagina, which in the majority of cases would be most satisfactory, unless we are dealing with an unusual situation. The Williams operation would be less traumatic to perform, and recovery would be more rapid, than with the McIndoe procedure. We must remember that this patient had an invasive cancer of the cervix treated by a radical Wertheim hysterectomy. Fibrosis and adhesions increase the risk of bladder or rectal perforation.

Ingram (5) has used specially designed dilators in the vagina with the use of a bicycle seat to exert pressure in dilating a stenosed or constructed vagina. This rationale is logical and workable, although I have no experience with this method.

Individualization cannot be overstressed in cases of this type. The gynecologist (2, 4) must continually involve himself or herself with the whole female patient as related to her life within her environment. Good dialogue with the patient and her mate before, during, and after surgery is mandatory, especially in dealing with a cancer patient. One must not treat the disease only at the expense of the patient. Long-term survival and cures are necessary goals in the surgical management of the patient, especially those in whom invasive malignant disease is diagnosed. They also need, more than others, the concerned understanding and honest dialogue of a compassionate physician who is interested in their overall well-being. Neglect, avoidance, or indifference on the part of the physician produces dire traumatic emotional consequences within the patient. No physician should be guilty of any such accusations.

REFERENCES

1. Abithol MM, Davenport JH: Sexual dysfunction after therapy for cervical carcinoma. *Am J Obstet Gynecol* 119:181, 1974.
2. Adelusi B: Coital functions after radiotherapy for carcinoma of the cervix uteri. *Br J Obstet Gynaecol* 87:821, 1980.
3. Decker WH, Schwartzman E: Sexual function following treatment for carcinoma of the cervix. *Am J Obstet Gynecol* 83:401, 1962.
4. Dennerstein L, Wood C, Burrows GD: Sexual response following hysterectomy and oophorectomy. *Obstet Gynecol* 49:92, 1977.
5. Ingram JM: The bicycle seat stool in the treatment of vaginal agenesis and stenosis: A preliminary report. *Am J Obstet Gynecol* 140:867, 1981.
6. McCall JL, Keaty EC, Thompson JD: Conservation of ovarian tissue in the treatment of carcinoma of the cervix with radical surgery. *Am J Obstet Gynecol* 75:590, 1958.
7. McIndoe A: Treatment of congenital absence and obliterative conditions of the vagina. *Br J Plast Surg* 2:254, 1950.
8. Nichols DH, Randall CL: *Vaginal Surgery*, ed. 2. Baltimore, Williams & Wilkins, 1983.
9. Siebel MN, Freeman MG, Graves WL: Carcinoma of the cervix and sexual function. *Obstet Gynecol* 55:484, 1980.
10. Siebel MN, Freeman MG, Graves WL: Hysterectomy for carcinoma-in situ and sexual function. *Gynecol Oncol* 11:195, 1981.
11. Vasicka A, Popovich NR, Brausch CC: Post-irradiation course of patients with cervical carcinoma: A clinical study of psychic, sexual and physical well-being of sixteen patients. *Obstet Gynecol* 11:403, 1958.
12. Williams EA: Congenital absence of the vagina: A simple operation for its relief. *J Obstet Gynaecol Br Commonw* 71:511, 1964.

Section II

Adnexal Surgery

16

Oophorectomy—Resection of Endometrioma with Discovery of a 5-cm Segment of Ureter in Wall of Specimen

David H. Nichols

Case Abstract

A 10-cm endometrioma was carefully dissected and removed intact from the right pelvic sidewall of a 29-year-old infertility patient. The unopened specimen was removed and handed off the table for examination by the pathologist. The pathologist opened the specimen, confirmed that it was a benign endometrioma, and identified a 5-cm segment of ureter attached to the wall of the specimen. This previously unsuspected ureteral defect was confirmed by exploration of the left retroperitoneal area.

DISCUSSION

Failure to recognize a missing segment of ureter is a life-threatening surgical disaster requiring reoperation and attempt at salvage. Its recognition emphasizes the importance of accounting for the integrity of the full length of the urinary tract with each pelvic surgical procedure. Once the problem is recognized at the time of the initial operation, the responsible surgeon has a number of problem-solving options or stages from which to choose, the choice reflecting the surgeon's experience and knowledge concerning repair of surgical damage to the urinary tract and the availability of competent and timely consultation. The following are among the surgical choices:

1. Reanastomosis of the ureter, probably over an indwelling stent of ureteral catheter (or lacking one, the substitution of a plastic pediatric feeding tube which is of about the same external diameter). For this to be successful and without probability of subsequent stricture, the ends of the ureter should be cut elliptically or spatulated for an anastomosis using interrupted fine sutures of polyglycolic acid placed through the ureteral muscularis. The anastomosis must be tension-free and the site drained extraperitoneally for several days through a separate stab wound, anticipating some transient urinary leakage, until drainage has ceased. Care should be taken that the end of the drain is not in physical contact with the anastomotic site lest fistula formation be invited. The ureteral stent should remain in place for 10 to 14 days, the distal end having been threaded through the urethra and taped to an indwelling Foley catheter or coiled within the bladder to be removed cystoscopically. A follow-up intravenous pyelogram should be performed at 3, 12, and 18 months postoperatively to ensure that no silent ureteral stricture has formed.

2. If the upper end of the transected ureter is close enough to the bladder, a ureteroneocystostomy can be performed through a transabdominal cystotomy using an incision through the full thickness of the bladder. The ureter is fed through a separate stab wound into the bladder, and the end spatulated or fish-mouthed so that it may be sewn to the mucosa and muscularis of the bladder by some interrupted intravesical polyglycolic acid sutures. The serosal surface of the bladder and of the ureter should be approximated by a few additional interrupted sutures to help remove the strain on the anastomotic suture line. The distal ureteral stump should be either ligated or excised. This site of anastomosis should be drained extraperitoneally for a few days to reduce the chance of urinoma or hematoma. Anastomotic tension can be further reduced by the use of a "psoas hitch," by which the bladder dome is elevated by one's fingers introduced through the temporary cystotomy and sewn to the fascia of the psoas muscle by a few interrupted sutures. An indwelling ureteral stent may be inserted for 10 to 14 days, if desired, and the cystotomy closed in two layers.

3. A wide-based flap of bladder (Boari flap) may be fashioned and folded into a tubular extension to function as distal ureter, the tip anastomosed to the free proximal end of the ureter, and the cystotomy closed with interrupted polyglycolic acid sutures. The width of the base of the flap should measure at least one-third the distance of the length of the flap to help preserve the vesical blood supply to the newly constructed tube, since postoperative necrosis of the tubular flap is a distinct risk. Use of the temporary ureteral stent is optional, and this site should be separately drained as described above.

4. If the proximal ureter is too short to use for anastomosis, a cross-vertebral ureteroureterostomy will permanently anastomose the proximal end of the transected ureter to the contralateral "normal" ureter. This does risk future stricture at the site of anastomosis, possibly damaging the function of each kidney, and would be most safely performed only by a surgeon experienced in this procedure.

If the surgeon is uncomfortable with any of the above choices, or an intraoperative consultant is not available, or the condition of the patient requires termination of the operation, there are several options that will temporarily salvage the affected kidney until competent help and reoperation are available:

1. Bridge the gap between the ends of the ureter with a stent (a ureteral catheter or pediatric feeding tube), making no attempt to anastomose the ends of the ureter.
2. Divert the urine to the outside by using a temporary percutaneous ureteral stent.
3. Perform a cutaneous ureterostomy.
4. Temporarily tie off each end of the severed ureter. The kidney, though soon hydronephrotic, will survive for several days with damage reversible once the obstruction has been surgically relieved.
5. If the planned reintervention is not possible within a few days, a percutaneous nephrostomy will drain the kidney almost indefinitely.

Other secondary procedures for use some days after the initial injury include the following:

1. The kidney may be permanently lowered by freeing its connective tissue attachments but preserving its blood supply, thus making possible a tension-free ureteroureteral anastomosis.
2. An ileal loop may be fashioned to bridge the gap between the cut ends of the ureter.
3. If kidney damage is severe and irreversible, nephrectomy might be necessary.

A primary goal, although occasionally painful for both the patient and operator, should be salvage of the patient's kidney function. The choice of procedure should be made according to the surgeon's experience and surgical background. Postoperatively the patient and her family must be given a full disclosure of damage, its immediate solution, and the possible complications of the complication, and a plan for further treatment, follow-up, or consultation disclosed. If only a temporary solution has been chosen, a qualified consultant should be engaged promptly to recommend or perform a permanent surgical remedy. The now stable patient can be transported to the consultant if the latter is unable to come to see the patient.

In the patient described, the author would recommend a ureteroneocystostomy with psoas hitch and possibly a Boari flap, if necessary.

17

Bilateral Ovarian Mature Cystic Teratomas in a Young Woman

James L. Breen
Julian E. De Lia
John T. Comerci, Jr.

Case Abstract

A 7-cm cyst of the left ovary was found in a 22-year-old para I. It was persistent and tender and at surgery was identified as a mature cystic teratoma that replaced much of the ovary. A similar smaller cyst was found in the opposite ovary.

DISCUSSION

In this case bilateral mature cystic teratomas were found in a young woman of low parity. A low transverse incision was performed in light of the low incidence of ovarian cancer found in this age group. Management consisted of bilateral oophorocystectomies with preservation of ovarian tissue. Attention was directed at utilizing surgical techniques that would ensure minimal interference with tubo-ovarian function and future fertility.

INTRODUCTION

The patient presented in this case represents a clinical situation seen commonly in patients with mature cystic teratomas. Preoperative evaluation and surgical management will vary according to the patient's age, physical findings, and reproductive desires. Three surgical decisions need to be addressed in this patient: (1) type of abdominal incision; (2) intraoperative management; (3) procedures to maximize future fertility.

Choice of Incision

A low vertical incision allows easier exploration of the upper abdomen and permits cephalad extension if it is necessary. Advantages of low transverse incisions (Pfannenstiel) include better cosmesis, lower infection and dehiscence rate, and less postoperative discomfort. Ultimately, the choice of incision is governed by the operative procedure envisioned and the potential problems to be encountered, most significantly ovarian malignancies.

66

The lowest incidence for malignant neoplasms occurs during the second to fourth decades of life. In childhood, one-third of ovarian neoplasms are malignant. After age 40 there is an increasing incidence of ovarian cancer, with 70% of ovarian malignancies occurring after 50 years of age.

Although immature elements of other germ cell tumors may coexist with mature elements in mature cystic teratomas, this is most commonly encountered under the age of 18, with less than 5% occurring in patients over 18 years of age (2,3,4). The incidence of malignant degeneration of mature cystic teratomas is approximately 1.7% (8) and occurs rarely in the first two decades of life, with 75% of cases detected between the ages of 30 and 70 years (17).

Of all ovarian tumors, the mature cystic teratoma is most amenable to a preoperative diagnosis. Approximately 50% of these neoplasms can be noted on a simple scout film of the abdomen. Computed tomography can accurately diagnose a teratoma because of the complex appearance of the mass, with dividing septa, internal debris, variable attenuation, and distinct calcifications (10). Ultrasonography usually shows highly reflective tissue interfaces with areas of acoustic shadowing that obscure the back wall of the cyst (17). Ultrasound may fail to detect cystic teratomas, since their strong attenuation of sound may cause them to mimic bowel (12). Magnetic resonance imaging (MRI) is probably the most accurate test available. The signal characteristics of hemorrhagic cysts, that is, endometriomas and lipid-containing cysts such as mature cystic teratomas, may be difficult to distinguish because they have the same signal intensity. The appearance of blood and lipid in ovarian tumors can be sufficiently different on lipid- and water-suppression MR images to allow an accurate distinction between the two (9).

Mature cystic teratomas have physical findings that are characteristic of both benign and malignant ovarian neoplasms. Their mobility, smoothness, cystic nature, and unilaterality suggest a benign nature. Torsion is the most common complication associated with mature cystic teratomas (11,15,16,13), with rates ranging from 3.2% to 16% (17,15,16,5,1). Torsion in and of itself argues against malignancy in that extremely large size, external excrescences, or extracystic invasive growth would impede rotation and hence torsion. In spite of this, the occasionally solid nature, large size, and bilaterality may suggest malignancy.

Judgment is required on the part of the surgeon to determine the need for additional studies or examinations prior to laparotomy, to aid in determining the nature of the adnexal mass. In general, studies that are helpful include an x-ray examination of the chest and abdomen, complete blood count, urinalysis, liver function tests, tumor markers such as CA-125, CEA, alpha fetoprotein, and serum chorionic gonadotropin. It should be noted that pure mature cystic teratomas, not associated with other germ cell tumors, have been associated with elevated levels of alpha fetoprotein (14). Extensive preoperative studies will not be necessary in most instances of unilateral or bilateral masses occurring in reproductive-aged patients similar to the one presented. Ultimate test selection, however, will be modified by the patient's age, history, and physical examination (7).

The final decision as to which incision to use can be made following a careful pelvic examination in the operating room, while the patient is under general anesthesia. Indeed, it should be a routine practice to reevaluate or confirm previous pelvic findings prior to making an incision for the treatment of pelvic masses. One may find that the situation is different from that noted previously. We feel, given a patient with the findings outlined in this case presentation, that a low transverse incision would be acceptable, realizing that it can be made much larger by converting it to a Cherney incision if necessary.

Intraoperative Management

Immediately upon entering the abdomen an evaluation is made to see if ascitic fluid is present and to determine the status of the abdominopelvic cavity serosal surfaces. Until the exact nature of the tumor is known, ascitic fluid or peritoneal washings should be collected, since these will be important in the proper clinical staging if the ovarian tumors are malignant. Once the exact nature of the tumor is determined, the above may not be necessary.

The exploration of the upper abdomen should precede the pelvic exploration. Particular attention is paid to the diaphragmatic surfaces, liver, gallbladder, kidneys, bowel surfaces, and periaortic nodes. With this completed, the bowel can now be gently packed away from the pelvis and the pelvic organs examined visually and manually to determine the nature of the tumor.

Mature teratomas are frequently found anterior to the uterus, a condition that may be due to the low specific gravity of the sebaceous material within the cyst or to the fact that its germ cell origin makes it, from an embryologic standpoint, a midline tumor.

Grossly mature cystic teratomas are usually globular or cystic structures. They possess a smooth, glistening capsule that is milky white in color unless an accumulation of fat or hair beneath the capsule is present, in which case it may appear yellow or gray. The contents are normally in a liquid state at body temperature; however, the cyst contents become semisolid upon cooling. The majority of cysts are unilocular. Rokitansky's protuberance is a rounded, white, shiny mass projecting from the wall toward the center of the cyst. When bone or teeth are present they are usually located in this area. Rokitansky's protuberance is a common site of malignant degeneration and should be well sectioned during pathologic analysis. The key to the diagnosis of type and the determination of the benign or malignant nature of the tumor often will depend on the appearance of its contents after it is opened in the operating room. It is a good principle not to rupture or open any tumor prior to its removal, to prevent intra-abdominal spill.

Since most patients with mature cystic teratomas are of reproductive age, treatment should be conservative whenever possible. Attempts should be made to completely remove the cyst to avoid recurrence. Oophorectomy is an acceptable mode of treatment with torsion and loss of viability when cystectomy is followed by uncontrollable hemorrhage, or when preservation of ovarian function is no longer a concern. Many times oophorectomies are performed because the surgeon is intimidated by the size of the tumor, a thin ovarian cortex, or risk of cyst rupture. However, not only may the removal of an affected ovary compromise a patient's fertility, but possible future pathology of the remaining contralateral ovary may cause the physician to regret the original procedure.

The laparoscopic management of mature cystic teratomas should be performed only by those who possess great facility with techniques of operative laparoscopy. Spillage of cyst contents intra-abdominally is difficult to irrigate adequately via the laparoscope. In addition, failure to remove the cyst in its entirety can lead to recurrence and/or infection with subsequent decreased fertility.

The patient presented was desirous of future fertility and had bilateral disease. Every attempt should be made, in such a patient, to excise benign solid tumors and cysts carefully, provided the remaining portion of the ovary can be preserved with an adequate blood supply. The ovary should be isolated from surrounding structures by packs to prevent spilling of the tumor's contents, which could lead to postoperative peritonitis or a chronic granulomatis response.

A shallow linear incision of the ovarian capsule is made far from the mesovarium and should be of sufficient length to allow for removal of the tumor. The tumor is then carefully shelled out from the remaining ovary. Bleeding, which is most prominent in the hilar region, may be controlled by fine suturing of individual vessels, by delicate electrocautery, or by running a horizontal mattress suture close to the hilum. Two rather broad flaps of ovarian tissue will remain. Care should be taken to reapproximate these flaps to achieve a repair free from abraded or raw edges.

The excised cyst should now be opened to verify its nature before addressing the opposite ovary. Occasionally, the exact nature may have to await a frozen section or permanent histologic evaluation. These tumors are known to occur in a mixed form with immature elements. A study by Yanai-Inbar and Scully (19), which examined 350 immature teratomas and 10 cases of dermoid cyst with microscopic foci of immature tissue, found that 26% of immature teratomas contained grossly visible dermoid cysts, 10% were associated with a dermoid cyst in the contralateral ovary, and 2.6% were preceded by resection of a dermoid cyst from the same ovary. Follow-up of 10 cases of dermoid cyst containing microscopic foci of immature elements revealed no evidence of recurrence 11 months to 7 years postoperatively.

When some confusion exists as to whether immature or other germ cell elements are present, it is best to continue along the conservative route and not extirpate the reproductive organs. One must maintain the willingness to reoperate, pending definitive histologic evaluation of the tumor on permanent sections.

In this patient the management of the opposite ovary was dictated by finding a cyst present on close inspection. This cyst should have been managed as outlined above. Not as clear is the management of the opposite ovary when it appears normal in the presence of a contralateral mature teratoma. The incidence of bilateral mature cystic teratomas is reported to be approximately 10% (16,5,1). In the past, the finding of small foci of mature teratomas on bivalving normal ovaries prompted the recommendation that routine wedge resection should be performed to exclude occult bilaterality whether the ovary appeared abnormal or not. The indiscriminate removal of ovarian tissue, however, causes follicle reduction as well as potential adhesion formation, hemorrhage, or infection (18). Studies have shown that histologic examination of a normal contralateral ovary identifies a teratoma in approximately 1% of cases (1,6). Suspicious contralateral cysts can be aspirated, and if the fluid is oily and immiscible with saline they should be removed. Although it cannot be denied that inspection and palpation may occasionally miss the small occult tumor, necessitating reoperation, we feel the risk of reoperation to restore fertility is greater in patients treated with wedge biopsy of a normal ovary.

Prophylaxis of Adhesions

A significant number of women presenting with infertility will give a history of prior pelvic surgery. Pelvic adhesions and anatomic distortion are undesirable sequelae of gynecologic surgery regardless of the indication for the initial surgery. These are particularly disconcerting when the patient is desirous of retaining her reproductive capacity. Since adhesion formation seems to be the result of trauma, major emphasis should be placed on the use of techniques that minimize adhesion formation. The advent of gynecologic microsurgery has considerably improved the outcome of adnexal surgery. Although it is unreasonable to suggest the use of magnification in ovarian tumor surgery, other principles can be adopted with potentially rewarding results. These include (1) careful washing of surgical gloves to remove talc and the use of lint-free swabs and packs; (2) elimination of sponging by use of irrigation and suction instead; (3) gentle handling of tissue by avoiding the use of instruments that traumatize tissue; (4) use of pinpoint electrocautery, bipolar tips, or very fine suture ligatures for hemostasis; (5) elimination of raw surfaces by careful reapproximation of cut surfaces; (6) use of fine nonreactive sutures with atraumatic needles for ovarian repair (no. 6–0 Dexon or Vicryl can be used without magnification); and (7) avoidance of prolonged drying of tissue. The time spent in instituting these techniques will be rewarded by a lowered incidence of iatrogenic infertility in the patient with benign disease.

REFERENCES

1. Ayhan A, Aksu T, Develioglu O, Tuncer ZS: Complications and bilaterality of mature ovarian teratomas (clinicopathological evaluation of 286 cases). *Aust NZ J Obstet Gynaecol* 31:83, 1991.
2. Breen JL, Bonamo JF, Maxon WS: Genital tract tumor in children. *Pediatr Clin North Am* 28:355, 1981.
3. Breen JL, Maxon WS: Ovarian tumor in children and adolescents. *Clin Obstet Gynecol* 20:607, 1977.
4. Breen JL, Neubecker RD: Malignant teratoma of the ovary. *Obstet Gynecol* 21:669, 1963.
5. Caruso PA, Marsh MR, Minkowitz S, Karten G: An intense clinicopathologic study of 305 teratomas of the ovary. *Cancer* 27:343, 1971.
6. Doss N, Forney JP, Vellios F, Nalick RH: Covert bilaterality of mature ovarian teratomas. *Obstet Gynecol* 50:651, 1977.
7. Johnson GH: Pelvic mass and the diagnosis of carcinoma of the ovary. *Clin Obstet Gynecol* 22:557, 1979.
8. Kelly RR, Scully RE: Cancer developing in dermoid cysts of the ovary. A report of 8 cases, including a carcinoid and leiomyosarcoma. *Cancer* 14:989, 1961.
9. Kier R, Smith RC, McCarthy SM: Value of lipid- and water-suppression MR images in distinguishing between blood and lipid within ovarian masses. *Am J Rad* 158:321, 1992.
10. Lakkis WG, Martin MC, Gelfand NM: Benign cystic teratoma of the ovary: A 6-year review. *Can J Surg* 28:444–446, 1985.
11. Matz MH: Benign cystic teratomas of the ovary. A review. *Obstet Gynecol Surv* 16:591, 1961.
12. Mitchell DG: Benign disease of the uterus and ovaries. *Rad Clin North Am* 30:777, 1992.
13. Pantoja E, Rodriguez-Ibanez I, Axtmayer RW, Noy MA, Pelegrina I: Complications of dermoid tumors of the ovary. *Obstet Gynecol* 45:89, 1975.
14. Perrone T, Stepper TA, Dehner LP: Alpha-fetoprotein localization in pure ovarian teratoma. An immunohistochemical study of 12 cases. *Am J Clin Pathol* 88:713, 1987.
15. Peterson WF: Malignant degeneration of benign cystic teratomas of the ovary. A collective review of the literature. *Obstet Gynecol Surv* 12:793, 1957.
16. Peterson WF, Prevost EC, Edmunds FT, Hundley JM, Morris FK: Benign cystic teratomas of the ovary. A clinico-statistical study of 1,007 cases with a review of the literature. *Am J Obstet Gynecol* 70:368, 1955.
17. Singh P, Yordan EL, Wilbabanks, Miller AW, Wee A: Malignancy associated with benign cystic teratomas (dermoid cysts) of the ovary. *Sing Med J* 29:30, 1988.
18. Toaff R, Toaff ME, Peyser MR: Infertility following wedge resection of the ovaries. *Am J Obstet Gynecol* 124:92, 1976.
19. Yanai-Inbar I, Scully RE: Relation of ovarian dermoid cysts and immature teratomas: An analysis of 350 cases of immature teratoma and 10 cases of dermoid cyst with microscopic foci of immature tissue. *J Gynecol Pathol* 6:203, 1987.

18

Unilateral Pelvic Abscess Following Removal of Intrauterine Device

Abe Mickal

Case Abstract

A 34-year-old divorced para II had been wearing an intrauterine device (IUD) for 2 years but was annoyed by persistent uterine tenderness and menorrhagia, although there was no history of fever. She requested permanent sterilization. At surgery, her physician removed the intrauterine device, performed a dilatation and curettage (D&C), and through the laparascope performed a bilateral tubal coagulation. Five days later the patient was seen in the emergency room with considerable pelvic discomfort, chills, and fever (103°F), and tachycardia (pulse 110). The uterus was quite tender, and it was evident that an adnexal fullness was present on the right side. The patient was given a prescription for ampicillin, 500 mg four times daily, and sent home.

One week later, her symptoms were unimproved, although her temperature rarely exceeded 101°F, and there was a distinct adnexal mass on the right side. The ampicillin was continued. When seen again 2 weeks later, the right adnexal mass was estimated at 6 cm in diameter and was exquisitely tender, but there was no fullness or bulging of the cul-de-sac. There was chronic low-grade body temperature that reached its highest point at 8 p.m. (101°F). The patient requested that she be seen by a consultant. A consultation was arranged. The consultant confirmed the above findings, discontinued the ampicillin, and placed the patient on chloromycetin, 250 mg four times a day. Her fever disappeared within 2 days and a leukocytosis and elevated sedimentation rate gradually subsided. The mass persisted, and 1 month later the patient was taken to surgery for laparotomy.

DISCUSSION

Was Pelvic Inflammatory Disease Present at the Time of Initial Surgery?

There are numerous reports in the literature regarding the effect of an IUD on intrauterine and tubal infections. Taylor et al. (12) reported unilateral tubo-ovarian abscess in IUD wearers. The reason for the unilaterally was imbedding of the IUD on the uterine wall, producing an infection at this site. This infection spread to the corresponding tube and ovary by direct extension or by lymphatic spread. Since this report there have been similar reports regarding unilateral tubo-ovarian abscesses in IUD wearers (8,10). The final answer to the exact impact of the IUD on tubo-ovarian disease is not yet in.

Edelman and Berger (3), in November of 1980, reported that their study did not support the concept that wearers of the IUD were more likely to have unilateral tubo-ovarian abscesses. They also concluded that further studies would be required to define more completely the relationship between IUD use and pelvic inflammatory disease.

Burkman (1) reported the results of case control studies in 16 hospitals in 9 cities in the United States regarding the association of IUDs and pelvic inflammatory disease. There were 1447 patients in the pelvic infections group and 3453 patients in the control group. Some of the conclusions reached in this study were:

1. There was an increased association for women aged 25 years or less and for nonblack women.
2. Recent insertion or reinsertion of an IUD was associated with an increased risk for pelvic infection, but duration of use was not.
3. The pelvic infection persisted several months after removal of the IUD.
4. The type of IUD does not markedly influence the risk.
5. The risk is greater when the IUD is compared to other forms of contraception or no contraception.
6. First-episode hospitalization of IUD users for pelvic infection is twice the baseline for pelvic infection alone. This is of great economic as well as health significance.

The association of an increased pelvic inflammatory disease rate with or without abscess formation has been fairly well substantiated. The original article by Taylor et al. in 1975 (12) implicated all types of IUDs in the development of pelvic infections or tubo-ovarian abscesses. The discontinuance of the IUDs with multifilament tails was of some value in reducing the risk of ascending infection, but a major problem still persists. Smith and Soderstrom (11) examined removed sections of fallopian tubes during sterilization and found a nonbacterial salpingitis rate of 47% in IUD users compared to less than 1% in nonusers. Eschenbach et al. (4) reported in 1977 that, of 500,000 cases of pelvic infections, 110,000 occurred in women with an IUD in place.

All of the previously mentioned information illustrates the fact that the IUD is a potential focus of infection. There should be a good doctor–patient dialogue and understanding of the IUD and its related problems and benefits. Many other factors may also predispose an individual to the development of pelvic infections. These factors include the sexual activity of the individual, multiplicity of sex partners, personal lifestyle and environment, history of previous pelvic problems, status of pelvic organs at time of IUD insertion (cervicitis, etc.), age and parity, and insertion problems (perforations, complete, or incomplete).

The Centers for Disease Control in Atlanta held a symposium on pelvic inflammatory disease in June, 1980. A brief summary of this meeting by Golden (6) was reported as follows:

1. In women who develop salpingitis, 20% become infertile.
2. Those who can conceive have a 6- to 10-fold increased risk of ectopic pregnancy.
3. In 1976, 35% of women in this country who used no contraception were involuntarily sterile, indicating the magnitude of the infertility problem.

4. One-half of the deaths from ectopic pregnancies can be attributed to the ectopic gestation resulting from scarring from bouts of salpingitis. (Deaths from ectopic gestations account for 11% of the maternal deaths in the United States.)
5. Direct and indirect costs of pelvic inflammatory disease amount to about $2 billion per year.

Powers (7) reported 204 ectopic pregnancies between 1974 and 1978. Twenty-one women (10.3%) had an IUD in place at time of diagnosis, and 18 (18.8%) had used IUDs in the past. It was interesting to note that only 27 (13.2%) patients had a record or history of salpingitis. Seventy-seven (37.7%) were nulliparous, and 66 of the 127 parous patients had only one delivery. The largest age group was between 25 and 29.

In summarizing the question relating to infection with the IUD, one must conclude:

1. Since most IUD wearers are young and of low parity, the long-term impact of the IUD on future reproductive capacity has not been fully assessed or reported.
2. There is an increased risk of pelvic infection. It may be subclinical and well within the tolerance of the individual to deal with it provided there is no superimposed infection or trauma.
3. There is a definite increased risk of ectopic pregnancies.
4. In young women nulliparous or of low parity, the IUD may not be the contraceptive of choice. The author does not recommend the IUD for young, single, or nulliparous patients except in unusual circumstances.

Surgical Procedures Done on This Patient

After removal of an IUD, D&C, and laparoscopic tubal sterilization, this patient developed complications—namely, a tubo-ovarian abscess. Therefore, one questions the advisability of doing all these procedures at the same time and in the order in which they were done.

The author's feeling is that the time to remove the IUD was when the patient was seen in the office and all aspects of the problem were discussed. This was not an emergency admission, and the patient would have been a better candidate for a diagnostic D&C for menorrhagia. Many IUDs are removed in the office without problems. The menorrhagia could have been a result of the IUD, and the removal may have been of some aid in determining this effect. A D&C would have been indicated for a final diagnosis on this patient's bleeding problems at the time of her hospitalization for the tubal sterilization 1 or 2 weeks later.

The need for antibiotics should also be determined at the time of the office visit and IUD removal. If on examination the patient has signs and symptoms of pelvic infection (leukocytosis, cervical–uterine pain, adnexal tenderness, etc.), then a 5- to 6-day course of oral antibiotics may be indicated. The author uses either doxycycline hyclate (Doxycycline), 100 mg bid, or erthyromycin stearate (Erythromycin), 500 mg tid.

This patient with persistent uterine tenderness was taken to surgery for the removal of the IUD, D&C, and laparoscopic tubal sterilization. No mention was made of short-term prophylactic antibiotics, and in the author's opinion they should have been used. All antimicrobial agents that have been used prophylactically have shown fairly good results. The Louisiana State University Ob-Gyn Service at Charity Hospital has had more experience with cephoxitin sodium (Mefoxin) and ticarcillin sodium (Ticarcillin), principally because the Ob-Gyn Service has had investigational studies related to these drugs. Metronidazole (Flagyl), doxycycline hyclate, and the second- and third-generation cephalosporins have been reported as being equally effective.

LAPAROSCOPIC TUBAL STERILIZATION: FIRST AND LAST

Another area of consideration in this patient is the chronologic order of procedures performed. There is no question that a subclinical salpingitis exists in most IUD wearers. However, the vast majority of IUD patients undergo laparoscopic tubal sterilization without major complications. This indicates that cauterization of the fallopian tubes seldom causes a preexisting salpingitis to flare up, or if it does, the body's host defense mechanisms can usually cope with it. When a laparoscopic tubal cauterization is done, the avenue for direct spread of an intrauterine infection to the ovaries is usually sealed off. If one contemplates doing a removal of an IUD and D&C and tubal sterilization, then doing the laparoscopic procedure first may reduce the chances for tubo-ovarian infection.

The author would choose the following order in which these procedures would be done: (a) office removal of IUD and short-term oral prophylactic antibiotics, 3 to 4 days; (b) tubal sterilization, and D&C when admitted to hospital in 2 weeks.

POSTOPERATIVE FOLLOW-UP

The patient was seen in the emergency room on the fifth postoperative day with considerable pelvic discomfort, chills, and fever (103° F), tachycardia (110), tender uterus, and adnexal fullness on the right side.

All of the above findings warrant immediate admission and evaluation of the patient for a possible tubo-ovarian abscess, with appendicitis to be ruled out. One of the major problems in treating moderate to severe pelvic infection with or without abscess formation is inadequate treatment. The fault lies equally with the patient and the physician. The patient delays in seeking help and the doctor, unfortunately, is disenchanted with the so-called PID (pelvic inflammatory disease) patient. This implied diagnosis does much to detract the physician from actively and aggressively evaluating and treating the patient. We are seeing less of this neglect now compared to 10 to 20 years ago, because sections of infectious diseases are being established in obstetrics and gynecology departments with marked emphasis on improved care and management of patients with pelvic infections. Postgraduate courses in pelvic infections and antibiotic therapy have also contributed to this improvement.

The best time to cure or alter the destructive course of inflammatory disease is at the time of original attack. Hospital cost is admittedly high, but inadequately treated infections are far more expensive and devastating to the individual's reproductive system.

One other possible consideration in the etiology of the patient's postoperative morbidity is bowel injury at the time of laparoscopic tubal cauterization. The fact that the patient's clinical course did not progressively worsen would indicate that bowel injury probably did not occur, but it must be part of the differential diagnosis.

CHOICE OF ANTIBIOTICS

Ampicillin trihydrate is a good oral antibiotic, but it alone is not adequate treatment for a patient presenting as this patient did in the emergency room. One week later, the patient was still febrile (101° F) with a distinct adnexal mass. Admission to the hospital was again justified but not done. Ampicillin trihydrate was continued, and the patient was not seen for 2 weeks. In neither instance was the best interest of the patient served. A delay of seeing such a sick patient for 2 weeks is also not appropriate management.

It must again be restated that in gynecologic and obstetric infection we are dealing with polymicrobial organisms (aerobes, anaerobes, and *Chlamydia trachomatis*), especially the *Bacteroides* species. Treatment should always be directed at all groups of organisms with special emphasis on the anaerobes. Their eradication early in the treatment phase is directly proportional to the speed of recovery and response of the patient. Specific coverage for *Chlamydia trachomatis* must be part of the treatment of pelvic inflammatory disease.

Plan of Management

1. Admit to hospital when first seen in the emergency room on the fifth postoperative day.
2. Complete evaluation: interval history, physical examination, including bimanual, rectovaginal, complete blood count, urinalysis, x-ray of chest and flat plate of the abdomen, and culdocentesis with culture.
3. Parenteral intravenous fluids supplementing oral fluids.
4. Antibiotics directed at polymicrobial nature of the disease. Coverage must be adequate for aerobes, anaerobes, and chlamydial infection. The majority of pelvic infections are polymicrobial and must be treated accordingly: cefoxitin sodium (Mefoxin) 2 g by intravenous piggyback every 6 hours with doxycycline hyclate 100 mg intravenously every 12 hours. Metronidazole (Flagyl) 500 mg every 6 hours can be added as the third drug of choice if needed.
5. Ultrasound of pelvic area: This is of diagnostic help in 70% to 75% of cases and offers good follow-up on progression or regression of the disease signs.
6. Daily monitoring of vital signs.
7. If response is noted with antibiotic regimen, then continue therapy as long as progress is noted.
8. Laparoscopy would be reserved as an added diagnostic aid when and if needed. The clinical response of the patient would be a determining factor. Cultures from the fallopian tubes and cul-de-sac should always be taken at time of laparoscopy.
9. If the patient's response is poor or her condition deteriorates, then physical reevaluation is done involving chest, kidneys, abdomen, pelvis, and extremities.
   (a) Add antibiotics for more intensive anaerobic coverage—clindamycin phosphate (Cleocin phosphate) 600 mg every 6 hours intravenously, or chloramphenicol sodium succinate (Chloromycetin) 2 g stat, then 1 mg, then 1 g every 6 hours intravenously, or metronidazole (Flagyl)

500 g every 6 hours intravenously. Any of the above can be combined with Mefoxin. Tobramycin sulphate or amikacin sulphate (Amikin) may also be added if indicated. Double- or triple-agent antibiotic therapy is often needed in severe infection.

(b) Supportive conservative treatment is continued as long as the patient is responding and progress is being made.

10. If after 8 to 10 days of therapy the patient is improved but an adnexal mass 8 to 10 cm persists and is identifiable by careful rectovaginal examination and ultrasound, then exploratory laparotomy is resorted to.

Surgery is indicated in patients who are not responding to aggressive medical management as indicated by the vital signs, abdominal pain and distention, and/or a progressively enlarging adnexal mass. It is better to explore the abdomen and remove an early unruptured tubo-ovarian abscess and preserve the remaining organs than await rupture and do a more extensive surgical procedure.

SURGICAL PROCEDURE DONE ON PATIENT

A right tubo-ovarian, unruptured abscess was removed. Culture of the abscess was positive for enterococcus and *Bacteroides fragilis*.

The culture reaffirms the problem of anaerobic organisms in pelvic infections and the need for antimicrobials to cover the aerobic and especially anaerobic organisms. If this patient had been admitted on the fifth postoperative day when her symptoms warranted admission, it is presumed that proper antibiotic therapy may have prevented the ultimate development of a frank tubo-ovarian abscess.

All patients with an initial diagnosis of tubo-ovarian abscess do not necessarily have a discrete abscess. This is a working and presumptive diagnosis and can only be proven by laparoscopy or laparotomy, especially early in the disease process, when rupture or leaking of the abscess has not occurred. The clinical impression of an adnexal mass (abscess) may be only an acute salpingo-oophoritis with adhesions to omentum or bowel giving rise to an ill-defined mass, often referred to as a tubo-ovarian complex. Many tubo-ovarian abscesses begin in this manner, with the ovary becoming later invaded by bacteria at an ovulatory site or by lymphatic or hematogenous spread. Early and aggressive conservative management with broad-spectrum antibiotics may be effective in treating the original infection before a true abscess develops. When dealing with pelvic infections with a questionable mass, it is best to consider the most potentially dangerous aspect of the problem and work in that direction rather than to minimize the situation. Too often the disease process develops faster than anticipated and we then must "catch up" and try to stem the tide.

The Louisiana State University Ob-Gyn Service (5) clinically diagnosed 247 tubo-ovarian abscesses between the years 1970 and 1979. Aggressive conservative management was instituted while at the same time preparations were made for surgery if it became indicated. Fifty-seven percent of these patients required surgery, and the other 43% were discharged as relatively cured after medical management. Unfortunately, we do not have adequate follow-up data on the fate of patients who were admitted with a clinical diagnosis of tubo-ovarian abscess and responded to aggressive medical management. In spite of this inadequate follow-up, the author still believes that this is the proper approach to patients presenting with this problem. The sooner the patient is admitted and treated the less the incidence of surgery. The longer the duration before treatment, the higher the incidence of surgery. Those medically treated are made aware of their condition and counseled regarding the future of the reproductive organs as well as hopefully being educated toward improved personal care and concern.

There is a changing philosophy toward surgery for tubo-ovarian abscesses. The Louisiana State University Ob-Gyn Service, along with many others (2, 9), has changed from an outright surgical approach after adequate medical management to a more aggressive medical management with surgery being reserved only for those patients who do not respond or in whom the disease process is not controlled. It has been the policy of the Ob-Gyn Service to remove only the infected organs, but it is difficult to adhere to this policy when surgery is done for ruptured abscesses with free pus in the pelvis or abdomen. There should be no hesitancy on the part of the gynecologist in removing unilateral tubo-ovarian abscess or severely diseased adnexa. This is an excellent time for full pelvic inspection and bacteriologic studies of the diseased organs, as well as cultures from the cul-de-sac and the ostia of the opposite fallopian tube. This is especially advocated in young patients, those of low parity, and patients who desire future pregnancies. The advances being made in antibiotic therapy, especially with regard to anaerobes, provide moral and therapeutic support in our management of patients with unilateral or bilateral tubo-ovarian disease problems. It is no longer necessary to feel that doctors may as well remove everything to prevent recurrence. The better understanding that now exists regarding organisms and their behavior as well as our improved bacteriologic techniques aided by adequate aggressive medical management warrants our conservative surgical approach, especially in those young patients desirous of future pregnancies. The success of in vitro fertilization demands that we counsel our patients about its potential and the possibility of preserving the uterus and an ovary if clinical conditions warrant. In such cases, the removal of diseased and distorted fallopian tubes and the preservation of the uterus and ovary are justifiable. This is also a good opportunity for cultures of the pelvic structures and institution of appropriate therapy. In some cases, aspiration of ovarian abscess and preservation of ovary is indicated. The risk is well worth taking by the conscientious physician who has developed a good rapport and dialogue with his or her patients.

REFERENCES

1. Burkman RT: Association between intrauterine device and pelvic inflammatory disease. *Obstet Gynecol* 57:269, 1981.
2. Cunningham FG, Mickal A: Pelvic infection. In: Benson RC (ed): *Current Obstetric and Gynecologic Diagnosis and Treatment*. Los Altos, CA, Lange, 1980.
3. Edelman DA, Berger GA: Contraceptive practice and tubo-ovarian abscess. *Am J Obstet Gynecol* 138:541, 1980.
4. Eschenbach DA, Harvisch JP, Holmes KD: Role of contraception and other risk factors. *Am J Obstet Gynecol* 128:838, 1977.
5. Ginsberg DS, Stern JL, Hamod KA, et al: Tubo-ovarian abscess: A retrospective review. *Am J Obstet Gynecol* 138:1055, 1980.
6. Golden: International Symposium of Pelvic Inflammatory Disease, I and II. *Am J Obstet Gynecol* 138:845, 1980.
7. Powers DN: Ectopic pregnancy: A five year experience. *South Med J* 73:1012, 1980.
8. Rickart RM: Ovarian abscesses in IUD wearers. Problem-patient conference. *Contemp Ob-Gyn* 17:141, 1981.
9. Rivilin ME, Hunt JA: Ruptured tubo-ovarian abscesses—is hysterectomy necessary? *Obstet Gynecol* 50:518, 1977.

10. Scott WC: Pelvic abscess in association with intrauterine contraceptive device. *Trans Pacific Coast Obstet Gynecol Soc* 45:43, 1978.
11. Smith MR, Soderstrom R: Salpingitis: A frequent response to intrauterine conception. *J Reproduc Med* 16:159, 1976.
12. Taylor ES, McMillan BE, Greer BE, et al: The intrauterine device and tubo-ovarian abscess. *Am J Obstet Gynecol* 123:338, 1975.

19

Bilateral Chronic and Symptomatic Salpingitis: Should Hysterectomy Be Performed?

Howard W. Jones, Jr.

Case Abstract

Bilateral, symptomatic, and recurrent pelvic inflammatory disease was identified in a 26-year-old nulligravid patient who was contemplating marriage and wondering about her future fertility. The patient was disabled by chronic pelvic pain and tenderness, worse around the time of her menstrual period, and had had frequent febrile flare-ups during the preceding year. Bilateral persistent, tender adnexal masses were identified, somewhat fixed in position and measuring 5 to 7 cm in diameter. Laparotomy, with probable salpingectomy and possible hysterectomy, was recommended. Preoperatively, the patient expressed her plans to marry someday and was visibly upset about her potential loss of fertility. She inquired whether it was necessary that her uterus be removed and whether she might be a future candidate for in vitro fertilization.

DISCUSSION

If it is necessary because of disease to remove the fallopian tubes, conventional wisdom has held that a total hysterectomy should also be done. This "incidental" hysterectomy is based on the simple concepts that, with no tubes, reproduction is impossible; that the uterus can therefore serve no reproductive purpose; and that in later years it can only be the source of difficulty, such as from functional bleeding, sarcoma of the uterus, adenocarcinoma of the corpus, cancer of the cervix, and so forth.

All of this has now changed. Reproduction is possible without fallopian tubes and, with the use of donor eggs, reproduction is also possible without ovaries. For patients without tubes, the possibility of pregnancy by in vitro fertilization approaches the expectancy of pregnancy occurring during any one menstrual cycle. The natural inefficiency of reproduction per cycle is overcome in normal reproduction because with normal tubes the opportunity to become pregnant repeats itself thirteen times each year. For the best possibility for pregnancy from in vitro fertilization, the ovaries need to be available, as they almost always are for ultrasound-guided harvest, and seem to produce eggs better if not involved in the consequences of extensive surface peritoneal inflammatory reaction.

At the time of surgery, when in vitro fertilization is contemplated for sometime in the future, there are special considerations. The ovaries, of course, should be preserved if possible. Salpingectomy should be carried out by removal of the tube in the standard method, but the traditional method of using a deep cornual wedge, with the removal of the interstitial portion of the tube, should no longer be employed. There have been reports of ruptures of the uterus during pregnancy at the site of cornual excision (2). This risk seems to increase when the procedure is carried out bilaterally. Therefore, in removing the tube from the uterus, either no wedge or a very superficial wedge should be used, enabling the approximation of the serosal surfaces in a delicate surgical fashion.

After removal of the tubes, attention should be given to removing, insofar as possible, any periovarian adhesions so that the surface of the ovary is as normal as possible.

With contemporary transvaginal oocyte harvest, it is not necessary to suspend the ovaries, as was formerly desirable, when oocyte aspiration by laparoscopy was the rule. In fact, there is some advantage for the contemporary technique of transvaginal oocyte aspiration to have the ovaries in or easily available through the cul-de-sac.

In the event, for any reason, the utero-ovarian ligament is severed, it is appropriate to refasten it to the uterus at a somewhat lower position than normal (Fig. 19.1).

While using transvaginal aspiration, it is sometimes necessary to traverse the uterus with the aspiration needle. Although this can usually be safely done, it is better to avoid it to minimize complications, and for this reason: if the uterus is in retroverted position, it is desirable at the time of operation to carry out a suspension by shortening the round ligaments by the method of Gilliam (1), or by some modification thereof.

If the ovary is largely destroyed or so intimately involved in the inflammatory process or its residua that it is no longer savable, this does not mean that in vitro fertilization is impossible for this patient, even if both ovaries are so involved. Therefore, hysterectomy may not be indicated, even if both ovaries are removed. If the uterus is normal, reproduction is theoretically and practically possible, provided that the patient is willing to accept a donor egg.

The practical point of the recent considerations is that it is incumbent upon the surgeon to be aware of the newer reproductive technologies and to discuss these possibilities at length with the patient prior to any operation that might involve an "incidental" hysterectomy.

As with all infertility surgery, routine antibiotics are indicated and should be used in a prophylactic manner if no organism can be identified, but obviously, if pus is encountered at the time of operation, a culture should be taken and the antibiotic therapy modulated depending upon the bacteriological findings.

There are very few circumstances in contemporary surgery where drainage of the abdomen is indicated. Even with a ruptured tubo-ovarian abscess with the removal of the adnexa, aspiration, and irrigation of the peritoneal cavity, drainage is not helpful. Indeed, drainage should be avoided unless there is some urgent indication for it, such as a raw oozing area of an unremovable abscess that was drained. In short, the objective of the surgery should be to leave the pelvis as clean as possible, with the thought that subsequently the ovaries could be approached for the purpose of harvesting mature eggs.

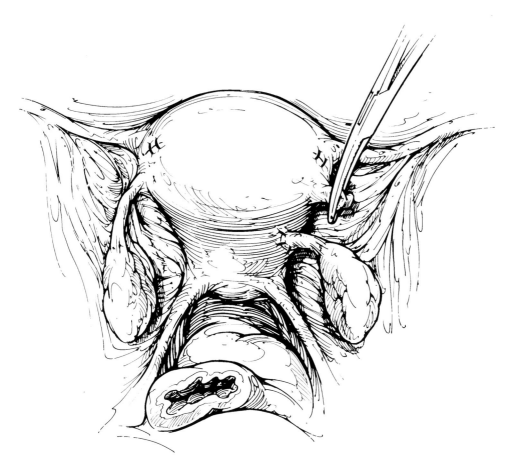

Figure 19.1.   Diagram showing appearance of pelvis following bilateral salpingectomy. Right utero-ovarian ligament has been clamped and cut to be reattached at level on the posterior wall of the uterus, as shown.

REFERENCES

1. Gilliam DT: Round-ligament ventrosuspension of the uterus: A new method. *Am J Obstet Gynecol* 41:299, 1900.
2. Mohlen J, Schortle B: Cornual resection as prophylaxis against interstitial pregnancy: Is it necessary or dangerous? A review of the literature. *Eur J Obstet Gynecol Reprod Biol* 17:155, 1984.

SECTION III

LAPAROSCOPIC AND FERTILITY SURGERY

20

Inability to Insufflate the Peritoneal Cavity at the Time of Laparoscopy

John O. L. DeLancey
William W. Hurd

Case Abstract

A 42-year-old gravida II, para II requested permanent irreversible sterilization and was taken to the operating room for a laparoscopic tubal ligation. She had no significant medical problems but was 5 feet 3 inches and weighed 240 pounds. The Veress needle was placed several times through an infraumbilical incision, but a "hanging drop" test and insufflation pressures indicated that the needle was not in an intraperitoneal position. Additional attempts both with and without elevating the abdominal wall were likewise unsuccessful. Faced with an anesthetized patient requesting sterilization and an inability to create a pneumoperitoneum, the surgeon reflected on what to do next.

DISCUSSION

Every experienced gynecologist has had occasional difficulty creating a pneumoperitoneum in preparation for laparoscopy. In a thin individual, conversion to open laparoscopic technique or performance of a minilaparotomy are acceptable alternatives when creation of a pneumoperitoneum cannot be achieved. This is also possible in a more obese patient (4), but a relatively large incision is required to gain access to the fascia. A short habitus, thick abdominal wall, and abundant preperitoneal adipose tissue not only make it difficult to successfully place the insufflating needle into the peritoneal cavity, but also make open laparoscopy or true minilaparotomy more challenging. In the obese woman, the abdominal wall may be so thick that a relatively long and deep incision may be required to visualize the fascia, and admission to the hospital after surgery may be necessary. Some authors have advocated direct insertion of the laparoscopic trocar (3,6) as a way to enter the peritoneal cavity, but in an obese individual, this may be met with the same problems as creating a pneumoperitoneum prior to trocar insertion (2).

Anticipating difficulty insufflating the abdomen may facilitate management and prevent the problems that arise once this problem has occurred. Any patient scheduled for laparoscopy should consent to laparotomy if the need arises, and this is especially true for individuals in whom difficulty in entering the abdominal cavity is expected. Recognizing this, several considerations should enhance the likelihood that the peritoneum will be successfully entered.

The best chance to enter the peritoneum may be on the first attempt. Once insufflation is begun with the needle in the preperitoneal space, the peritoneum is pushed away from the abdominal wall, making subsequent entry more difficult. Therefore, the surgeon should focus on maximizing the chance that the first attempt at insufflation is successful. The first step in preventing preperitoneal insufflation is to have the right equipment available, and to confirm that it is working properly. In obese individuals, having a 15-cm Veress needle available rather than the usual 12-cm needle will often be the difference in preperitoneal versus intraperitoneal placement. Second, the needle must be clear of debris. If a piece of lint or old clot is present, the higher insufflation pressure may appear to indicate preperitoneal position when the needle is actually in the abdominal cavity. If the needle is not completely screwed onto the obturator, the hole in the needle may be partially covered and the pressures similarly artificially elevated. To avoid these problems, one should attach the needle to the insufflation machine and confirm that the measured pressures are low prior to inserting it into the abdomen.

Confirming the intraperitoneal position of the needle before insufflation begins prevents the displacement of the peritoneum away from the inner surface of the abdominal wall by the insufflating gas. A "hanging drop" technique may be used to see if the needle is intraperitoneal prior to beginning insufflation. One should place a 5-cc syringe filled with saline on the Veress needle and remove the plunger so that it acts as a funnel, then lift forcefully on the abdominal wall. Since the peritoneal space is a potential space, lifting on the abdomen creates a negative pressure there and will suck the saline out of the syringe. In the preperitoneal area, the fibers of the transversalis fascia connect the peritoneum with the undersurface of the rectus muscles, and upward traction of the abdominal wall simply lifts the peritoneum without creating a significant negative pressure there. Some small amount of saline may be drained from the syringe even if it is located in the preperitoneal space, but experience with this technique will indicate the greater degree of suction present when the needle tip is intraperitoneal.

The distance between the abdominal skin and the peritoneal cavity varies with body mass (5), as does the distance between the abdominal wall and the aorta, vena cava, and iliac vessels. In slender individuals it is necessary to place the needle at a sufficiently oblique angle that it misses the aorta, vena cava, and iliac vessels (see Fig. 21.1, p. 92). In obese individuals, however, the abdominal wall is so far from these vessels that this is not necessary. In very obese individuals, the distance between the skin and the peritoneum may be greater than the longest Veress needle and therefore insertion at this angle will not enter the peritoneum successfully. Therefore, in obese women a carefully performed vertical insertion using a 12-cm needle may be safe. When this is properly selected and carefully performed, peritoneal entry can be achieved. The judgment of the surgeon concerning the patient's body habitus in this approach is important.

The peritoneum is attached to the base of the umbilicus. This anatomic point may be used to facilitate entry into the peritoneal cavity (Fig. 20.1). Placing the Veress needle directly through the base of the umbilicus traverses the shortest distance available on the abdominal wall. The skin in this area is sometimes tough, and a sharp needle may be necessary. A small superficial stab incision with a no. 11 blade may facilitate entry. Since the peritoneum is relatively fixed in this position, this is an ideal technique to try when preperitoneal insufflation has already occurred, since the peritoneum here is less likely to have been pushed away from the abdominal wall.

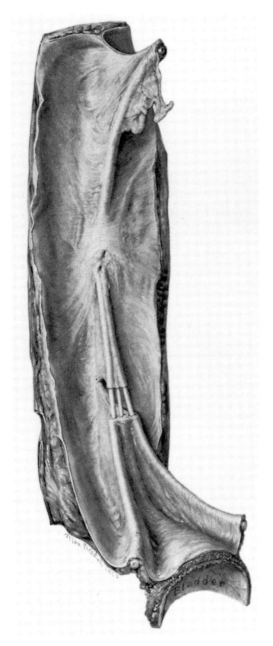

Figure 20.1.   Illustration showing the insertion of the obliterated umbilical ligaments and the urachus inserting into the inner surface of the umbilicus. (By Brodel M. With permission, the Department of Art As Applied to Medicine, Johns Hopkins Hospitals, Baltimore, MD.)

Despite all precautions, preperitoneal insufflation does occasionally occur and successful management of this situation is important to complete the planned procedure. In thin women, an open laparoscopy technique may be adopted, or a minilaparotomy performed. In obese women, we have found it preferable to stay with the closed laparoscopic approach except when previous surgery suggests the presence of adhesions to the anterior abdominal wall. Preperitoneal insufflation is recognized when insertion of the trocar and laparoscope reveals the typical appearance of the preperitoneal space. At this point several liters of CO_2 have dissected the space open. It is sometimes possible in these instances to locate a transparent window of peritoneum, and the laparoscope may be bluntly advanced through the peritoneum. This should only be attempted if the surgeon has adequate visualization and can see through the peritoneum to be sure that no bowel will be injured. Similarly, a Veress needle can be placed and, again, if visualization is possible, used to enter the peritoneum (7). If these direct techniques for entry are not possible or if they prove unsuccessful, one should deflate the preperitoneal space prior to removing the trocar, since if the gas is left in place it will continue to hold the peritoneum away from the abdominal wall and make entry more difficult. Once the preperitoneal space has been evacuated, a Veress needle placed through the middle of the umbilicus, because of its attachment to the peritoneum, is sometimes more successful. Once the preperitoneal space has been dissected, the peritoneum is no longer attached to the underside of the rectus sheath, and insufflation pressures and the hanging drop technique are no longer able to differentiate intraperitoneal from preperitoneal insufflation.

The cul-de-sac of Douglas offers an ideal site for insufflation when attempts to obtain a pneumoperitoneum through the abdominal wall of obese women have failed, since fat does not occur between the vaginal wall and the peritoneum here. Using a technique identical to culdocentesis, the Veress needle may be inserted directly through the posterior vaginal wall into the cul-de-sac and insufflation begun (1). The pressure created in the abdominal cavity by insufflation through the cul-de-sac will press the peritoneum against the abdominal wall so that the laparoscopic trocar may be successfully inserted. When preperitoneal insufflation has been noted with the laparoscope, the trocar should be left in place and the valve opened to allow the preperitoneal gas to escape as the cul-de-sac insufflation proceeds. After one has filled the abdominal cavity and evacuated the preperitoneal space, the trocar may be inserted.

The cul-de-sac extends for several centimeters along the posterior vaginal wall (8), and so an ample area for needle insertion is present even when the peritoneum has been dissected off of the inner surface of the abdominal wall (9). Prior to performing this technique, however, the cul-de-sac should be palpated to ensure that it is not distorted by endometriosis. If nodularity or scarring is detected, the rectum may have become adherent to the cervix and vagina due to endometriosis, and an alternative technique should be adopted. Experience with knowing where to insert the needle in future cases may be gained during any laparoscopy by laparoscopically viewing the location of a probe placed vaginally. The vaginal wall behind the uterus can be pushed with this probe while one watches on the video monitor to see the relationship between the sound, cervix, and posterior vaginal wall. In addition, in instances where cul-de-sac insufflation has been required, insight into the performance of this technique may be gained if the Veress needle is left in place until after the laparoscope is inserted. This will allow its position to be noted relative to surrounding structures and provide valuable information to guide entry to the cul-de-sac when the situation arises in future patients. If cul-de-sac insufflation fails, then direct insertion through the fundus of the uterus may be attempted (10). Although some use this technique routinely, we have chosen to use it when other techniques have failed.

Instances will arise when all the resourcefulness of the surgeon in applying these and other techniques fails to produce a pneumoperitoneum. Sound judgment about when to abandon attempts to create a pneumoperitoneum and when to proceed to minilaparotomy or laparotomy is essential. The surgeon's pride in proving that he or she can create a pneumoperitoneum should never overshadow concern for the patient's overall safety. Unrecognized abdominal wall tumors, unsuspected malignancy affecting the abdominal cavity, adherence of bowel to the abdominal wall, and other factors may make creation of a pneumoperitoneum unsafe or impossible. When reasonable attempts to create a pneumoperitoneum have failed, reexamination of the patient under anesthesia should be undertaken and serious consideration given to abandoning the closed laparoscopic procedure in favor of open laparoscopy or laparotomy.

REFERENCES

1. Ansari AH: The cul-de-sac approach to induction of pneumoperitoneum for pelvic laparoscopy and pneumography. *Fertil Steril* 21:599–605, 1970.
2. Byron JW, Fujiyoshi CA, Miyazawa K: Evaluation of the direct trocar insertion technique at laparoscopy. *Obstet Gynecol* 74:423–425, 1989.
3. Copeland C, Wing R, Hulka JF: Direct trocar insertion at laparoscopy: An evaluation. *Obstet Gynecol* 62(5):655–659, 1983.
4. Holtz G: Laparoscopy in the massively obese female. *Obstet Gynecol* 69:423–424, 1987.
5. Hurd WH, Bude RO, DeLancey JOL, Gauvin JM, Aisen AM: Abdominal wall characterization with magnetic resonance imaging and computed tomography: The effect of obesity on the laparoscopic approach. *J Reprod Med* 36:473–476, 1991.
6. Jarrett JC II: Laparoscopy: Direct trocar insertion without pneumoperitoneum. *Obstet Gynecol* 75:725–727, 1990.
7. Kabukoba JJ, Skillern LH: Coping with extraperitoneal insufflation during laparoscopy: A new technique. *Obstet Gynecol* 80:144–145, 1992.
8. Kuhn RJP, Hollyock VE: Observations on the anatomy of the rectovaginal pouch and septum. *Obstet Gynecol* 59:445–447, 1982.
9. Neely MR, McWilliams R, Makhlouf HA: Laparoscopy: Routine pneumoperitoneum via the posterior fornix. *Obstet Gynecol* 45:459–460, 1975.
10. Wolfe WM, Pasic R: Transuterine insertion of Veress needle in laparoscopy. *Obstet Gynecol* 75:456–457, 1990.

21

Arrhythmia and Drop in Blood Pressure During Inspiration with the Veress Needle

William W. Hurd

Case Abstract

Diagnostic laparoscopy was being performed on a 23-year-old nulligravida for pelvic pain. A Veress cannula was placed through an infraumbilical skin incision at 45° from horizontal. The tubing from the insufflator to the Veress cannula had been attached to the cannula prior to placement. Insufflation was begun at 1 L/min, and when the pressure was found to be less than 10 mmHg, insufflation was increased to 6 L/min. When 2.5 L of gas had been delivered, the pressure suddenly increased to >30 mmHg. Simultaneously, the anesthesiologist noted the sudden onset of ventricular tachycardia and a "sloshing" sound from the precordial stethoscope. The Veress cannula was immediately removed. Within seconds, the patient became profoundly hypotensive and both the pulse and blood pressure became undetectable.

The cardiac monitor initially showed ventricular tachycardia, followed within two minutes by ventricular fibrillation.

DISCUSSION

Injury to major retroperitoneal vessels is one of the least common but most serious complications of the closed laparoscopic technique, occurring in approximately 3 per 10,000 laparoscopies (9). This includes both vessel perforation by the Veress needle with intravascular insufflation and vessel laceration by the 10-mm primary trocar.

Theoretically the blind placement of sharp instruments through the umbilicus aimed toward the pelvis should rarely, if ever, result in vessel injury because both the aorta and inferior vena cava bifurcate near the level of the umbilicus. Unfortunately, in many cases the aortic bifurcation is at or below the level of the umbilicus, and in most patients the left common iliac vein crosses the midline below the umbilicus (5). Furthermore, the margin of error may be small, especially in thin patients, where the anterior-posterior distance from the umbilicus to the retroperitoneal vessels may be as little as 2 to 3 cm (Fig. 21.1) (4).

The primary strategy to minimize the risk of vessel injury is the use of proper placement techniques for the Veress needle. Because of the significant changes in anterior wall anatomy associated with increasing weight, it is important to understand these changes and adjust technique accordingly.

In patients who are of normal weight or who are overweight but not obese (i.e., less than 200 lb), a standard technique for closed laparoscopy can be used. The first step is to transabdominally palpate the sacral prominence, which may be surprisingly close in thin patients. In an effort to maximize the distance between the umbilicus and major vessels, the abdominal wall is elevated by grasping the skin and subcutaneous tissue midway between the symphysis pubis and the umbilicus. The Veress needle is inserted through the base of the umbilicus at 45° from horizontal.

The spring-loaded guard of the Veress needle automatically retracts as the fascia is perforated. However, care should be used to keep the guard extended after the tip has entered the abdominal cavity. This maneuver makes inadvertent retroperitoneal puncture extremely unlikely since vessel puncture by the blunt guard would be difficult. Unfortunately, this is not possible when using a disposable Veress needle. This inability to keep the guard extended, coupled with the extreme sharpness of disposable Veress needles, may represent additional hazards when using this type of equipment.

Regardless of the type of Veress needle used, verification of needle location prior to insufflation is extremely important. First, the lateral mobility of the needle should be verified, since posterior retroperitoneal penetration of the needle will prevent lateral mobility. Second, a syringe should be used to aspirate through the needle to make sure that blood cannot be aspirated. Finally, a "hanging drop" test should be performed, in which a drop of saline placed on the hub of the needle is pulled into the hub of the needle when the abdominal wall is elevated. If any of these tests are not reassuring, the needle should be removed and replaced into the peritoneal cavity.

Once the Veress needle appears to be properly placed, insufflation at a low rate (1 L/min) should be begun while watching the intra-abdominal pressure monitor. Only after insufflation of approximately 0.5 to 1 L of CO_2 with an acceptable pressure of less than 15 to 20 mmHg should a high flow rate (6 to 10 L/min) be used.

In the obese patient (> 200 lb), the thickness of the abdominal wall requires an alteration of the approach for inserting the Veress needle. If the needle is placed through the base of the umbilicus at 45°, it may not reach the peritoneal cavity (Fig. 21.1). For this reason, it has been suggested that the Veress needle be placed at nearly 90° from horizontal (4,8). To minimize the risk of vascular injury, the umbilicus is elevated (i.e., supported to avoid depression) using towel clips placed through the skin near the umbilicus. A standard-length Veress needle is then inserted in a somewhat more vertical orientation than normal (Fig. 21.1C) and checked for location as described above. Following insufflation, a primary 10-mm trocar is similarly inserted.

Extra-long instruments are unlikely to be an advantage with this approach since the average vertical distance from skin to peritoneum is only 4 cm in obese patients (Fig. 21.1). These longer instruments may actually increase the risk with this vertical approach since the major vessels lie immediately beneath the umbilicus in many patients (5).

A final strategy to avoid the risk of intravascular insufflation is the exclusive use of an open technique. Although techniques for open laparoscopy have been available for years (3), most laparoscopic procedures continue to be performed using a closed rather than an open technique (12). This may be because open techniques are perceived as slower and more difficult to perform since special instruments and fascial sutures are required to ensure an airtight seal at the relatively large fascial opening (7). Although techniques have been developed that avoid the use of both a Veress needle and a sharp

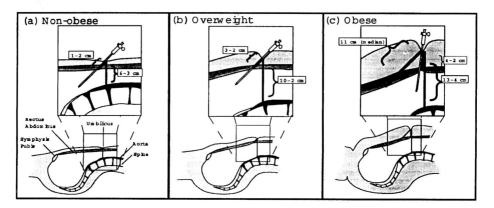

Figure 21.1.   Diagram of representative sagittal views of a patient from three groups: **A.** Nonobese: body mass index (BMI) <25 kg/m² (*N* = 14). **B.** Overweight: BMI 25–30 kg/m² (*N* = 9). **C.** Obese: BMI >30 kg/m² (*N* = 10). A 11.5-cm Veress needle is superimposed on each view for comparison. (Adapted from Hurd et al: The relationship of the umbilicus to the aortic bifurcation: Implications for laparoscopic technique. *Obstet Gynecol* 80(1):48–51, 1992.)

trocar, and avoid carbon dioxide leakage without the use of fascial sutures (7,6), the ultimate utility of these techniques has yet to be determined.

Certainly, intravascular insufflation with the Veress needle is an extremely rare event when the proper technique is used. However, each laparoscopic surgeon should be prepared to deal with this potentially fatal complication since immediate recognition and treatment may be life-saving (2).

It is important to keep in mind that the first signs of intravenous placement of the Veress needle may be subtle. Because the venous system is a low-pressure system, the initial insufflation pressure will remain low when the needle tip is intravascular. The first sign of intraperitoneal insufflation may be an abnormal precordial sound representing intravascular bubbles (2). This may be followed by a sudden increase in insufflation pressure as the entire venous system is filled with CO_2 (10).

At this point, the most common cardiac arrhythmia will be ventricular tachycardia (2,10). This is usually followed by profound hypotension and cyanosis. These events are probably the result of a gas-lock in the right side of the heart, resulting in both pulmonary outflow obstruction and obstruction of venous return to the heart (1).

The cornerstone of management for gas embolism is immediate recognition and treatment. After removal of the Veress needle, initial treatment consists of hyperventilation with 100% oxygen and treatment of cardiac dysrhythmias. Hypotension should be treated with external cardiac massage. This may serve the dual function of restoring circulation and breaking up the gas embolus (10). In some cases, aspiration of the gas embolus may be necessary to restore circulation. This is performed by placing the patient in a left lateral decubitus position and performing aspiration through a central line placed via the external carotid vein (1).

After the patient is stable hemodynamically, laparoscopy should be performed using an open technique to evaluate the patient for intraperitoneal hemorrhage or retroperitoneal hematoma formation requiring laparotomy and repair. In the absence of these problems, laparoscopic surgery can be performed as originally planned. However, close observation postoperatively in an intensive care setting is important because delayed vascular collapse after intravascular insufflation is possible (11).

Although intravascular insufflation can almost always be avoided by proper technique, technical difficulty due to obesity, anatomic variation, or inexperience may result in this rare complication. Immediate recognition and appropriate treatment may be life-saving in these cases.

In the case presented, external cardiac massage was begun. Defibrillation resulted in temporary sinus rhythm on each attempt, but reverted to ventricular fibrillation within seconds. Despite heroic resuscitative efforts, neither pulse nor measurable blood pressure could be restored and the patient was pronounced dead 1 hour after the start of the procedure.

REFERENCES

1. Alvaran SB, Toung JK, Graff TE, Benson DW: Venous air embolism: Comparative merits of external cardiac massage, intracardiac aspiration, and left lateral decubitus position. *Anesth Analg* 57:66–70, 1978.
2. de Plater RM, Jones IS: Non-fatal carbon dioxide embolism during laparoscopy. *Anaesth Intensive Care* 17:359–361, 1989.
3. Hasson HM: Open laparoscopy vs closed laparoscopy: A comparison of complication rates. *Adv Plann Parent* 13:41, 1978.
4. Hurd WW, Bude RO, DeLancey JOL, Gauvin JM, Aisen AM: Abdominal wall characterization by magnetic resonance imaging and computed tomography: The effect of obesity on laparoscopic approach. *J Reprod Med* 36(7):473–476, 1991.
5. Hurd WW, Bude RO, DeLancey JOL, Pearl ML: The relationship of the umbilicus to the aortic bifurcation: Implications for laparoscopic technique. *Obstet Gynecol* 80(1):48–51, 1992.
6. Hurd WW, Ohl DA: Use of a blunt trocar for open laparoscopy without facial sutures. *Surg Gynecol Obstet* (in press).
7. Hurd WW, Randolph JF Jr, Holmberg RA, Pearl ML, Hubbell GP: Open laparoscopy without special instruments or sutures: A comparison to a closed technique. *J Reprod Med* (in press).
8. Loffer FD, Pent D: Laparoscopy in the obese patient. *Am J Obstet Gynecol* 125:104–107, 1976.
9. Mintz M: Risk and prophylaxis in laparoscopy: A survey of 100,000 cases. *J Reprod Med* 18:269–272, 1977.
10. Morison DH, Riggs JR: Cardiovascular collapse in laparoscopy. *Can Med Assoc J* 111:433–437, 1974.
11. Root B, Levy MN, Pollack S, Lubert M, Pathak K: Gas embolism death after laparoscopy delayed by "trapping" in portal circulation. *Anesth Analg* 57:232–237, 1978.
12. Yupze AA: Pneumoperitoneum needle and trocar injuries in laparoscopy: A survey on possible contributing factors and prevention. *J Reprod Med* 355:485–490, 1990.

22

Injuries to Abdominal Wall Blood Vessels at Laparoscopy

William W. Hurd

Case Abstract

A laparoscopic myomectomy was being performed on a 32-year-old nulligravida for symptoms of menorrhagia and infertility. A 10-mm laparoscope had been placed through an infraumbilical port using a standard closed technique. In order to use larger instruments, including a morcellator, a 12-mm disposable trocar was placed 5 cm to the left of midline and 3 cm above the symphysis. Brisk bleeding was immediately noted from the trocar site. The trocar was removed and a chromic suture on a large tapered needle was placed through the incision into the abdominal cavity. A laparoscopic needle holder was used to direct the needle out of the abdominal cavity through the incision, and the ligature was tied. This transabdominal suture resulted in good hemostasis, with a blood loss to this point of approximately 200 mL. Twenty minutes after the procedure, symptoms of hypovolemic shock and abdominal distention were noted.

DISCUSSION

Vascular injury at laparoscopy may include either injury to the major retroperitoneal vessels during placement of the Veress cannula or primary trocar placement (see Chapter 21), or injury of the abdominal wall vessels during lateral trocar placement. Abdominal wall vessel injuries were rare in the past during procedures such as diagnostic laparoscopy and tubal ligation because trocars were placed almost exclusively in the relatively avascular midline (4). However, abdominal wall vessel injuries, as illustrated in the case abstract above, have become more common with the development of more complicated operative laparoscopic procedures that place large trocars laterally (2).

Avoiding vessel injury requires knowing which vessels are at risk and visualizing them prior to trocar placement, when possible. Anterior abdominal wall vessels can be divided into superficial and deep vessels based on their location.

The most consistent superficial vessels of the abdominal wall are the superficial epigastric and superficial circumflex iliac arteries. These both originate from the femoral artery and course cephalad through the subcutaneous tissue, branching as they go. Fortunately, these vessels can often be seen, and thus avoided, by transilluminating the abdominal wall with the laparoscope. This is especially true in light-skinned and thin women.

The deeper, and largest, vessel of the anterior abdominal wall is the inferior epigastric artery. This vessel, often referred to as the "deep" epigastric artery, originates from the external iliac artery and is accompanied bilaterally by the inferior epigastric veins. It courses cephalad along the abdominal wall peritoneum until midway between the symphysis pubis and the umbilicus, where it blends into the body of the rectus abdominis muscle. Because of its deep location, this vessel cannot be seen by transillumination. However, this vessel can often be seen laparoscopically, and thus avoided, as it courses along the peritoneum between the obliterated umbilical ligaments and the insertion of the round ligament into the inguinal canal.

Another method to avoid injury is to know the most likely location of the anterior wall vessels, and to place lateral trocars accordingly. This method is important because the vessels are often not visible either by transillumination or by laparoscopic visualization.

Immediately above the symphysis, both the superficial and inferior (deep) epigastric arteries are located approximately 5.5 cm from the midline (Fig. 22.1) (1). Surprisingly, this location corresponds very closely to the traditional location used for lateral trocar placement (3), and vessel injury as described above may result from trocars placed in this area. Therefore, a more lateral approach should be used. However, at this level, the superficial circumflex iliac artery is approximately 7 cm from the midline, so a more lateral approach may increase the risk of injuring this vessel.

A safer location may be 8 cm or more above the symphysis pubis and 8 cm from the midline (point A, Fig. 22.1). At this level, the epigastric arteries are more medial and the circumflex iliac artery is more lateral. Even at the level of the umbilicus, 8 cm from the midline appears to be an ideal location for lateral trocars since this roughly correlates to the somewhat less vascular lateral margin of the rectus muscle.

Unfortunately, anatomic variation and anastomoses between vessels make it impossible to know the exact location of every vessel in the abdominal wall. For this reason, other strategies should also be used to avoid vessel injury. One strategy is the exclusive use of trocars with conical tips rather than pyramid tips.* Conical tips have a smooth surface and may decrease the risk of vessel injury compared to pyramid tips (3). Another strategy is to place only smaller trocars lateral to the midline, placing larger trocars in the relatively avascular midline whenever possible. Not only are smaller trocars less likely to encounter blood vessels, but vessels that can be displaced laterally by smaller trocars may be unable to accommodate larger trocars without rupturing.

Despite the use of the strategies outlined above, occasional vessel injury is inevitable. Therefore, a plan of management for vessel injury should be developed prior to trocar placement. Because the deep vessels (i.e., the inferior epigastric arteries) are usually much larger than the superficial vessels, management can be divided into two approaches based on the vessel injured.

If the inferior epigastric artery is injured, brisk intra-abdominal bleeding will usually be immediately visible from the wound approximately 5 cm lateral to the midline. Although transabdominal suturing has been suggested for this condition (3), as illustrated by the case above, this inexact method of hemostasis may loosen during patient movement, with potentially catastrophic results.

Another approach is to selectively ligate the bleeding vessel. However, in order to obtain temporary hemostasis while the surgical team is preparing for a larger incision, a Foley catheter technique may be used. For this technique, a Foley catheter (10

---

*The three sharp edges of pyramidal trocars may slice the side of a vessel they pass by.

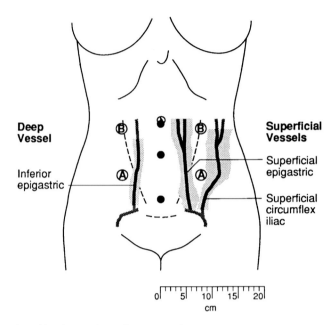

Deep Vessel

Inferior epigastric

Superficial Vessels

Superficial epigastric

Superficial circumflex iliac

Figure 22.1.   Location of the deep and superficial vessels of the anterior abdominal wall, frontal view. Black vessels with gray shadows represent mean ± SD for data from abdominal computer tomograms. Vessels shown without SD are extrapolated locations. The dashed lines indicate the relative location of the rectus abdominis muscle lateral margin and the symphysis pubis. The solid circles indicate standard sites for midline laparoscopic trocar placement, and the open circles indicate the recommended locations for lateral trocar placement 8 cm from midline at levels 8 cm above symphysis (A) and at the level of the umbilicus (B). (Adapted from Hurd WW, et al: The location of abdominal wall blood vessels in relationship to abdominal landmarks apparent at laparoscopy. *Am J Obstet Gynecol* [in press].)

French or larger) is placed through the trocar sleeve and the balloon is filled with 10 mL of fluid. The sleeve is then removed from the abdomen and traction placed on the Foley catheter. This traction can be maintained by cross-clamping the catheter near the skin with hemostatic forceps.

When the surgical team is prepared for laparotomy, the transverse skin incision above the vessel injury can be enlarged to approximately 3 to 4 cm, and taken down through the subcutaneous tissue and the rectus fascia. The rectus muscle can then be retracted medially with a small retractor and the epigastric artery visualized as it courses cephalad from its origin from the external iliac artery. The vessel can then be clamped with forceps and tied with a ligature. If the vessel cannot be visualized at this point, the incision can be enlarged until the vessel can be seen. Because of the vascular anastomoses, the vessel should be ligated cephalad as well. Laparotomy can be used if necessary, but may be avoided in many cases.

Injury of a superficial vessel may be less life-threatening but may result in significant hematoma formation with associated discomfort and risk of abscess formation (2). For this reason, any persistent bleeding from the trocar site should be dealt with when discovered. If any bleeding is noted from the trocar site after removal of the trocar sleeve, the subcutaneous tissue should be explored for the site of bleeding. When possible, the injured vessel should be grasped with Crile hemostatic forceps and sealed with electrocautery. On occasion, extension of the incision will be necessary to localize the site of bleeding. In cases where bleeding is less brisk and the vessel cannot be identified, the use of a pressure dressing followed by reevaluation of the patient in the immediate postoperative period may be adequate. Should a significant hematoma result, conservative management is appropriate in most cases, with local application of a pressure dressing and heat and close observation for signs of infection.

Knowledge of the location of vessels at risk during laparoscopy and attempts to visualize of them prior to trocar placement may minimize the risk of vessel injuries. However, because of anatomic variation, other strategies for vessel injury prevention and contingency plans for expedient treatment of these injuries should be familiar to every laparoscopist.

In the case presented, the patient was returned to surgery, where laparotomy revealed a severed and actively bleeding inferior epigastric artery and a 1500-mL hemoperitoneum. The artery was ligated both distally and proximally and the patient recovered without further complication.

REFERENCES

1. Hurd WW, Bude RO, DeLancey JOL, Newman JS: The location of abdominal wall blood vessels in relationship to abdominal landmarks apparent at laparoscopy. *Am J Obstet Gynecol* (in press).
2. Hurd WW, Pearl ML, DeLancey JOL, Quint EH, Garnett B, Bude RO: Laparoscopic injury of abdominal wall vessels: A report of three cases. *Obstet Gynecol* 82:673–676, 1993.
3. Semm K: *Operative Manual for Endoscopic Abdominal Surgery*. Chicago, Yearbook, 1987, pp. 130–151.
4. Yuzpe AA: Pneumoperitoneum needle and trocar injuries in laparoscopy: A survey on possible contributing factors and prevention. *J Reprod Med* 34:485, 1990.

23

Laparoscopy with Unexpected Viscus Penetration

Alan H. DeCherney

Case Abstract

Diagnostic closed laparoscopy was planned for a 26-year-old infertility patient. Insufflation of gas through the Veress needle was apparently uneventful, but after the operator had introduced the laparascope into the abdomen, she found she was viewing a mucous membrane of a large cavity strongly resembling the interior of the stomach. The anesthetist reported that gas was now coming from the patient's mouth, even though the trachea had been intubated.

DISCUSSION

Perforation of an intra-abdominal viscus by the Veress needle in preparation for laparoscopy is a common occurrence of little serious consequence. The diagnosis is made by either eructation or flatus occurring during the procedure. This depends on what part of the gastrointestinal tract is perforated, with the stomach yielding eructation and the colon leading to flatus production. If the diagnosis of the perforation of the viscus is made when only the Veress needle has penetrated the organ, one should remove the Veress needle and proceed with the laparoscopy after reinsufflation through another site. The surgeon must keep in mind, though, that this perforation might be the result of adhesions of the viscus to the anterior abdominal wall, and not just the result of a random puncture. Proceeding with open laparoscopy might be a wise choice at this juncture. Another alternative would be using the "needlescope" so as to advance the needle to insufflate and inspect at the same time.

Once the laparoscope is in place, the site of puncture by the Veress needle should be inspected, but usually this does not require any further surgical intervention. It is not known how often this happens. Puncture of the bladder by the Veress needle requires the same conservative approach as would apply to any other viscera.

The approach used for a needle perforation is not appropriate when the *trocar* penetrates an intra-abdominal viscus. Unfortunately, this is a more commonly diagnosed entity, since it is often difficult to tell if only the Veress needle has penetrated a viscus, but it is easy to tell that the trocar has penetrated a viscus. When the laparoscope itself is introduced, one views a mucosal surface. Once this occurs and has been identified, the gynecologist should *leave the laparoscope in place*, do a laparotomy, identify the defect, and close that defect in an appropriate manner after the laparoscope has been removed. The laparoscope is left in place to seal the puncture and also to allow identification of the site of trauma.

Bowel should be repaired by a purse-string or double-layered suture closing if the laceration is less than one-half the diameter of the lumen of the bowel. If the laceration exceeds one-half the diameter of the lumen (as it might since these lacerations sometimes are oblique), then a segmental resection and anastomosis should be performed. Also of paramount importance is maintaining the blood supply to the traumatized area; if the mesenteric blood supply is interrupted by the puncture, then a resection must be done no matter what the size or length of the laceration. It is appropriate to have a general surgeon as a consultant in this type of surgery.

The trocar or Veress needle may go through the bladder. Routinely, the intraumbilical puncture site is too high for this to occur. In this case the second puncture may go into the bladder, the operative field being obscured by massive pelvic adhesions. Occasionally this must be confirmed by cystoscopic examination, but in any event, if the defect leaks urine into the peritoneal cavity, the bladder should be repaired in a purse-string or two-layered suture fashion. It is appropriate to have urologic consultation if this occurs.

There are ways by which these complications can be prevented, and certainly most important is patient selection. Patients who have had previous bowel surgery should have an open laparoscopy rather than a closed laparoscopy. On the other hand, it is difficult to tell which patients who have had previous pelvic surgery should have an open laparoscopy. An alternative to the routine procedure is to use a small-gauge laparoscope such as the needlescope, with a 2- to 3-mm-diameter endoscope to identify intraperitoneal structures before the incision is made, and actually advance the needle and insufflate under direct visualization.

Any patient who has had a bowel or stomach perforation by the trocar should be treated in the same manner as anyone who has had bowel surgery, including nasogastric tube, prophylactic antibiotic coverage, and a prolonged period of putting the intestine to rest. The same goes for laceration of the bladder—the Foley catheter should be left in for the full 7 days, and the patient should be placed on prophylactic antibiotics.

Veress needle perforations require no special postoperative orders other than observation for the development of either chemical or bacterial peritonitis, of which the patient must be advised. They require no increase in usual hospital stay.

24

Cystic Adnexal Mass

William D. Schlaff

Case Abstract

A 32-year-old G4 P3ab1 female who had her last menstrual period 1 week earlier presented for laparoscopic tubal ligation. She was currently using condoms and foam for birth control, and had regular menses. Preoperative urine pregnancy test was negative. She was 5'1" tall and weighed 170 pounds. Preoperative examination under anesthesia was normal; however, it was limited by her weight. At the time of laparoscopy, the patient was found to have a 5 × 5 cm dark, possibly hemorrhagic cyst on her right ovary. Laparoscopic tubal banding was performed without complication.

DISCUSSION

Adnexal masses are caused by a variety of physiologic and pathophysiologic processes. Follicular or corpus luteum cysts represent a continuum of ovarian cyclic function, and are the predominant adnexal masses found in adult women. Neoplastic cystic adnexal processes found in young women are likely to be benign and include ovarian cystadenomas or benign teratomas. However, age alone does not exclude a malignant ovarian process. Endometriomas of the ovary can occur at any age, but are far and away most common in reproductive-age women. Adnexal masses in postmenopausal women often represent epithelial cell neoplasms and are the most worrisome. Thus, the clinical importance of an adnexal mass is closely related to the age and reproductive status of the patient.

When ovarian masses are found during routine office examination in reproductive-age women such as the patient presented above, the mass is commonly assumed to be a functional ovarian cyst. Ultrasound examination can be performed, and the finding of a unilocular cyst in the absence of ascites is reassuring. Functional ovarian cysts have commonly been managed with estrogen/progestin therapy, presumably causing regression by suppressing pituitary gonadotropins. However, in a randomized study of patients with sonographically confirmed unilocular adnexal cysts of ≥ 1.5 cm in mean diameter, norethindrone 1 mg and mestranol 0.5 mg (Ortho Novum 1/50®) was no more effective than simple observation in producing regression (4). On the other hand, patients with adnexal masses that persisted for as long as 9 weeks were found to have significant pathology at the time of surgical exploration. Thus, when we identify a unilocular cyst in an outpatient, we recommend simple observation for at least 6 weeks rather than hormonal suppression.

On occasion, an adnexal mass is unexpectedly found at the time of laparos-copy. Whether or not to intervene in this situation depends on a variety of factors. Signs suggesting malignancy such as ascites, papillations of the tumor, or excrescences on the ovarian surface preclude laparoscopic management. Consultation with a gynecologic oncologist should be sought when available, and laparotomy with full staging for suspected malignancy is mandated. At the other end of the spectrum, if the cyst appears unilocular, clear, and less than 6 cm, it is likely self-limited and therapy is rarely required.

The etiology and optimal management of the mass that does not fall into either of the above categories are far less straightforward. It is perplexing to manage the adnexal mass that appears complex rather than unilocular, dark rather than clear, or semisolid rather than cystic. Aspiration with cytologic examination of the cyst fluid has often been advocated in the management of these masses of uncertain etiology. However, studies correlating cyst fluid cytology with final histologic diagnosis have confirmed that the vast majority of cystic masses contain only benign cells (91%), but fluid from cystad-enomas and endometriomas may contain atypical cells which are interpreted as possibly malignant (9). Recurrence, which has been reported in 30% of cysts that are aspirated, is another problem with this technique. Given the potential for misdiagnosis as well as the high incidence of recurrence, we do not recommend simple diagnostic aspiration of such masses. Instead, we feel that one should either remove the cyst intact or defer surgical management to a later time after a full preoperative evaluation.

If a decision is made to treat the unexpected mass found at the time of surgery, the technique used should be tailored to the nature of the mass and the experience of the surgeon. In general, simple aspiration of a clear, unilocular cyst can be performed through a single accessory trocar in the lower abdominal midline. For any significant surgical procedure such as ovarian cystectomy, we recommend using three accessory trocars across the lower abdomen for those surgeons who are experienced enough with laparos-copy to manage cystectomy, or conversion to laparotomy for those who aren't. Fenestra-tion of a simple, unilocular cyst may be used for either ovarian or parovarian masses. A window is made in the wall of the cyst using either sharp dissecting scissors or electro-cautery. Laser can also be used to make this incision. These masses rarely bleed, and excessive energy use should be avoided. At the very least, biopsy of the cyst wall should be performed, though removal is preferable.

If bloody or chocolate-color material is aspirated, the cyst is probably a corpus luteum or endometrioma. Although a neoplastic process is possible, it is not likely. When this type of material is obtained, it is prudent to proceed with cystectomy. An incision is made in the ovarian capsule, generally with electrosurgery or a laser. The cyst wall is dissected bluntly off the ovarian cortex, and can usually be easily removed in its entirety. It is often difficult to differentiate a corpus luteum from an endometrioma. However, if multiple implants of endometriosis are present in the pelvis, the latter diagnosis is more likely and a more aggressive approach to laparoscopic resection should be considered. In the absence of endometriotic implants, the mass is more likely to be a corpus luteum. Should one obtain mucinous fluid or sebaceous material from the cyst after the initial aspiration, this more likely represents a mucinous adenoma or benign teratoma. Again, the cyst should be removed with aggressive irrigation of the pelvis to minimize the risk of peritoneal inflammation.

Dermoid cysts can sometimes be suspected because of sebaceous material visible through the capsule. In this circumstance, the decision to remove the masslaparoscopically or by laparotomy is a difficult one. If one decides to proceed laparoscopically, the ovary should be incised on the antitubal portion if at all possible. Ideally, the cystic mass can be dissected out of the ovary without perforation or rupture. A "endo-bag" can be used to isolate the ovary or the cystic mass from the remainder of the pelvis. This may also allow decompression of the mass once it has been removed from the ovary so that the material can all be removed from the abdomen without spillage. As with a ruptured corpus luteum or endometrioma, the pelvis should be copiously irrigated to minimize the risk of reaction to the foreign tissue.

If the cystic mass being considered is adherent to adjacent structures or to the sidewall, one should strongly reassess the advisability of performing the procedure laparoscopically. This type of surgery requires a degree of comfort with retroperitoneal dissection and treatment in and around major vessels or the ureter. One should be comfortable with opening the pelvic sidewall and using hydrodissection or direct visual inspection to identify all of these important pelvic structures and be certain that the procedure can be performed safely. Oophorectomy rather than cystectomy is rarely indicated for a histologically benign mass. Therefore, if the surgeon is contemplating oophorectomy because cystectomy may be excessively difficult laparoscopically, strong consideration should be given to abandoning the laparoscopic approach and performing the type of surgery that would allow conservation of the ovary. This is particularly true in the case where the ovarian cystectomy may be complicated by adherence to adjacent structures.

Perhaps the most worrisome aspect of the laparoscopic management of an ovarian cyst is the threat of spilling the contents of a malignant tumor into the pelvis. In a retrospective survey of the Society of Gynecology Oncologists, 42 cases of malignant ovarian neoplasms managed laparoscopically were reported (3). Unfortunately, close to one-third of these adnexal masses were less than 8 cm, unilateral, and unilocular, all characteristics suggestive of benignity. The authors observed that laparoscopic management of these cases resulted in inadequate resection and delay in definitive therapy, and expressed their concern that laparoscopic management of any undiagnosed mass may prove dangerous. Another recent analysis of patients with stage I epitheal ovarian cancer concluded that rupture of the tumor during laparotomy was not important prognostically but, rather, the histologic grade of the tumor and degree and density of adhesions to adjacent structures were found to be important (2). These conflicting results reinforce the uncertainty of how best to manage the patient with the unexpected adnexal mass from the standpoint of risk of tumor spread.

Ideally, unexpected adnexal masses at the time of other laparoscopic surgery could be avoided altogether. Unfortunately, given that the bimanual pelvic exam is far from perfect, this would almost certainly require routine ultrasonography prior to surgery. This option seems quite expensive and impractical. Thus, we will likely be left with the occasional conundrum of the unexpected adnexal mass. Most will be obviously benign, and a few obviously malignant. The most difficult to manage are those of uncertain etiology. Hopefully, new techniques such as intracorporeal ultrasound probes that may be passed through a 10-mm laparoscopy sheath will help us to reduce the uncertainty of management in those worrisome masses that do not fall into the category of clearly benign or clearly malignant.

REFERENCES

1. Davila RM: Cytology of benign uterine cystic masses. *Acta Cytologica* 37:385–390, 1993.
2. Dembro AJ, Davy M, Stenwig AE, Berie EJ, Bush RS, Kjorstad K: Prognostic factors in patients with stage I epithelial ovarian cancer. *Obstet Gynecol* 75:263–273, 1990.
3. Maiman M, Seltzer V, Boyce J: Laparoscopic excision of ovarian neoplasms subsequently found to be malignant. *Obstet Gynecol* 77:563–565, 1991.
4. Steinkampf MP, Hammond R, Blackwell RE: Hormonal treatment of functional ovarian cysts: A randomized, prospective study. *Fertil Steril* 54:775–777, 1990.

25

Ectopic Pregnancy in an Infertility Patient with Coexistent Chronic Pelvic Inflammatory Disease

Celso-Ramón García
Phillip C. Galle

Case Abstract

A laparoscopy was performed on a 28-year-old nulligravid, infertility patient because of a suspected ectopic pregnancy. At laparoscopy, the diagnosis was confirmed, in addition to the presence of many adhesions from previous pelvic inflammatory disease. The opposite tube was thickened and clubbed, and the fimbriated end was occluded.

DISCUSSION

Ectopic pregnancy continues to challenge the gynecologic surgeon. The treatment of ectopic pregnancy includes laparotomy, operative laparoscopy, and chemotherapy. The type of procedure depends on the condition of the patient, the condition of the fallopian tube, and her desire for future fertility. With the current techniques and instruments available for operative laparoscopy, laparoscopy is assuming a greater role in the treatment of ectopic pregnancy as well as other types of gynecologic surgery. The patient described above provides the opportunity to review the options regarding types of treatment for ectopic pregnancy, the role of immunization, and postoperative human chorionic gonadotropin (HCG) surveillance. It also affords the opportunity to discuss the treatment of a hydrosalpinx.

Diagnosis

The key to the management of the patient with an ectopic pregnancy lies in early diagnosis. To do this, one must maintain a high index of clinical suspicion. With more sensitive assays for HCG, ultrasound, and endoscopy, an early diagnosis is facilitated. With the combination of ultrasound and HCG levels, often intrauterine pregnancies can be confirmed and thus rule out ectopics. Definitive diagnosis is the presence of a fetal heart activity demonstrated on ultrasound. However, earlier diagnosis of a viable intrauterine pregnancy utilizes the ultrasound appearance of a gestational sac and HCG level. With abdominal ultrasound and HCG levels of 6500 mIU/ml or greater, a discriminatory zone has been described to identify early intrauterine pregnancies (8). With transvaginal ultrasound, the resolution is better for both intrauterine and extrauterine visualization. With an HCG level of 2000 mIU/ml or more one should be able to identify a gestational sac with the most normal intrauterine pregnancies. If one fails to visualize a sac, the diagnosis of an ectopic is very likely.

If the HCG level is less than 2000 mIU/ml, close follow-up is essential and includes the presence of symptoms, repeat ultrasound, and HCG levels. Abnormalities on ultrasound in patients with ectopic pregnancies are described, but the exact diagnosis ultrasonographically depends on the experience of the ultrasonographer and the resolution of the equipment.

Although there are no long-term prospective studies on culdocentesis, we believe that it rarely influences management. Moreover, it could increase the risk of intraperitoneal contamination with vaginal or other flora. A positive culdocentesis would not exclude an etiology of less significant intraperitoneal bleeding that might be managed with laparoscopy, nor does a negative test preclude further diagnostic procedures. Although aggressiveness in intensity and promptness of the diagnostic review should be emphasized, the least invasive approaches should be selected relative to the patient's condition. With surgical management a laparoscopy will confirm the diagnosis and can be used to treat a significant number of patients. A laparoscopy should not be performed when a patient is in shock, nor probably in the situation where ultrasonographic findings and clinical symptoms suggest the diagnosis of significant tubal rupture.

Management

Management may vary depending on the patient's age, her desire for future fertility, and other gynecologic data, such as a history of abnormal cytology or pelvic infections, the location and the severity of the ectopic pregnancy, and the condition of the patient. When an ectopic pregnancy is suspected, the patient or couple should be informed of the range of treatment modalities, which include conservative tubal surgery, medical treatment, or extirpative surgery, which might include salpingectomy, salpingo-oophorectomy, and even hysterectomy. Hysterectomy would probably only be indicated if there is a major problem in obtaining hemostatis with an interstitial ectopic pregnancy, if there is extensive pelvic inflammatory disease, or if the patient's underlying condition is grave. With adequate information the patient can assume a more active role in her management. She should be cautioned that even with conservative surgery the risk of another ectopic pregnancy remains elevated. In patients who desire future fertility, conservative surgery allows the best opportunity to preserve reproduction function. Conservative surgery includes expression of products of conception, linear salpingostomy, or tubal resection. Since future fertility is dependent on the procedure as well as adhesion formation, there should be gentle handling of tissue, copious irrigation and suction, meticulous hemostasis, and, if sutures are used, fine nonreactive sutures.

A laparoscopic approach can be used to treat a significant number of ectopic pregnancies. Laparoscopic treatment includes expression, linear salpingostomy, segmental resection, and salpingectomy. Prerequisites for laparoscopy are experience with operative laparoscopy and adequate instrumentation. There are certain limitations to laparoscopic treatment. Contraindications to this approach would include the patient who is hemodynamically unstable, tubes that are ruptured with significant damage, the size of the ectopic pregnancy, tubes that are not accessible, or inadequate visualization of other pelvic structures such as the contralateral tube and ovary. The upper limit of size recommended is 3 to 5 cm (14).

The unruptured ectopic pregnancy presents a compromised organ, but the ruptured ectopic pregnancy offers an even poorer prognosis dependent on the degree of damage related to hemorrhage and disruption of the oviduct. If tubal reconstruction can be accomplished, it is advisable. It should be emphasized that even in the presence of a "normal"-appearing contralateral tube, it is impossible to rule out occult tubal pathology.

In the patient who is hypovolemic and unstable, secondary to blood loss, there is little controversy as to the best management. Here, the main objective involves obtaining prompt hemostasis, fluid and electrolyte replacement, and appropriate blood transfusion. Stabilization and prompt intervention are essential to control the bleeding. If the gestation is located in the distal portion of the tube or with a tubal abortion, removing the pregnancy tissue and securing adequate hemostasis may be all that is needed. When the ruptured segment presents in the midportion with the distal portion of the tube and fimbria intact, the products of conception and damaged portion of the tube may require resection, leaving as much normal tissue as possible if conservation is desired. After a period of convalescence, an elective tubal reconstruction procedure can be scheduled. Resection and anastomosis have been suggested at the time of initial therapeutic surgery, but the patient's condition and the anatomic distortion may not support such operative reconstruction. Those that are done may not be successful because of the luminal and anatomic discrepancies secondary to the ectopic changes in the tube, precluding a meaningful anatomosis.

Special Clinical States

Controversy arises in the patient with an ectopic tubal pregnancy and tubal pathology. There are authors who, on the basis of an early series of ectopic pregnancies treated with laparotomy, advise restoration of the contralateral tube (3,10,14). Most authors, including ourselves, currently recommend delaying other infertility surgery (2,12).

In order to outline the management of an ectopic pregnancy and coexistent chronic pelvic inflammatory disease with a hydrosalpinx, we will consider several aspects. With current advances in operative laparoscopy, neosalpingostomies can be performed laparoscopically for the treatment of distal tubal disease. In a review of 199 cases of laparoscopic neosalpingostomies, the pregnancy rate was 32% and the term pregnancy rate 21% (4,5,6,7,9). These results compare favorably with results reported with an abdominal approach. One needs to be cautious with advocating widespread utilization of laparoscopy for distal tubal disease. In most series where neosalpingostomies are subdivided into categories by extent of disease, there is significant difference in outcome. With laparotomy neosalpingostomy the pregnancy rate and term pregnancy rate with mild disease are 64% and 46%; with moderate disease, 38% and 20%. There is a concern that the milder cases of hydrosalpinx are more amenable to laparoscopic treatment and that some series may have a predominance of milder cases. In order to compare laparoscopic with laparotomy neosalpingostomy more objectively, additional data are necessary regarding results of laparoscopic treatment according to a standard classification of disease. Because of these concerns we rarely perform laparoscopic neosalpingostomies.

In the patient described the approach would depend on the condition of the patient, the characteristics of the ectopic pregnancy, and the extent of pelvic inflammatory disease. If the patient is hemodynamically stable, and the ectopic pregnancy amenable to laparoscopic treatment, this would be undertaken. If the hydrosalpinx was mild to moderate, we would not correct the tube at the time of laparoscopy. The follow-up would depend on the type of procedure performed. If linear salpingostomy had been performed, and the patient had not established a pregnancy within 6 months to 1 year, a laparoscopy and hysterosalpingogram would be scheduled to evaluate the tubes prior to a major surgical procedure to resect or reconstruct the damaged portion of the ectopically treated tube, if necessary, and correct the hydrosalpinx on the other tube.

If a laparotomy is necessary to treat the ectopic pregnancy, whether to correct the hydrosalpinx would depend on many variables. Tubal surgery performed as an emergency yields poorer results of varied success. The adnexal structures are often edematous and hyperemic, posing suboptimal time for reconstruction as well as predisposing to adhesion formation. Since the pregnancy rates are highest with the initial operative procedure, a neosalpingostomy would not be undertaken. An exception to delaying a neosalpingostomy at the initial laparotomy would be the patient with minimal tubal disruption and minimal peritoneal bleeding who is treated with expression or linear salpingostomy. In most cases we would remove the ectopic pregnancy by techniques which would preserve as much of the tube as feasible, and then repair the tube. Following a linear salpingostomy, if the patient did not become pregnant in 6 months to 1 year, a laparoscopy and hysterosalpingogram would be scheduled to evaluate the tubes prior to a major surgical procedure. The major surgical procedure would include repairing the tube that had the ectopic pregnancy if necessary, and a neosalpingostomy on the tube with the hydrosalpinx. If a segmental resection or salpingectomy had been performed, a laparotomy would be performed at a later date. With a resection, an anastomosis would be done together with a neosalpingostomy on the contralateral tube.

Postoperative Management

Rho-immunoglobulin should be given to unsensitized Rh-negative patients. The dose recommended is 50 mg prior to 13 weeks gestation, and 300 mg for gestations of 13 weeks or greater (1).

In patients undergoing conservative surgery, follow-up HCG levels should be carried out postoperatively to confirm adequate removal of products of conception. In asymptomatic patients whose levels persist, we would favor either initial therapy with one course methotrexate or surgery. In the patient with coexistent chronic pelvic inflammatory disease, we would wait for complete resolution and healing of the tube with the ectopic pregnancy prior to further evaluation and treatment.

One should be aware that in an infertility patient temporary contraception may be necessary. Often patients or couples need to grieve and emotionally resolve the loss associated with the pregnancy prior to attempting another pregnancy. Since approximately 70% of patients will have ovulated within 2 weeks following an ectopic pregnancy, contraception should be started early (11).

Summary and Conclusion

For an ectopic pregnancy in an infertility patient with chronic pelvic inflammatory disease and a contralateral hydrosalpinx, the operative procedures would depend upon the location of the pregnancy, the extent of tubal damage, and the hemodynamic status. Initially a laparoscopic approach would be attempted, unless the patient was not hemodynamically stable, the tube had significant damage, the ectopic pregnancy exceeded 3 to 5 cm in size, or the tube was not accessible. In these instances or if there were complications encountered laparoscopically, a laparotomy would be performed. At a later date, both the effects of the inopportune gestation and preexisting adnexal disease could be approached. With conservative procedures postoperative levels of HCG should be followed until negative. If the levels fail to drop, then treatment such as methotrexate therapy or additional surgery should be initiated.

REFERENCES

1. American College of Obstetricians and Gynecologists: Technical Bulletin 61, March, 1981.
2. Bruhat MA, Manhes H, Mage G, et al: Treatment of ectopic pregnancy by means of laparoscopy. *Fertil Steril* 33:411, 1980.
3. Bukosky I, Langer R, Herman A, et al: Conservative surgery for tubal pregnancy. *Obstet Gynecol* 53:709, 1979.
4. Canis M, Mage G, Pouly JL, et al: Laparoscopic distal tuboplasty: Report of 87 cases and a 4 year experience. *Fertil Steril* 56:616, 1991.
5. Daniell JF, Hebert CM: Laparoscopic salpingostomy utilizing the CO_2 laser. *Fertil Steril* 41:558, 1984.
6. Dubuisson JB, de Joliniere JB, Aubriot FX, et al: Terminal tuboplasties by laparoscopy: 65 consecutive cases. *Fertil Steril* 54:401, 1990.
7. Fayez JA: An assessment of the role of operative laparoscopy in tuboplasty. *Fertil Steril* 39:476, 1983.
8. Kadar N, Romero R: HCG assay and ectopic pregnancy. *Lancet* 1:1205, 1981.
9. Mettler L, Giesel H, Semm K: Treatment of female infertility due to tubal obstruction by operative laparoscopy. *Fertil Steril* 32:384, 1979.
10. Skulj V, Pavlic F, Stoiljkovic C, et al: Conservative operative treatment of tubal pregnancy. *Fertil Steril* 15:634, 1964.
11. Spirtos NM, Spirtos TW, Inouye C, et al: Resumption of ovulation after ectopic pregnancy. *Obstet Gynecol* 69:933, 1987.
12. Swolin K: A tubal surgeon's recommendation for the surgical treatment of ectopic pregnancy. *J Reprod Med* 25:38, 1980.
13. Thornton KL, Diamond MP, DeCherney AH: Linear salpingostomy for ectopic pregnancy. *Obstet Gynecol Clin NA* 18:95, 1991.
14. Vehaskari A; The operation of choice for ectopic pregnancy with reference to subsequent fertility. *Acta Obstet Gynecol Scand* 39:3, 1960.

26

Missing Needle

Ray V. Haning, Jr.

Case Abstract

Following a microsurgical tuboplasty the surgeon had broken scrub, and as the first assistant was preparing to close the peritoneal cavity, the circulating nurse reported the needle count as one missing, a microsurgical needle. A flat plate obtained on the operating room table failed to reveal the needle.

DISCUSSION

Finding the Lost Needle

Standard x-ray techniques are of great assistance in locating or ruling out the intra-abdominal location of needles for no. 6-0 or larger sutures. Microsurgical needles are too small to be visualized by standard x-ray techniques. Even using a Bucky tray and a small field (24 × 30 cm) to cut down on scatter, we were unable to visualize no. 7-0, 8-0, or 9-0 needles (Ethicon TG140-8, formerly GS9) placed on a patient's abdominal wall at the time of a hysterosalpingogram scout film. We had no trouble visualizing the no. 6-0, 5-0, or 4-0 needles (Ethicon taper RB-1) or larger needles in the x-ray department (technique: 1.2 mm focal spot, 60 kv, 8 mAs). A portable abdominal flat plate film (35 × 43 cm, focal spot approximately 2 × 2 mm) obtained in the operating room with a grid to cut down on scatter would provide even poorer resolution. This is because an increase in the size of the focal spot increases the size of the penumbra, and as the x-ray field becomes larger, the scatter problem increases, producing still poorer resolution. Although it is possible theoretically to increase the resolution of x-ray techniques by using smaller fields and smaller focal spots, instruments with smaller focal spots are not readily available in the operating room, limiting their utility. The use of multiple small fields presents problems in ensuring that the needle will not be missed between the fields surveyed. Thus, in the operating room, techniques for finding the missing microsurgical needle are realistically limited to visual search of the operative site and the use of strong magnets to locate the needle lost elsewhere. A strong magnet in a sterile drape could theoretically be used to check the superficial areas of the operative field, but, again, such magnets are not readily available in the operating room. Strong magnets are not able to assist in finding a needle that has gained access to the abdominal cavity and that is not superficial in its location. Although the lost needle should be retrieved if possible, the microsurgical needle lost in the operative site is unlikely to be harmful to the patient because of its small size. Thus, the microsurgeon must ultimately make a decision either to stop the search or to continue the search for the missing needle. Such a decision is based on the risk-benefit ratio. If a needle is lost and cannot be found, the patient should be informed of the status of the needle count, the steps that were taken to locate the needle, and the rationale for stopping the search at the point where it was stopped.

Prevention of Needle Loss

Since locating a lost microsurgical needle is so difficult, it is useful to discuss techniques for prevention of microsurgical needle loss. There are three possible prospective approaches that can be of use: (1) careful needle handling, (2) careful draping and packing of the microsurgical field to limit access of the dropped needle in the abdominal cavity to only the small microsurgical field itself, and (3) careful measures by the scrub nurse and circulator to make sure that the used needles are stored securely to prevent loss on the instrument table and to make sure that the number of all types of needles used on the case is known so that in the event that the count is one missing, it can be immediately determined what size of needle is being sought.

A little recognized problem in dealing with the microsurgical needle is the visual acuity of the scrub nurse. Many people over 40 years of age have begun to lose some ability to accommodate visually. This results in loss of visual acuity for close work, making it difficult for them to see microsurgical needles or suture without corrective lenses such as bifocals. Such individuals should wear appropriate corrective lenses if they are to work with microsurgical sutures.

NEEDLE HANDLING

The needle should be handled in such a way as to minimize the chance of dropping it or dislodging it from the suture prematurely. Thus, in addition to receiving it from and passing it back to the scrub nurse always grasped in the jaws of the needle holder or grasped by the suture in a rubber-shod clamp, care should be taken not to weaken the fine suture by holding it in metallic clamps or the needle holder. Small rubber-shod clamps should be used to hold untied sutures if the needles are still attached, and care should be taken not to place such clamps near the attachment of the suture to the needle because this can promote premature separation of the suture from the needle. Once the needle is back on the instrument table the scrub nurse must take equal care to see that the needle is not lost there since loss on the instrument table will result in an incorrect needle count at the end of the case. In spite of all these precautions, the occasional loss of a microsurgical needle will continue to occur.

Laparoscopic Hysterectomy — Ureter Transected

Harry Reich
Sheila E. Buchbinder

Case Abstract

A 53-year-old woman underwent laparoscopic hysterectomy for a 12-week-size leio-myomatous uterus and severe menometrorrhagia, necessitating two emergency room visits for hypovolemic shock. At the time of laparoscopic hysterectomy with ureteral catheters in place, both ureters were dissected to the point of passage under the uterine blood vessels. On the right side, the area was noted to be fibrotic. The MULTI-Fire Endo GIA 30 stapler was used for ligation of the uterine vessels. Near the conclusion of the procedure, the right ureteral stent could not be removed. Inspection revealed that the right ureteral wall and stent were entrapped by the staple line approximately 5 cm above the ureterovesical junction.

DISCUSSION

Definition

Ureteral injury occurs in approximately 0.5% to 1% of pelvic operations (2). The risk of ureteral injury during laparoscopic hysterectomy using the Endo-GIA is well documented (10,1).

There are a variety of operations where the laparoscope is used as an aid to hysterectomy. It is important that these different procedures are clearly delineated:

Diagnostic laparoscopy with vaginal hysterectomy indicates that the laparo-scope is used for *diagnostic* purposes, when indications for a vaginal ap-proach are equivocal, to determine if *vaginal hysterectomy* is possible (4). It also ensures that vaginal cuff and pedicle hemostasis is complete and allows clot evacuation.

Laparoscopic-assisted vaginal hysterectomy (LAVH) is a vaginal hysterectomy after laparoscopic adhesiolysis, endometriosis excision, or oophorectomy (9). Unfortunately, this procedure is also used inappropriately in place of vaginal hysterectomy to staple-ligate the upper uterine blood supply of a relatively normal uterus.

Laparoscopic hysterectomy (LH) denotes laparoscopic ligation of the uterine arteries by electrosurgery desiccation, suture ligature, or staples. All maneuvers after uterine vessel ligation can be done vaginally or laparoscopically, including anterior and posterior vaginal entry, cardinal and uterosacral ligaments division, uterine removal intact or by morcellation, and vaginal closure vertically or transversely. Ureteral isolation has always been advised (7,8).

Total laparoscopic hysterectomy (TLH) is a laparoscopic-assisted abdominal hysterectomy. Laparoscopic dissection continues until the uterus lies free of all attachments in the peritoneal cavity. The uterus is removed through the vagina with morcellation if necessary. The vagina is closed with laparoscopically placed cuff suspension sutures incorporating the uterosacral ligaments (8).

Laparoscopic supracervical hysterectomy (LSH) has recently regained advocates after suggestions that total hysterectomy results in a decrease in libido. The uterus is removed by morcellation from above or below.

Prevention of Ureteral Injury

The laparoscopic surgeon must rely almost entirely on visual recognition to identify normal structures in the abdomen and pelvis. Nowhere does this create more difficulties than with identification of the ureter. When open abdominal hysterectomy is done for benign pathology, the ureters can be palpated in the broad ligament and avoided as the infundibulopelvic ligaments or adnexa are clamped. The method of clamp placement used to divide the uterine arteries and cervical ligaments ensures that only tissues directly adjacent to the cervix, and therefore medial to the ureters, will be divided. These options are not available to the laparoscopic surgeon, and the ureter has to be identified and often partly mobilized to make many laparoscopic operations safe. Ureteral isolation should be an integral part of laparoscopic hysterectomy procedures, and bulky staplers should rarely be used for uterine vessel ligation.

LAPAROSCOPIC TECHNIQUES TO IDENTIFY THE URETER

Three approaches have been used for laparoscopic ureteric identification, which may be called medial, superior, and lateral (5,3). Ureteral dissection is preferable to visualizing the ureter through the peritoneum early in the case, since bleeding, although rarely sufficient to be of concern, stains the surrounding tissues, making it very difficult to identify the underlying ureter and hypogastric artery during the process of ligating the uterine vessels.

The Medial Approach

If the uterus is anteverted, the ureter can usually be easily visualized in its natural position on the medial leaf of the broad ligament. This allows the peritoneum immediately above the ureter to be incised to create a "window" in the peritoneum, which makes for safe division of the infundibulopelvic ligament, the utero-ovarian ligament, and the uterine vessel pedicle.

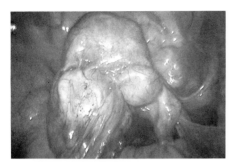

Figure 27.1. Extensive adnexal and cul-de-sac adhesions are present.

Immediately after exploration of the upper abdomen and pelvis, each ureter is isolated deep in the pelvis, if possible. This is done early in the operation before the pelvic sidewall peritoneum becomes edematous and/or opaque from irritation by the CO_2 pneumoperitoneum or aquadissection and before ureteral peristalsis is inhibited by surgical stress, pressure, or Trendelenburg's position. The left ureter is dissected first because it is usually more difficult to find. The ureter and its overlying peritoneum are grasped deep in the pelvis on the left below the lateral rectosigmoid attachments at the pelvic brim. Atraumatic concave grasping forceps are used to grab the ureter and its overlying peritoneum on the pelvic sidewall below and caudad to the ovary, lateral to the uterosacral ligament. Scissors are used to divide the peritoneum overlying the ureter and are inserted into the defect created and spread. Thereafter one blade of the scissors is placed on top of the ureter, the buried blade visualized through the peritoneum, and the peritoneum divided down to the deep pelvis where the uterine vessels cross the ureter (Fig. 27.2). Connective tissue between the ureter and the vessels is separated with scissors. Often the uterine artery is ligated at this time to diminish backbleeding from the upper pedicles (Fig. 27.3).

The Superior Approach

The superior approach entails dissecting the rectosigmoid off the left side of the pelvic brim and freeing the infundibulopelvic ligament vessels from the roof of the broad ligament to allow the ureter that lies below it and the superior rectal artery to be identified. The ureter is then reflected off the broad ligament and traced into the pelvis. Although this has been used very effectively by the author, it is being replaced by the

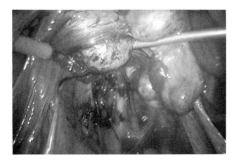

Figure 27.2. Peritoneum is opened to identify left ureter and ureteral artery after adnexal mobilization.

Figure 27.3.   Left uterine artery ligature secured. Ureter can be well visualized on medial leaf of broad ligament.

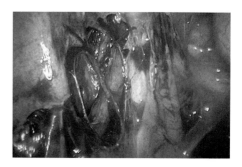

medial and lateral approaches, especially for difficult hysterectomies where the adnexa are adherent to the pelvic wall and uterus and during radical pelvic surgery. This approach allows a more systematic development of the retroperitoneum.

The Lateral Approach

The triangle of the pelvic sidewall is delineated by displacing the uterus to the contralateral side. The base of this triangle is formed by the round ligament, the lateral border by the external iliac artery, the medial border by the infundibulopelvic ligament, and the apex by where the infundibulopelvic ligament crosses the common iliac artery. The peritoneum in the middle of the triangle is incised with dissecting scissors and the broad ligament opened by bluntly separating the extraperitoneal areolar tissues. Small vessels are coagulated because the slightest amount of bleeding stains the extraperitoneal areolar tissues and may obscure the view of the underlying structures. The peritoneal incision is extended first to the round ligament, which is *not* divided at this time, and then to the apex of the triangle, lateral to the infundibulopelvic ligament. On the left side, congenital rectosigmoid adhesions are separated from the underlying peritoneum, and the pelvic sidewall triangle is opened near its apex.

The infundibulopelvic ligament is pulled medially with grasping forceps to expose the ureter at the pelvic brim where it crosses the common or external iliac artery. It may be necessary to reflect the ureter off the medial leaf of the broad ligament for a short distance to aid in its identification, although this is not always required. The ureter does not have to be peeled off the broad ligament for its entire pelvic course to be visible. The dissection of the apex is more difficult on the left side partly because the ureter is covered by the mesentery of the sigmoid colon, but mainly because it crosses the iliac vessels higher (more cephalad), and consequently lies more medial than the right ureter.

The dissection is carried bluntly underneath and caudad to the round ligament, until the obliterated hypogastric artery is identified extraperitoneally and traced to the origin of the uterine artery. If any difficulty is encountered, the artery should be first identified intraperitoneally where it hangs from the anterior abdominal wall (obliterated umbilical artery), traced to where it passes behind the round ligament. Then with both its intraperitoneal portion and the dissected space under the round ligament in view, the intraperitoneal part of the ligament is moved back and forth. It will almost always be possible to detect corresponding movements in the extraperitoneal portion of the ligament.

The obliterated hypogastric arteries are next traced proximally to the uterine artery origin, and the pararectal spaces opened by blunt dissection proximal and medial to the uterine vessels, which lie on top of the cardinal ligaments. Once the pararectal spaces have been opened, the ureter is easily identified on the medial leaf of the broad ligament, which forms the medial border of the pararectal space. The uterine artery and cardinal ligament at the distal (caudal) border of the space and the internal iliac artery on its lateral border also become clearly visible. The uterine artery can easily be ligated at this time (Fig. 27.4).

Treatment Options for Ureteral Transection

Most surgeons use no. 4–0 absorbable suture (chromic, Vicryl, or Monocryl) on a small tapered atraumatic needle. Nonabsorbable suture is not used because of its propensity for stone and crust formation. A simple stitch is used, although occasionally a stay suture is required. Ideally a "no touch" technique is employed: the suture is placed to approximate mucosa to mucosa, without holding the ureter. If the ureter is transected, a half-spatulated anastomosis is performed from the tip of one end to the apex of the other. Any kind of soft stent (Bard, Cook, Meditech, or Microvasive) can be placed cystoscopically and removed 3 weeks later. Patency is confirmed by either ureterogram or IVP. Ureteroneocystostomy is done if anastomosis is not possible.

Author's Choice

In the case described at the beginning of this chapter, an additional midline suprapubic 5-mm trocar was added to the existing two lower abdominal trocar sites. The surrounding tissue at the site of injury was separated from the ureter with scissor dissection. One centimeter of ureter encompassing the staples and the original stent was excised, since it was not possible to pull the staples out. A double-pigtail stent was placed transurethrally with laparoscopic guidance prior to the removal of the original stent. After spatulation (oblique division of the ureter to increase luminal size), the ureter was reapproximated with four no. 4–0 Vicryl (J-304H taper RB-1, Ethicon) sutures for a tension-free anastomosis. Intracorporeal knot tying was used. The knots were further secured with individual hemoclips. A Jackson-Pratt drain was placed through the trocar sheath, properly positioned, and left alongside the repair site for 48 hours. After minimal drainage, the drain was removed and the patient was discharged on the morning of the

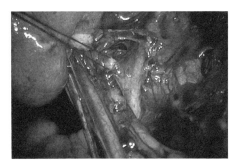

Figure 27.4. The extraperitoneal portion of the right obliterated hypogastric artery is identified. Uterine artery is seen crossing right ureter after its origin from the hypogastric artery. Ligature is seen on right uterine artery at its origin.

third postoperative day. She returned to work within a 2-week period. The stent was removed in the office after 5 weeks and IVP study at 3 months was normal. Six-month follow-up identified no complications.

The ability to suture laparoscopically greatly enhances the surgeon's ability to repair visceral injury (6). Laparoscopic staplers are presently too bulky for uterine vessel ligation. Stents are not protective because they frequently cannot be seen in the cardinal ligaments.

This author is committed to prevention of ureteral injury intraoperatively by ureteral dissection. Stents are not used. Postoperatively, early recognition of insult to ureteral integrity is done by obtaining a single-shot IVP on anyone reporting lateralized pain of any kind—abdominal, flank, or back. The bottom line is that an aggressive approach to ureteral protection can reduce but not eliminate ureteral injury. However, prompt recognition and management can prevent multiple surgical procedures and significant patient morbidity, including organ loss.

REFERENCES

1. Alderman B: Letter to the editor: Ureteric injury. *Gynaecol Endosc* 2:186, 1993.
2. Daly J, Higgins KA: Injury to the ureter during gynecologic surgical procedures. *Surgery, Gynecol & Obstet* 167(1):19–22, 1988.
3. Kadar N, Reich H: Laparoscopically assisted radical Schauta hysterectomy and bilateral laparoscopic pelvic lymphadenectomy for the treatment of bulky stage IB carcinoma of the cervix. *Gynaecol Endosc* 2:135–142, 1993.
4. Kovac SR, Cruikshank SH, Retto HF: Laparoscopy-assisted vaginal hysterectomy. *J Gynecol Surg* 6:185–189, 1990.
5. Reich H: Pelvic sidewall dissection. In: Hulka J and Reich H: *Textbook of Laparoscopy*, ed. 2. New York, W.B. Saunders, 1994, p. 245.
6. Reich H, Clarke HC, Selek L: A simple method for ligating in operative laparoscopy with straight and curved needles. *Obstet Gynecol* 79:143–147, 1992.
7. Reich H, DeCaprio J, McGlynn F: Laparoscopic hysterectomy. *J Gynecol Surg* 5:213–216, 1989.
8. Reich H, McGlynn F, Sekel L: Total laparoscopic hysterectomy. *Gynecol Endosc* 2:59–63, 1993.
9. Summit RL, Stovall TG, Lipscomb GH, Ling FW: Randomized comparison of laparoscopy-assisted vaginal hysterectomy with standard vaginal hysterectomy in an outpatient setting. *Obstet Gynecol* 80:895–901, 1992.
10. Woodland MB: Ureter injury during laparoscopy-assisted vaginal hysterectomy with the endoscopic linear stapler. *Am J Obstet Gynecol* 167:756–757, 1992.

Endometriosis of the Rectovaginal Septum in an Infertility Patient with Rectal Penetration at the Time of Surgery

John J. Mikuta

Case Abstract

A 36-year-old gravida 0 para 0 was evaluated for an infertility problem over 10 years previously. Laparoscopic examination at that time revealed the presence of small endometrial implants on the uterosacral ligaments and the posterior surface of the lower uterine body, as well as minor implants on the right ovary. In other areas there was evidence of powder burn on the bladder peritoneum and along the left infundibulopelvic ligament. The patient was encouraged to attempt pregnancy. She was unsuccessful. She subsequently was lost to follow-up but after 5 years was again seen, having remarried and again requesting fertility evaluation. At this time pelvic examination revealed findings of extensive involvement of the cul-de-sac area with endometriosis and also in other areas of the peritoneum, including the fallopian tubes. The ovaries were found to be relatively free and the fimbriated ends of the fallopian tubes were mobile and normal appearing. The patient was again advised to try pregnancy. This she did for several months without success. She returned for a trial of hormonal therapy. This was carried out and the patient was placed on danazol (Danocrine) for a period of 6 months. Several months following the completion of danazol therapy she again tried to conceive. She was again unsuccessful and was experiencing increased pelvic pain along with dyspareunia. She was again lost to follow-up for approximately 18 months and when seen in the office there was evidence of extension of the endometriosis into the rectovaginal septum with some anterior dissection of the cul-de-sac in the upper rectovaginal area. After extensive discussion with the patient and her husband, it was recommended that laparoscopic examination be again performed and, depending on the extent of the disease in the pelvis, a decision be made whether further conservative surgery could be carried out or whether it would be advisable to sacrifice some of the pelvic reproductive organs, including, if necessary, hysterectomy.

At the time of the laparoscopy there was extensive involvement of the pelvis with adhesions. The cul-de-sac was obliterated from the lower portion of the uterus and this whole area was adherent to the rectum. Both tubes and ovaries were involved in a mass of adhesions with endometrial implants apparent bilaterally. A decision was made to carry out a total abdominal hysterectomy and bilateral salpingo–oophorectomy. At the time of the procedure, after the adnexa had been freed by retroperitoneal dissection and after the uterine vasculature had been secured and the bladder flap taken down, efforts to free the posterior portion of the uterus, which was densely involved with endometriosis in the area of the anterior rectal wall, led to an entry into the rectum. This was approximately 2 cm in length in a slight diagonal fashion. There was no evidence of any fecal contamination of the surrounding area, and the mucosa was noted to be clean.

DISCUSSION

This patient presents with obvious evidence of progressive involvement of the pelvic structures with external pelvic endometriosis. The classic spread to the cul-de-sac and the uterosacral ligaments as well as to the adnexa is not unexpected. Patients who are followed for long periods of time with known endometriosis, particularly when there is episodic care at irregular intervals, may frequently end up with the kind of situation described here. The management in this case as described should be very simple and safe. A small rent into the rectum, particularly where the bowel is relatively free, can be readily repaired with a double-layer closure of the bowel wall. After removal of the uterus, irrigation of the pelvic cavity should provide adequate cleansing of the peritoneal cavity and reduction of the bacterial contamination, and allow good primary healing. To drain or not to drain at this point is a somewhat unsettled matter. If there was some fecal contamination, particularly with liquid feces in an unprepared bowel, the repair should primarily be carried out followed by thorough cleansing and irrigation of the peritoneal cavity, with continued postoperative antibiotics and drainage of the pelvic area with Jackson-Pratt drains.

If there is an extensive tear of the rectum, particularly an irregular one, this would be handled in one of two ways, depending on circumstances. In the absence of a prepared bowel and gross contamination the safest and most expeditious approach is to do a primary-end colostomy with resection of the injured bowel and to perform the Hartmann pouch procedure. After ample recovery time reanastomosis of the bowel can be carried out. The second approach is to do a primary resection of the injured bowel with a primary end-to-end hand-sewn anastomosis, or for lower-level anastomoses an EEA stapler could be used. The use of the EEA stapler provides one with the opportunity to perform very low anastomoses and to be able to avoid a temporary colostomy. In patients who have had many prior surgical procedures this is a distinct advantage.

Prevention

In patients who are known to have extensive pelvic disease, whether it be endometrosis, pelvic inflammatory disease, ovarian tumor masses, or ovarian remnant syndrome, preparation of the bowel is of vital importance. Mechanical cleansing alone is a great asset to the surgeon, both because it removes the bulk of intestine to be dealt with and because it reduces the amount of bacterial contamination in the large intestine. The use of antibiotics such as cephalosporins and/or metranidazole is also helpful in reducing the contamination of the peritoneal cavity should injury occur. A second point is that it is helpful to have some idea of the internal character of the bowel, particularly in the area of possible involvement such as that adjacent to the cul-de-sac and higher up in the pelvis. This also helps to rule out possible polyps or malignancy and may allow the surgeon to determine the degree of mobility of the structures prior to surgery. The third point concerns dealing with intestinal adhesions; whether they are large or small intestinal adhesions, it is wisest to use sharp scissors dissection along the line of the obvious adhesions whenever possible. This is particularly important when one is dealing with markedly adherent portions of intestine near the posterior surface of the uterus, the upper portion of the cul-de-sac, and the area below the cervix along the uterosacral ligaments. Blunt dissection and sponge dissection should not be attempted since tearing into the surrounding structures, particularly the rectum, is much more likely to occur. The fourth point is that it may be more feasible to carry out dissection of the anterior (ventral) portion of the uterus, taking down the bladder flap and identifying and securing the uterine vessels before dealing with the cul-de-sac problem. The vagina may be entered anteriorly, and then by placing one's finger against the posterior vaginal wall toward the cul-de-sac, one can accomplish sharp dissection of the bowel from the cervix and upper vagina more readily.

Finally, in the patient who insists on preserving the pelvic structures at all costs, conservative surgery even in patients such as described here may be a possibility. The patient should be warned that conservative surgery may be fraught with dangers, such as the risk of developing further pelvic masses from residual endometriosis, the possibility of endometriotic and other ovarian cysts, and the potential for ovarian remnant syndrome. With very aggressive follow-up and with the availability of treatment with the oral contraceptive pills, danazol, or GnRH agonists, the patient may be spared the need for extensive surgery in the future.

SELECTED READINGS

Mikuta JJ: Extensive pelvic disease and the difficult hysterectomy. In Nichols DH: *Gynecologic and Obstetric Surgery*. St. Louis, CV Mosby, 1993.

Schwartz SI: Surgery of the colon, incidental to gynecologic surgery. In Nichols DH: *Gynecologic and Obstetric Surgery*. St. Louis, CV Mosby, 1993.

William TJ: Endometriosis. In: Thompson JD, Rock JA (eds): *Te Linde's Operative Gynecology*, ed. 7. Philadelphia, JB Lippincott, 1992.

Williams TJ, Pratt JH: Endometriosis in 1,000 consecutive celiotomies: Incidence and management. *Am J Obstet Gynecol* 129:245–250, 1977.

SECTION IV

ENDOSCOPIC SURGERY

29

Hysteroscopy — Hysteroscopic Resection of Intrauterine Septum Progresses to Perforation of the Uterine Fundus

John F. Randolph, Jr.

Case Abstract

Hysteroscopic metroplasty was being performed on a 31-year-old G3 P0 with the diagnosis of a müllerian anomaly made preoperatively by hysterosalpingography and confirmed as a resorption defect, or septum, on simultaneously performed laparoscopy. An 8-mm recirculating resectoscope was being utilized with video monitoring providing good visualization. The uterine cavity was noted to be symmetric with both ostia clearly visualized and a broad-based septum noted to extend to the lower uterine segment. With the resectoscopic knife the septum was incised in a transverse motion with progressive division of the septum and separation of the anterior and posterior endometrial surfaces. After the surgeon extended the knife just medial to the right tubal ostia and began to incise the midline, there was a sudden loss of pressure within the uterine cavity with clear flow of distending medium to the area of incision and collapse of the cavity.

DISCUSSION

Inadvertent perforation of the uterine fundus at the time of hysteroscopic metroplasty, or resection of a uterine septum, is a generally avoidable problem that has been encountered by nearly all gynecologic surgeons who perform the procedure on a regular basis. Fortunately, since uterine septa are midline structures away from major blood vessels and are less vascular than fundal myometrium, the risk of significant bleeding resulting from the perforation is relatively small. The two most significant concerns at the time of the perforation are the possibility of injury to an extrauterine structure such as the bowel, and the likelihood that the procedure will need to be terminated because of loss of visualization. In addition, perforation will open some myometrial vascular spaces and increase the likelihood of extravasation of distending medium with resultant risk of water intoxication. In the unacceptable situation where visualization has been inadequate and the perforation is not in the relatively safe area between the tubal ostia, the risk of bleeding from uterine vessels or damage to ureters or pelvic vessels becomes a major concern.

Appropriate preparation of the patient prior to surgery to optimize visualization and the application of methodical technique will significantly decrease the likelihood of uterine perforation. As with other hysteroscopic surgical procedures, such as myomectomy or endometrial ablation, preoperative preparation to minimize endometrial growth is advantageous. The author has found that 8 weeks of therapy with a gonadotropin-releasing hormone agonist provides excellent endometrial suppression. Other authors have described the use of Danocrine, continuous progestins, or oral contraceptives. Suction curettage of the endometrial surface prior to initiating the metroplasty has been advocated by some and found by the author to be of advantage with many hysteroscopic procedures. However, there is some difficulty in obtaining adequate curettage near the tubal ostia in women with uterine septa.

Adequate visualization requires appropriate surgical instruments. Modern recirculating operative hysteroscopes or resectoscopes provide the optimal visualization necessary to safely perform this procedure. Currently the most commonly used distending medium for resectoscopic surgery is a 1.5% solution of glycine that is hypo-osmolar and nonconductive. However, uterine septa can be incised with flexible and rigid hysteroscopic scissors and fiberoptic lasers utilizing a variety of solutions, including high-molecular-weight dextran, sorbitol, and mannitol. Whatever is chosen, a solution optimizing visualization must be used and meticulous monitoring of fluid intake and output must be maintained.

A methodical strategy for incising the septum should be utilized. Defining the boundaries of the incision by scoring the endometrium over the septum should be the initial step in the procedure. Great care must be taken to avoid damage to the tubal ostia, and therefore the incision should end just medial to these two landmarks. The body of the septum should then be serially incised, resecting from side to side so as to allow the endometrial surfaces to separate from the distending pressure as the septum is incised.

The most difficult decision is to determine when the procedure is completed. The observation of increased bleeding from the incised surface suggests that the less vascular septum has been resected and the more vascular myometrium has been entered. Resectoscopic and laser techniques cauterize smaller myometrial vessels and diminish the utility of this technique. It is important to remember that the uterine fundus may appear convex even at the completion of the procedure.

It is imperative that some surveillance of the external uterine fundus be maintained throughout the procedure. Traditionally this has been done with laparoscopy to allow immediate recognition of perforation and to inspect other pelvic structures following a perforation to assess for possible injury. A less utilized option is to perform simultaneous real-time ultrasonography to provide a three-dimensional view of the uterus and to warn the surgeon of impending perforation. A useful technique to determine complete resection of the septum when a laparoscope is in place is to observe the external uterine fundus with the laparoscopic light turned off and to pass the end of the hysteroscope over the incised septum from cornua to cornua to visualize for uniform transillumination. When there is no longer decreased transfundal light transmission in the midline, the procedure is completed.

At the time of a recognized perforation the surgeon has one requirement followed by a therapeutic decision. The perforation site must be inspected laparoscopically for location and bleeding and all adjacent pelvic structures must be inspected for possible injury. This is particularly critical with resectoscopic or laser techniques, where thermal injury to adjacent structures may be encountered. Any fluid in the pelvis must be aspirated and appropriate irrigation utilized to optimize visualization of pelvic structures.

If inspection of the perforation site reveals significant bleeding, therapy will be dictated by location of the perforation and extent of the bleeding. Most perforations occur in the superior fundus between the cornua away from major vessels and will not bleed extensively. Bleeding of concern can generally be controlled by laparoscopic electrocautery. Surgeons capable of endoscopic suturing may utilize this technique if electrocautery fails, but most practitioners today will need to perform open suturing through a minilaparotomy incision. A perforation lateral to the cornua in the area of major vessels must be carefully observed for occult bleeding as evidenced by hematoma formation. Obvious or occult bleeding in this area will generally require a laparotomy to control bleeding without damaging other adnexal structures and imperiling future fertility.

The surgeon must then decide whether the procedure should be terminated or whether an attempt can be made for completion. Most perforations occur late in the procedure when the bulk of the septum has been resected, and should usually be managed by discontinuing the procedure. This is often necessary because loss of intrauterine pressure results in lack of visualization and the inability to complete the procedure. With the use of hysteroscopic pumps a procedure may be completed if adequate intrauterine distention can be maintained to allow visualization and safe incision. However, the risk of extravasation of fluid is high, and meticulous maintenance of fluid status must be carried out. If the perforation occurs early in the procedure, it is prudent to discontinue the procedure and return at a later date to perform the operation.

In the author's experience, in scenarios such as the one described the most prudent course of action is to terminate the procedure and reassess the uterine cavity by hysterosalpingography at a later date. However, if there has been careful maintenance of fluid status and no evidence of fluid overload, completion of the procedure can be undertaken if there is minimal tissue left to be incised.

SELECTED READINGS

1. Chervenak FA, Neuwith RS: Hysteroscopic resection of uterine septum. *Am J Obstet Gynecol* 141:351, 1981.
2. Daly DC, Walters CA, Soto-Albors CE, Riddick DH: Hysteroscopic metroplasty: Surgical technique and obstetric outcome. *Fertil Steril* 39:623, 1983.
3. Edstrom KGB: Intrauterine surgical procedures during hysteroscopy. *Endoscopy* 6:175, 1974.
4. Siegler A, Valle RF, Lindemann HJ, Mencaglia L: Therapeutic hysteroscopy—indications and techniques. St. Louis, CV Mosby, 1990, pp. 36–52.
5. Witz CA, Silverberg KM, Burns WN, Schenken RS, Olive DL: Complications associated with the absorption of hysteroscopic fluid media. *Fertil Steril* 60:745, 1993

30

Hysteroscopy — 400-Pound Patient with Uncontrollable Genital Hemorrhage — Emergency Care? Long-Term Care? Endometrial Ablation? Hysterectomy?

James A. Roberts

Case Abstract

A 44-year-old female was seen in consultation during an emergency room visit for vaginal hemorrhage. She had been experiencing irregular vaginal bleeding over the last several years but this episode was heavier than any she had had in the past. An examination revealed that she was 350+ lb. (The emergency room scale did not measure a weight above this level; she recalled that she weighed 423 lb the last time she was able to weigh herself.) Her blood pressure was stable but low at 85/53. Her pelvic exam was limited by her obesity but seemed normal except for a large amount of clot in the vagina and cervical os. After a negative pregnancy test result was received, an endometrial biopsy was performed which produced a large amount of tissue and clot. A dose of 25 mg of conjugated estrogen was given via slow intravenous push. Six hours later, her examination revealed that the vaginal bleeding had stopped. The pathology report from the endometrial biopsy returned showing endometrial hyperplasia.

DISCUSSION

Extremely obese women will often present with a history of irregular heavy vaginal bleeding. This is the result of androstanediol conversion to estriol in the massive amount of adipose tissue these women have. The resulting high level of unopposed estrogen will produce an environment that can cause uncontrollable vaginal bleeding from either endometrial hyperplasia or adenocarcinoma. The endometrial biopsy result obtained in this case should report the absence of an adenocarcinoma with 95% accuracy. If there is some additional concern about the presence of an adenocarcinoma or if the bleeding does not subside with the use of intravenous estrogen, a dilatation and curettage would be an excellent approach to this woman's bleeding problem. This procedure could be augmented by the addition of a hysteroscopy to identify any isolated areas in the endometrial cavity that may demonstrate an abnormality, such as a malignant degeneration or a vascular abnormality. Unfortunately, hysteroscopy will be very difficult in a woman such as this because of the large amount of blood that will be found in the endometrial cavity. In addition, hysteroscopy will often be more difficult in a woman who is as obese as this patient because of some obstruction to scope movement caused by the enlarged vulva.

When faced with a problem such as that outlined above, the clinician may consider the use of a hysterectomy as a solution to this complex situation. Although this may be appropriate in some circumstances, a minimally stable woman is not the best candidate for major abdominal surgery. This is particularly true for the massively obese woman. The report by Pitkin (2) outlines the added operative risks seen in obese women. These added risks make an abdominal hysterectomy a somewhat radical approach for the woman described in the case abstract. It is appropriate to consider the use of a vaginal hysterectomy for this woman, but again this is not without some significant risk. First, with the large amount of blood present, visualization of the operative structures can be quite limited. Second, although vaginal surgery is an excellent approach for the obese woman, reports from Pratt and Daikoku (4) and Pitkin (3) have found that, when compared to normal-weight women, obese women have a longer operative time and a greater blood loss. Therefore, this approach in the minimally stable obese woman would result in unacceptable risks and should not be considered until this woman is completely stable.

Therefore, it is best, in the emergency situation, to approach this woman with a combination of stabilizing techniques (i.e., blood and fluid replacement) and hemorrhage control with hormone manipulation. Only if these approaches do not provide improvement does one go to an operative intervention. All operative efforts should be carried out with the intent to do as little as possible but at the same time stop the hemorrhage. In most cases this would be a standard dilatation and curettage. The use of more invasive techniques, such as hysterectomy or angiographic embolization, should be reserved for those women who fail to respond to this less aggressive operative approach.

Once the emergent condition has been successfully treated, one must concentrate on the chronic nature of this problem. This woman presented with vaginal hemorrhage because of the anovulatory nature of her menstrual cycle. If nothing is done after the acute treatment is completed, she will almost certainly return with the same or a worse problem (i.e., adenocarcinoma). Since the basic problem is anovulation and nonproduction of progesterone, this woman should be treated chronically with cyclic replacement of progesterone. She can be given medroxyprogesterone acetate 10 mg or megestrol acetate 40 to 80 mg per day for 10 days of each month. This can be expected to induce regular endometrial shedding, which will eliminate both the problem of vaginal hemorrhage and the possible development of endometrial adenocarcinoma. Continuous treatment with progesterone can be used, but it is associated with increased appetite and weight gain. Under most circumstances, weight gain is not important, but in this woman the gain may be large and most significant. Intramuscular administration of progesterone has been used, but it has proven to be a problem when long-term use (over several decades) is necessary, which is likely in this woman. Other drugs, such as gonadotropin-releasing hormone agonists, have also been used effectively but they are more costly and cause more significant side effects.

In some cases, the use of progesterone is not effective or tolerated and another form of management is needed. In the past this has been either repeated dilatation and curettage or hysterectomy. Both of these approaches require that this high-risk woman be subjected to operative and anesthetic risks. In 1981, Goldrath et al. (1)

reported on the result of 22 women with severe menorrhagia who had their endometrium destroyed by means of a hysteroscopically directed Nd:YAG laser beam. Their initial results were very good, with 21 women experiencing either no menstrual flow or only slight vaginal spotting. They and others have suggested that although this approach is effective, it requires that the individual be treated first with an agent that will result in endometrial atrophy. Several reagents, such as danazol, have been successfully used for this purpose, but they must be given for 1 to 3 weeks prior to and after the endometrial ablation. This requirement disqualifies this modality as a way to treat these women in the acute phase of their disease. Therefore, this procedure should be considered only after the acute phase of the vaginal hemorrhage has been controlled.

Several follow-up studies have supported the initial success of this approach and have even suggested that PMS symptoms may decrease after this treatment. However, there are many who have found that this treatment fails after 5 or more years of patient follow-up. For this reason, it has been suggested that this procedure be restricted to those women who are expected to undergo menopause within 5 years. It is possible to repeat this treatment modality if bleeding recurs, so this 5-years-to-menopause rule is not a strict one, but it is good to follow because repeat endometrial ablation is more difficult and can be expected to be less successful. There are two additional problems with this approach. First, a Nd:YAG laser is required for this procedure. This is an expensive piece of equipment that may not be available at all hospitals. Second, the Nd:YAG beam is delivered via a quartz fiber, which cannot come into contact with the tissue being treated. This is somewhat difficult to do through the hysteroscope and can add a significant amount to the operative time. It also can result in an uneven treatment throughout the endometrium, which may explain the late failures seen by some investigators. In answer to these problems, Vancaillie (5) has described the use of the roller ball electrode. This approach requires a relatively small investment for equipment. The contact nature of this modality makes it easier to perform and should be more successful. The shorter operative time will decrease the chance of the woman experiencing fluid overload from a prolonged hysteroscopic procedure. However, this procedure still suffers from the same limitations of endometrial thickness, so it cannot be used in the acute phase of this illness. Long-term follow-up studies are not available, so it is not possible to know if this approach is going to be successful or if it will be limited to those women who are within 5 years of menopause.

In the woman described above, there are several options that must be considered before a hysterectomy is performed. If these are put into use, most of these women will be able to solve their hemorrhage problem with a minimum amount of morbidity and/or mortality.

References

1. Goldrath MH, Fuller TA, Segal S: Laser photovaporization of endometrium for the treatment of menorrhagia. *Am J Obstet Gynecol* 140:14–19, 1981.
2. Pitkin RM: Abdominal hysterectomy in obese women. *Surg Gynecol Obstet* 142:532–536, 1976.
3. Pitkin RM: Vaginal hysterectomy in obese women. *Obstet Gynecol* 49:567–569, 1977.
4. Pratt JH, Daikoku NH: Obesity and vaginal hysterectomy. *J Reprod Med* 35:945–949, 1990.
5. Vancaillie TG: Electrocoagulation of the endometrium with the ball-end resectoscope. *Obstet Gynecol* 74:425–427, 1989.

Section V

Vaginal Surgery

31

McIndoe Procedure with Rectal Penetration

John D. Thompson

Case Abstract

A McIndoe-type construction of a neovagina was being performed on an 18-year-old female with Mayer-Rokitansky-Käuster-Hauser syndrome. The skin grafts from the buttocks had already been taken and sewn to the outside of a rubber-covered stent. The surgeon had dissected the tunnel between the urethra and rectum, and was making a special effort to avoid unwanted penetration of the bladder. The dissection had proceeded about one-half the distance from the vulva to the estimated site of the abdominal peritoneum when it was evident that a two-finger-breadths longitudinal rent had been torn through the anterior wall of the rectum. This was confirmed by a rectal examination.

DISCUSSION

Organs derived from the müllerian ducts in the female include the fallopian tubes, uterus, and most of the vagina. Abnormal müllerian duct embryogenesis with failure of development of the vagina is usually associated with absence of a midline uterus. The uterus is usually represented by rudimentary bulbs on the lateral pelvic sidewalls. Fallopian tubes are attached to these small lateral muscular structures. The ovaries are normal structurally and functionally since their embryologic formation is from the genital ridge. Therefore, such patients are phenotypically female with perfectly normal female secondary sexual characteristics. A normal female body contour with normal breast development occurs at the usual age. The external genitalia are normal female. The karyotype is 44 XX, indicating a normal genetic female.

This condition is known as the Mayer-Rokitansky-Käuster-Hauser syndrome. These young girls are usually brought to the physician by their mothers because of amenorrhea. They may also present themselves later because of difficulty with intercourse. On examination, the vagina is absent except for a small dimple above the hymenal ring which represents that part of the vagina that forms from the urogenital sinus. Other anomalies, especially skeletal and urologic, may be found. Approximately 40% of these patients will be found to have major anomalies of the upper urinary tract, including absent kidney, pelvic kidney, crossed ectopy, and others. An intravenous pyelogram should always be done to assess upper urinary tract structure and function.

The unfortunate embryologic omission of the vagina has stimulated the inventive genius of gynecologic surgeons for almost a century. Although some still advise a nonoperative intermittent pressure technique to create a canal for intercourse, the resulting vagina may be inadequate in depth and caliber. Of all the surgical procedures devised, most gynecologic surgeons now use the Abbe-Wharton-McIndoe operation. The operation consists of three cardinal principles: dissection of an adequate space between the urethra and bladder anteriorly and the rectum posteriorly; insertion of a split-thickness skin graft over a suitable form; and continuous dilatation of the space until the constrictive phase of healing is complete. The first and second principles were advocated by Abbe in 1898. The first and third principles were advocated by Wharton in 1938. All three principles were advocated by McIndoe in 1938.

Dissection of an adequate space is usually not difficult in a patient who has not had previous surgery. However, if scarring from a previous surgical attempt is present, finding a proper plane for dissection may be more difficult. The dissection usually begins with a transverse incision in the vaginal mucosa at the apex of the dimple above the hymenal ring. Using blunt and sharp dissection with scissors, a Kelly clamp and Hegar dilators, one can develop channels on each side of a median raphe (Fig. 31.1). The result is reminiscent of a müllerian duct on each side divided by a midline septum. A finger can be inserted on each side. Exerting pressure in a posterior direction will allow the operator to divide the septum between the urethra and bladder anteriorly and the rectum posteriorly without injury to either of these important structures. If the dissection is difficult, a finger may be inserted into the rectum through the anus or an instrument placed through the urethra into the bladder. These simple maneuvers will help the operator determine the proper plane of dissection. The space should be developed superiorly to the peritoneal reflection of the lower cul-de-sac. The transverse diameter of the space can be enlarged by cutting the medial fibers of the puborectalis muscles bilaterally (Fig. 31.2).

For cosmetic reasons, the split-thickness skin graft should be taken from the buttocks. The skin of the buttocks is also thicker. Balsa wood is used for the form since it can be shaped to fit any space size. It should be covered with foam rubber and a rubber sheath before the skin graft is sewed over it. The form should not make undue pressure in any direction, and it should be larger in the transverse dimension than in the AP dimension.

A penetration into the rectal lumen such as described in this patient is most unfortunate since there is a greater risk of postoperative complications, especially infection. Hopefully, the rectum has been emptied previously with an enema and gross fecal contamination of the operative site will not occur. A broad-spectrum antibiotic should be given at once, if not previously administered. The edges of the rectal entry should be carefully delineated and closed with a series of interrupted no. 000 polyglycolic acid-type (Vicryl or Dexon) sutures. Even though the rectal laceration is longitudinal, it should be closed transversely. The initial mucosal closure should be reinforced by two additional layers of interrupted no. 000 polyglycolic acid-type (Vicryl or Dexon) sutures, folding the rectal wall transversely over the initial suture line. Dissection should be redirected in the proper plane and the space fully developed. The balsa wood form should be fashioned very carefully to fit in the space without placing pressure on the suture line in the anterior rectal wall. The skin graft should be sutured over the form and the form placed in the vagina (Fig. 31.3) to be left in for at least 1 week before it is removed the first time. The patient is then instructed in the use of the form until the constrictive phase of healing is complete. This usually requires at least 6 months and sometimes longer.

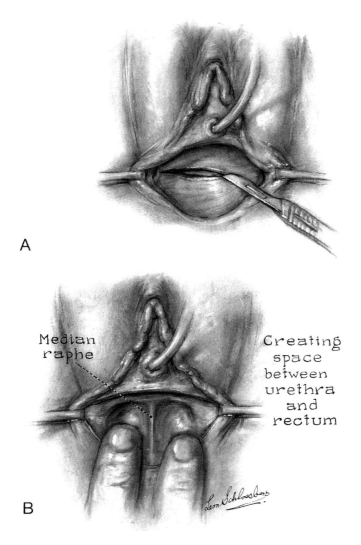

Figure 31.1. The McIndoe procedure. **A.** A traverse incision is made in the apex of the vaginal dimple. **B.** A channel can usually be dissected on each side of a median raphe. The median raphe is then divided. Careful dissection will present injury to the bladder and rectum. (Reproduced with permission from Mattingly RF, Thompson JD: *Te Linde's Operative Gynecology*, ed. 6. Philadelphia, JB Lippincott, 1985.)

Postoperative care of this patient is similar to that of any patient following repair of a rectal injury or a rectovaginal fistula. My personal preference is for a liquid diet for several days followed by a low-residual diet and stool softeners. The patient may be allowed to eat a regular diet after 3 weeks. Since the rectal injury occurred in healthy tissue, there should be no difficulty with healing and a colostomy should not be necessary. Of course, a colostomy may be required if primary healing does not occur.

If the injury had been sustained in the bladder instead of the rectum, the same general principles would be applicable. The margins of the bladder laceration should be

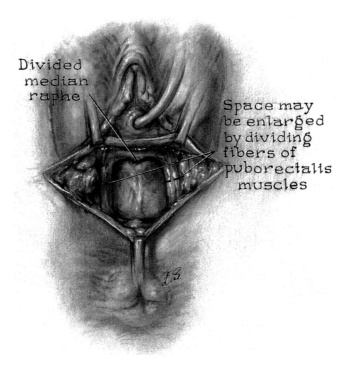

Divided
median
raphe

Space may
be enlarged
by dividing
fibers of
puborectalis
muscles

Figure 31.2.   A space between the urethra and bladder anteriorly and the rectum posteriorly is dissected until the undersurface of the peritoneum is reached. Incision of the medial margin of the puborectalis muscles will enlarge the vagina laterally. (Reproduced with permission from Mattingly RF, Thompson JD: *Te Linde's Operative Gynecology*, ed. 6. Philadelphia, JB Lippincott, 1985.)

carefully delineated and the bladder mucosa closed securely using interrupted no. 000 polyglycolic acid-type (Vicryl or Dexon) sutures. The security of the first layer should be tested by instilling 200 cc of a weak methylene blue solution transurethrally into the bladder. Any leakage should be stopped with reinforcing mattress sutures. Two additional layers of interrupted no. 000 polyglycolic acid-type (Vicryl or Dexon) sutures are used to approximate broad surface to broad surface without tension. Again, the form covered with the split-thickness skin graft should be fashioned carefully to avoid undue pressure on the suture line. In this situation, a transurethral Foley catheter should not be used. Instead, bladder drainage is provided for at least 2 weeks with a suprapubic catheter. Since the injury occurred in healthy tissue, primary healing should occur.

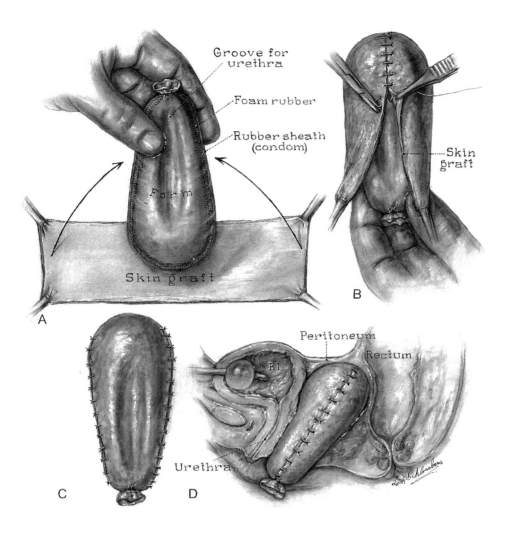

Figure 31.3. **A.** The form may be constructed of a central core of balsa wood covered by foam rubber and an outer rubber sheath (condom). A groove can be made to accommodate the urethra. The outer skin surface should be placed against the form. (**B** and **C**). The edges of the graft are sutured with no. 5–0 polyglycolic acid interrupted sutures. **D.** The form should fit the new vaginal space exactly, without undue pressure at any points. The bladder may be drained suprapubically. (Reproduced with permission from Mattingly RF, Thompson JD: *Te Linde's Operative Gynecology,* ed. 6. Philadelphia, JB Lippincott, 1985.)

SELECTED READIINGS

Abbe R: New method of creating a vagina in a case of congenital absence. *Med Rec* 54:836, 1898.

Evans TN, Poland ML, Boving RL: Vaginal malformations. *Am J Obstet Gynecol* 54:126, 1981.

Fore SR, Hammond CB, Parker RT, et al: Urologic and genital anomalies in patients with congenital absence of the vagina. *Obstet Gynecol* 46:410, 1975.

Garcia J, Jones HW Jr: The split-thickness graft technique for vaginal agenesis. *Obstet Gynecol* 49:328, 1977.

Griffin JE, Edwards C, Madden JD, et al: Congenital absence of the vagina. *Ann Intern Med* 85:224, 1976.

Ingram JM: The bicycle seat stool in the treatment of vaginal agenesis and stenosis: A preliminary report. *Am J Obstet Gynecol* 140:867, 1981.

Mattingly RF, Thompson JD: *Te Linde's Operative Gynecology*, ed. 6. Philadelphia, JB Lippincott, 1985, Chap. 15.

McIndoe AH, Banister JB: An operation for the cure of congenital absence of the vagina. *J Obstet Gynaecol Br Empire* 45:490, 1938.

Rock JA, Reeves LA, Retto H, et al: Success following vaginal creation for müllerian agenesis. *Fertil Steril* 39:809, 1983.

Thompson JD, Wharton LR, Te Linde RW: Congenital absence of the vagina. *Am J Obstet Gynecol* 74:397, 1957.

Wharton LR: A simple method of constructing a vagina. *Ann Surg* 107:842, 1938.

32

Postoperative Vaginal Fibrosis and Contracture Following Abbe-McIndoe Procedure

David H. Nichols

Case Abstract

In a 14-year-old patient with vaginal agenesis, a neovagina was created by the Abbe-McIndoe technique using a split-thickness skin graft. The patient did not wear the obturator regularly postoperatively, and now, at the age of 21 and contemplating marriage, she had a scarred and narrow vagina scarcely 1 finger breadth in diameter and measuring but 3 inches in depth. The patient requested relief. What options were available to her?

DISCUSSION

Failure to keep the Abbe-McIndoe-type neovagina dilated by an appropriate obturator will most inevitably result in stricture and fibrosis that will stubbornly resist stretching and dilation, and the amount of fibrosis increases with time. The importance of wearing an appropriate obturator following discharge from the hospital for an indefinite time must be thoroughly understood by the patient at the time of surgery in order to prevent this dreaded complication. Once initial surface healing of the vagina has been completed, the patient should be given a penile-sized rigid obturator to wear at bedtime for 3 months, the cavity size tested periodically by reinsertion. If it is found at any time to be tight, obturator wearing is reintroduced for as often as necessary. This "routine" is to be followed until such time as the patient becomes sexually active, in which event frequent coitus will preserve the size of the neovagina.

Once postoperative contracture has developed, however, remedies should be promptly initiated. If the patient is very well motivated and willing to undergo a long term of self-inflicted discomfort, she can use gradually increasing sizes of either the Frank-Ingram dilators or the erect organ of a patient and persistent sexual partner—anticipating that the gradual resolution of the problem by gradual dilatation may require up to a year or so of daily pressure.

An alternate surgical approach may be by the use of the Vecchietti operation (1), whereby a transabdominal long needle is passed through the length of the site of the neovagina. A strong suture is passed through the eye of the needle at the perineum, threaded through a plastic "olive," rethreaded through the eye of the needle, and the latter withdrawn. This brings the free ends of the sutures into the abdominal cavity, where they are threaded onto a ligature carrier that follows the path of each respective round ligament, and made to exit the skin of the abdomen at a site lateral to each rectus muscle. After the abdominal incision has been closed, the suture ends are threaded onto the springs of the metal Vecchietti frame and tension applied to the sutures. Sufficient daily traction is made to the end of each suture so as to advance the plastic olive a distance of 1 cm daily along the path of the neovagina. Sufficient depth for future coitus can be expected in about 1 postoperative week of traction, whereupon the olive, the metal frame, and the sutures are removed. The patient must wear progressively wider obturators for a total of about two hours daily until adequate coital width has been developed. The vaginal depth and width should be maintained by periodic wearing of the dilator until such time as the patient becomes sufficiently coitally active that depth and width will be maintained.

Alternatively, if the neovagina will admit two finger widths, bilateral relaxing incisions (at the 3 and 9 o'clock positions of the vagina) will restore diameter without sacrificing length, to be followed by wearing of a suitable rigid obturator daily during the initial healing phase and nightly for the period following.

If the scarred vagina has shrunk to a diameter of less than two finger breadths, one surgical alternate is that of vaginectomy followed by construction of a vagina. Because the connective tissue of the pelvis has been heavily infiltrated by fibrous tissue, the patient may be a candidate for a transplant of a segment of right colon obtained by elective transabdominal bowel resection as the substance with which to line the neovagina. This is particularly useful if the patient is in a situation where it may be socially difficult for her to wear the necessary obturator postoperatively. If she is able to wear the obturator postoperatively, as described above, another surgical alternate is vaginectomy followed by a new Abbe-McIndoe operation, though special care must be taken during the vaginec-tomy (Foley catheter in the bladder, operator's finger in the rectum) to avoid visceral penetration. The patient must understand the importance to her of wearing the obturator for an indefinite period of time postoperatively, as described above, to avoid a repetition of this most troublesome complication.

REFERENCE

1. Lang N: Vaginal aplasia. In: Knapstein PG, Friedberg V, Sevin BU (eds.): *"Reconstructive Surgery in Gynecology"* Thieme, NY, 1990, pp. 84–86.

33

Inability to Find an Enterocele That Was Suspected Preoperatively

John O. L. DeLancey

Case Abstract

A 68-year-old woman presented with a protruding vaginal wall some years after an abdominal hysterectomy had been performed for leiomyomas. A deep cul-de-sac was noted at the time of her hysterectomy, and a Marion–Moschcowitz culdoplasty was performed. She presented because of difficulty emptying her rectum and the need to reduce the prolapse to defecate. The examiner found that the anterior vaginal wall was normally supported but that there was a large rectocele. The vaginal apex lay just above the hymenal ring, and the bulge extended below this point. The examiner thought she could feel small bowel between the vagina and rectum above this. A transvaginal operation was undertaken beginning with a posterior colporrhaphy incision. The entire posterior wall was opened and the enterocele sought. There was a large quantity of adipose tissue, and despite extensive dissection the enterocele sac could not be located.

DISCUSSION

Failure to identify an enterocele during an operation for genital prolapse is one of the common reasons for operative failure (7). Although a large pulsion enterocele may be obvious during pelvic examination, this is not always the case. Rectovaginal examination usually reveals intestine between the rectum and vagina, and peristalsis of the small bowel may even be visible through the vaginal wall or bowel sounds may be audible. These enteroceles are also usually easy to find in the operating room and pose no particular difficulty in dissection. Certain cases arise, however, that challenge the most experienced vaginal surgeon, both in making the diagnosis of enterocele preoperatively and in locating the enterocele in the operating room.

When a surgeon is uncertain about the existence of an enterocele associated with uterine prolapse during preoperative examination, this situation may be resolved in the operating room. The cul-de-sac is always opened at the beginning of vaginal hysterectomy and a finger can be inserted into the pouch of Douglas to determine its depth and to see if an enterocele is present. Examination of the cul-de-sac should be a routine part of vaginal hysterectomy so that an enterocele does not go undetected and become a postoperative problem. When present, the enterocele should be repaired with one of the techniques that has proven effectiveness in treating enteroceles associated with uterine prolapse (6,8).

In patients with a prolapse who have previously had a hysterectomy it is sometimes more difficult to detect an enterocele in the examining room and the operating room. When the uterus is present it divides the anterior and posterior walls so that the distinction between a cystocele and enterocele is obvious. In women in whom the uterus was previously removed this distinction is not always obvious. Furthermore, because the cul-de-sac is not routinely opened during an operation for prolapse in a woman who has previously had a hysterectomy, intraoperative examination of the cul-de-sac is not always performed. Finally, previous culdoplasty may distort the normal anatomic relationships, making identification of the cul-de-sac difficult.

The key to identifying an enterocele begins with careful preoperative examination. If the surgeon is confident that an enterocele is present based on the preoperative examination, then dissection will be continued during surgery until the enterocele sac is identified and this element of the prolapse corrected. If, on the other hand, the presence or absence of an enterocele is unknown and identification during the operation is not easy, the search for an enterocele may be terminated prematurely out of concern for bowel or bladder injury. Since the patient cannot strain during the operation, identification of an enterocele may be more difficult intraoperatively than it is when the patient is awake. Therefore, whenever possible, the diagnosis of an enterocele should be confirmed when the patient is awake and can cooperate with examination so that the operative plan may be established.

Examining patients to detect an enterocele when the uterus is absent requires skill and careful observation. The nature of a prolapse changes depending on how forcefully a patient is straining. In a patient with uterine prolapse, for example, the protrusion of the cervix may not be obvious. When the patient is told to strain, a cystocele may at first be visible. With encouragement, and more forceful Valsalva, a rectocele may begin to protrude. It may only be with strong coughing that the cervix can be seen to separate the labia and become visible below the introitus. Similarly, an enterocele present in a woman who previously had a hysterectomy may not be evident until the patient strains forcefully and the prolapse is developed to its maximum extent. To be sure that an enterocele has not been missed, the examiner must decide if the prolapse has been placed under enough stress that all elements of the prolapse are evident. This is usually possible in the lithotomy position, but when a woman has trouble straining forcefully enough, examination in the standing position should be performed. Although some physicians worry that patients may object to this type of examination, patients with prolapse are actually more concerned when their physician has *not* examined them standing, because they know that when they lie down the prolapse often recedes into the pelvis and disappears. They know that it is only when they stand that their prolapse is the largest and fear that the physician has missed something by not examining them in the upright position.

Once the prolapse has been developed to its largest extent, the hysterectomy scar in the vagina should be located. This scar indicates the location of the vaginal apex, and its position denotes the degree of vaginal prolapse that is present (2). Since posthysterectomy enterocele and vaginal prolapse frequently coexist, this part of the examination is important. In addition, the location of the bulge relative to the hysterectomy scar may help provide information about the type of prolapse present. During a hysterectomy, the bladder extends to the vaginal cuff anteriorly, but posteriorly there are 3 to 4 cm of peritoneum covering the vaginal wall in the cul-de-sac (3.) This means that a bulge anterior to the vaginal cuff after a hysterectomy is usually a cystocele, whereas one that begins immediately posterior to the vaginal cuff is an enterocele. A bulge that begins immediately posterior to this scar is likely to be an enterocele but must also be differentiated from a high rectocele.

The distinction between a high rectocele and an enterocele is made on rectovaginal examination. This examination must be accomplished with the prolapse maximally developed. With finger in the rectum the examiner may trace out the contour of the anterior rectal wall and compare it with the visible contour of the posterior vaginal wall. When an enterocele is present, the vaginal wall and the rectal wall will be separated by the bulging mass of the enterocele. It should be reiterated that if the patient is not straining forcefully enough for the enterocele to be filled with intestinal contents, and the peritoneal cavity is collapsed and devoid of small intestine, that the enterocele will be missed. The presence of the enterocele may be confirmed by placing the index finger in the rectum and the thumb in the vagina so that the contents of the space between the rectum and vagina may be palpated. When doubt about the presence of an enterocele persists, examination in the standing position should be carried out.

Various technical means have been described to assist in diagnosing an enterocele. Some authors have used radiographic means to opacify the vagina, rectum, and small bowel for the purpose of defining a prolapse (5) and specifically for identifying an enterocele (4). It has also been suggested that a light be placed in the rectum to illuminate a rectocele, but not an enterocele (1). It seems likely that an enterocele large enough to be detected with transillumination will be obvious on pelvic examination. These techniques are helpful in visualizing the enterocele but, like pelvic examination, will only reveal an enterocele if the patient is straining forcefully enough to fill the enterocele sac with small bowel. Therefore, the same care with examination must be exercised with this as with other techniques of diagnosis.

When an enterocele has been detected in the office, it must be found in the operating room. Although this is easiest during an abdominal operation, transvaginal repair of enterocele is preferred by the author, not only because it is associated with more rapid recovery for the patient and avoids complications that arise from an abdominal incision, but also because it facilitates repair of any concomitant cystocele or rectocele. To approach enteroceles transvaginally, the surgeon must become familiar with their identification.

Two different approaches can be taken to the enterocele. A full-length posterior colporrhaphy incision can be made, or the enterocele may be approached directly through an incision over the enterocele in the upper vagina. In either event, dissection of the enterocele is similar.

Enteroceles usually occur between the fascial layer of the rectovaginal septum and the rectum. Therefore, the rectovaginal space, which lies between the fascia and the rectum, should be entered. Once this space has been entered and mobilized, a search for the enterocele sac should begin adjacent to the vaginal apex. Tissue in this region may be lifted, checked to make sure it is not a visceral wall, and transected. If a smooth surface similar to the peritoneum is identified, intraperitoneal position may be confirmed by identifying small intestine or omentum.

When identification of the enterocele sac is difficult, several maneuvers may be helpful. Along the posterior wall of the cul-de-sac, the peritoneum is attached to the rectosigmoid. Performing a rectal examination and pulling the rectosigmoid down into the vaginal incision will therefore pull the peritoneal reflection down and facilitate its identification. Some authors use a ring forceps or sponge stick inserted into the rectum for this same maneuver. In addition to bringing the cul-de-sac peritoneum closer to the surgeon, it identifies the location of the rectum and reduces the likelihood that it will be inadvertently injured.

An enterocele sac may sometimes be identified by inserting a Veress needle under the umbilicus and creating a pneumoperitoneum. The abdominal wall can then be compressed and the intraperitoneal pressure increased to fill the enterocele and make it visible. Although this is theoretically attractive and often works, the results of this maneuver are variable. Laparoscopy is also possible at the same time to try to visualize the enterocele. If the pneumoperitoneum has not distended the enterocele, however, laparoscopy may not add much information. Although the cul-de-sac is easily visible in women with normal support, the downward descent of the pelvic floor in women with prolapse places it far away from the surgeon. It is possible, however, that some of the long instruments usually used through an operative laparoscope could be placed through a suprapubic trocar and could reach the enterocele sac behind the pubic bone and define the cul-de-sac. However, one rarely needs to resort to these lengths.

If the peritoneum can still not be found, having the anesthesiologist lighten the anesthesia to the point where the patient "bucks" occasionally will allow the enterocele to fill and its location to become evident. Anterior retraction of the vaginal apex at the same time helps open the space where the enterocele will develop and facilitates its identification. Achieving this type of Valsalva, however, is far from predictable.

Some reasons for difficulty in locating an enterocele should be kept in mind. In some patients, adhesions of the small bowel to the cul-de-sac peritoneum are responsible for obliteration of the peritoneal cavity in this location and for difficulty in entering the peritoneal cavity, and this should be kept in mind during dissection. In this instance the peritoneal surface may be identified, but no free space is present. This is especially true in patients with enterocele after previous surgery. It is then appropriate to dissect the bowel adhesions sufficiently to elevate the small bowel and to close the space. Occasionally a mass of adipose tissue fills the space between the bowel and vagina, presenting as a mass but not an enterocele. This can only be verified once the peritoneum has been entered above this level and found to be in a normal position. In the end, it is the experience of the operator and careful, meticulous dissection that allows the peritoneal cavity to be entered.

With careful attention to these details, the problems that arise from missing an enterocele at the time of surgery may be avoided and the return of a prolapse soon after the patient leaves may be avoided.

REFERENCES

1. Altchek A: Diagnosis of enterocele by negative intrarectal transillumination. *Obstet Gynecol* 26:636–639, 1965.
2. DeLancey JOL. Anatomic aspects of vaginal eversion after hysterectomy. *Am J Obstet Gynecol* 166:1717–1728, 1992.
3. Kuhn RJP, Hollyock VE: Observations on the anatomy of the rectovaginal pouch and septum. *Obstet Gynecol* 59:445–447, 1982.
4. Lash AF, Levin B: Roentgenographic diagnosis of vaginal vault hernia. *Obstet Gynecol* 20:427–433, 1962.

5. Lazarevski M, Lazarov A, Novak J, Dimcevski D: Colpocystography in cases of genital prolapse and urinary stress incontinence in women. *Am J Obstet Gynecol* 122:704–716, 1975.
6. McCall MD: Posterior culdeplasty: Surgical correction of enterocele during vaginal hysterectomy, a preliminary report. *Obstet Gynecol* 10:595–602, 1957.
7. Symmonds RE, Williams TJ, Lee RA, Webb MJ: Posthysterectomy enterocele and vaginal vault prolapse. *Am J Obstet Gynecol* 140:852–859, 1981.
8. Torpin R: Excision of the cul-de-sac of Douglas for the surgical cure of hernias through the female caudal wall: Including prolapse of the uterus. *J Med Assoc Ga* 36:396–406, 1946.

34

Prolapse Subsequent to Le Fort Partial Colpocleisis

John O. L. DeLancey

Case Abstract

A 74-year-old woman sought the advice of her gynecologist because of recurrent uterine prolapse. One year previously she had had a Le Fort partial colpocleisis performed for procidentia. Her symptoms had initially resolved, but over the last 3 months she noted a mass protruding through her introitus. She had no incontinence or problems with defecation but was significantly troubled by the bulge (Fig. 34.1). She presented with a request that something be done about the prolapse. Her past medical history included chronic obstructive pulmonary disease, a myocardial infarction 6 years ago, and stabile angina. In addition, she had been troubled by constipation for many years and sometimes spent 20 to 30 minutes straining at stool to have a bowel movement.

DISCUSSION

Partial colpocleisis is an excellent treatment for uterovaginal prolapse in women who no longer are interested in being sexually active. Although this is an extremely effective treatment (3,2), prolapse may occasionally recur. When the patient's prolapse returns, the etiology for the failure will often determine the course of treatment that is appropriate. Before considering the management of this specific patient, a look at the factors that increase the likelihood that a colpocleisis will be successful may reduce the number of patients experiencing recurrent prolapse.

Two factors influence the strength and durability of a colpocleisis: the size of the areas on the vaginal walls that are brought into contact with one another and the size of the introitus below the repair. The larger the size of the rectangles that are denuded and sewn together at the time of the original colpocleisis, the greater the area which can resist break down of this repair. In the patient described above, review of the initial operative report revealed that a 2-cm-wide strip was taken off the anterior and posterior vaginal wall. This was not sufficient to hold up against the forces of the chronic cough from the patient's chronic obstructive pulmonary disease. A broader area of attachment, leaving only enough mucosa to keep the lateral channels patent, would provide a more durable repair. The prolapses that occur after this type of repair present few problems with subsequent surgery since the repair most often is completely disrupted and all that remains of the previous operation is the scar from the site of the original denudations. The repair of these lesions will be considered later.

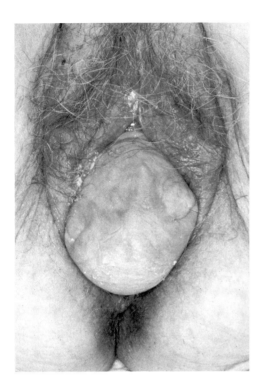

Figure 34.1. Prolapse after Le Fort colpocleisis. Note the stretched scar that indicates the lower margin of the previous repair. (Copyright 1994, John O. L. DeLancey.)

In individuals with a greatly enlarged hiatus, the colpocleisis is unsupported and is subjected to almost constant tension. Over the course of time, this can pull the repair apart and cause the prolapse to return. In this instance, the lower parts of the vagina prolapsed again, but the bulk of the colpocleisis remained intact. This poses a surgical challenge because the uterus is not visible above the repair. At the time of a colpocleisis, consideration should be given to performing a perineorrhaphy. By bringing the levator ani and the often separated tissues of the perineal body together in the midline, a solid shelf can be created on which the colpocleisis can rest. Since intercourse is not an issue for women after colpocleisis, the dyspareunia associated with tight perineorrhaphy is not of concern. Unless the patient's medical condition is so fragile that saving a few extra minutes in the operating room is critical, adding a perineorrhaphy to a colpocleisis is a prudent step.

Several options are available when colpocleisis has failed. If the repair has completely broken down, the prolapse can be managed like any other case of procidentia. If review of the first operative report reveals that the original operation was not correctly performed, then properly performing the colpocleisis is acceptable. If, however, the first operation was properly performed, repeating it is illogical. When the first repair has completely come apart and the cervix is visible, then vaginal hysterectomy and complete colpectomy are appropriate (1). Once the uterus has been removed, it is not necessary to leave channels on the side for mucous secretion or bleeding from the uterus. Complete obliteration of the vaginal canal provides more secure support for the pelvic organs, and is less likely to break down. As previously mentioned, perineorrhaphy is appropriate.

If the repair has not come apart, but rather the intact colpocleisis has prolapsed, then the surgical approach is less obvious. In these situations, the scar at the lower margin of the colpocleisis is visible at the bottom of a prolapsed portion of the vagina. The colpocleisis will have remained intact, but the portion of the vagina below the repair has everted. Our approach has been to perform a vaginal hysterectomy and complete colpectomy. To do this, the lateral channels can be used as a guide while the colpocleisis is taken down. This exposes the uterine cervix and recreates the rectangular flaps originally created during the first operation. At this point a vaginal hysterectomy may be performed. The remaining mucosa can then be removed and the vaginal canal obliterated, as is usually done when performing a complete colpocleisis. It is wise to leave a vaginal drain in place to avoid collection of fluid or blood after this type of operation. Again, a perineorrhaphy is appropriate.

If the patient's condition is so grave that a rapid operation is imperative, the surgeon may give a local anesthesic, and begin at the bottom of the previous colpocleisis, extending the colpocleisis to obliterate the prolapsed tissue, and sew the levator ani muscles together below the repair. This has the advantage of lower morbidity when compared with vaginal hysterectomy and total colpocleisis. We have no experience as yet with this approach.

REFERENCES

1. Adams HD: Total colpocleisis for pelvic eventration. *Surg Gynecol Obstet* 92:321–324, 1951.
2. Falk HC, Kaufman SA: Partial colpocleisis: The Le Fort procedure. *Obstet Gynecol* 5:617–627, 1955.
3. Ridley JH: Evaluation of the colpocleisis operation: A report of 58 cases. *Am J Obstet Gynecol* 113:1114–1119, 1972.

35

Uterovaginal Prolapse That Is Difficult or Impossible to Reduce

John O. L. DeLancey

Case Abstract

An 85-year-old homebound woman had been aware of a protruding mass between her legs but was too embarrassed to tell anyone about it. One day she was no longer able to push the softball-sized mass back into her vagina and became concerned. Soon she was unable to urinate normally and could only dribble small amounts of urine into the toilet, gaining little relief. Finally, she called her daughter, who came over and brought her to the hospital emergency room. An examination revealed a large, congested, peeling mass protruding between her legs. Catheterization at first yielded only 100 cc of turbid urine. Manipulation of the catheter into the dependent prolapse returned an additional 600 cc. A gynecological consultation was requested.

DISCUSSION

True incarceration of the uterus is uncommon, yet most gynecologists will encounter instances in which replacing a large prolapse proves to be difficult. Although women with this problem usually present acutely, the prolapse may have been irreducible for as long as a year before the patient seeks help (7). The dividing line between a large but reducible prolapse and one that is truly incarcerated is blurred. Initial management of women whose prolapses do not readily reduce involves assessing the reducibility of the mass, looking for possible reasons that the prolapse cannot be returned to the pelvis, evaluating possible problems that may have arisen from the prolapse, and, finally, evaluating the patient's overall health, since these prolapses often occur in older women who may have neglected routine health care.

Initial examination of the prolapse should determine its state and reducibility. Ulcerations should be examined to determine if biopsy is needed to detect malignancy, especially when they involve the transformation zone of the cervix. Infected ulcerations should be studied and the depth of their inflammation assessed. Although ulceration is common with uterovaginal prolapse, individuals who have allowed a prolapse to get to the point of being difficult to reduce often have avoided routine gynecologic care or cervical cytology studies. The possibility of cancer should be kept in mind. Urination with this size prolapse will be difficult, and a large residual urine volume should be expected. A catheterized urine for urinanalysis and for determining the postvoid residual urine volume should be obtained along with urinalysis to detect infection or blood.

When the prolapse cannot be replaced in the pelvis, the reason for its incarceration should be sought. Bladder calculi may make it difficult or impossible for the prolapse to be replaced in the pelvis (4,3). Urinalysis may reveal hematuria in this instance, and the stones may be visible on a standard radiograph (1) (Fig. 35.1) and may be palpable on examination if the prolapse is not too edematous. Other conditions should be kept in mind when considering the management of these prolapses. The bowel may be included in the incarcerated prolapse and may be necrotic from strangulation. This is suggested by evidence of intestinal obstruction and should be considered when planning operative management since laparotomy may be needed to repair the injured intestine (2,6). Cul-de-sac abscess may occur with incarcerated procidentia, and this diagnosis should be considered during initial evaluation since overly vigorous attempts at reduction might rupture the abscess and cause widespread peritonitis (5). Since bimanual vaginal examination is impossible in these women, rectal examination should be performed and the pelvis carefully palpated. A pelvic mass such as a leiomyoma of the uterus that prevents reduction of the prolapse, or a pelvic tumor, should also be considered.

The general medical condition of the patient should be assessed. Specifically, the potential for renal damage secondary to ureteral obstruction by the prolapse should be assessed with a creatinine and BUN level. If these tests are normal, there is little need for an IVP since the prolapse will be reduced either surgically or by means of a pessary. However, if the prolapse is reducible and the patient wishes to delay therapy, then obtaining an IVP prior to conservative follow-up to make sure that ureteral dilatation is not present would be prudent. This study should include films in the standing position since supine images, when the prolapse is not extra-abdominal, may fail to reveal the degree of obstruction present when the woman is upright.

Figure 35.1.   Radiograph showing bladder calculi outlining the contour of a prolapsed bladder. (Reproduced with permission from Chambers CB: Uterine prolapse with incarceration. *Am J Obstet Gynecol* 122:459–462, 1975.)

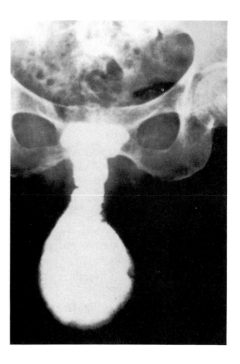

Reduction in the Clinic

Once the overall status of the patient and the nature of the prolapse have been evaluated, an attempt should be made to reduce the prolapse. One must make sure that the bladder has been emptied and that a pelvic mass or infection, which may make reduction dangerous, is not present. The key to reduction is patience and gentle but firm pressure. The negative intra-abdominal pressure caused by the knee-chest position may assist in replacing the prolapse and can be considered if initial attempts in the lithotomy position fail. Sometimes squeezing the prolapse to get some of the edema fluid out of it or temporarily wrapping it in an elastic bandage may reduce its size and facilitate its replacement. If the patient is uncooperative or the attempts at replacement too painful, sedation under careful monitoring can be considered. This should only be done if the patient's overall medical condition will permit it to be done safely.

If it is possible to temporarily reduce the prolapse, then several options must be considered for long-term management. If surgery is planned, it is best to allow the prolapse to remain in situ long enough for the edema to resolve, infections to be treated, and the patient's general status to be improved. When a family member or other caregiver can attend to the patient daily, the patient may be placed on a home care plan. A soft inflatable pessary can be fitted and the caregiver instructed in its placement and removal. Removal of the pessary daily followed by a cleansing tap water douche and application of topical estrogen cream (and antibiotics when needed) prior to replacing the pessary is ideal. The patient should be seen in the first few days after the pessary is inserted to make sure that it is not causing pressure ulceration. Once a program of care is initiated, a choice can be made between further use of the pessary and surgical cure. Occasionally, if the pessary cannot at first be retained, one or two sutures can be placed posteriorly in the outpatient clinic to narrow the introitus.

Reduction in the Operating Room

It is occasionally necessary to take a patient to the operating room to reduce the prolapse under anesthesia (Figs. 35.2, 35.3). Sometimes light sedation is all that is necessary, but the patient should be prepared for general or spinal anesthesia. Once the prolapse is reduced, the vagina can be packed to hold it in place and the patient returned to her room. The prolapse should remain reduced for several (3 to 5) days to allow the edema to resolve and the state of the tissues to improve. The labia must sometimes be sewn together to hold the packing in place in elderly uncooperative women. During this time, the patient may be kept sedated in bed to prevent the prolapse from being pushed out again. Low-dose subcutaneous heparin should be administered to prevent venous thrombosis. After several days have passed, the packing can be removed and the tissues examined. Once the tissues are amenable for surgery, the prolapse may be surgically corrected.

Definitive Treatment

Several surgical approaches can be considered in correcting the prolapse. It is rare for a prolapse to become incarcerated in a sexually active woman and so colpocleisis is often the operation chosen. The patient's acceptance of the loss of sexual function should not be assumed, however, and if the patient is able to understand her situation, this

Figure 35.2.   Photograph of an encarcerated posthyster- ectomy vaginal prolapse that required reduction under anesthesia.

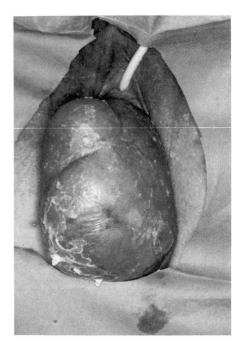

should be discussed with her prior to closing the vagina. If the patient is debilitated and a short operation is of the essence, then a partial colpocleisis is ideal. We usually add a tight perineorrhaphy to this if an extra 10 minutes of surgery is not a problem, since this provides a shelf for the colpocleisis to rest on and will decrease the possibility that the prolapse may return.

If the patient is healthy enough for a vaginal hysterectomy to be performed, this is preferable, since it removes the uterus as a potential source of bleeding or cancer. The ovaries in these patients can usually be removed, further reducing their risk of malignancy. Following hysterectomy, steps must be taken to suspend the vagina. A high McCall culdeplasty, fixation to the iliococcygeus fascia, or other technique familiar to the surgeon should be performed at the same time. We have also had experience with complete colpectomy after vaginal hysterectomy. This provides simple and effective res- olution of the problem.

If, despite all efforts, the prolapse cannot be reduced, then a vaginal hyster- ectomy and repair are indicated. When bladder stones are present, consultation with a urologist is advisable. If the stones are too large to be removed cystoscopically with or without fragmentation, then a a cystotomy may be accomplished and the stones removed. If there is little edema present and the tissues are in good condition, then vaginal hyster- ectomy and repair at the same time are appropriate. If significant infection and edema are present, it may prove wiser to allow the cystotomy to heal and to perform the hysterectomy at a later date. Complete colpectomy at the same time has been performed (7), and the actual operation carried out will depend on the surgeon's experience with various oper- ative procedures. It should be emphasized, however, that simply removing the uterus without taking steps to resuspend or obliterate the vagina is likely to result in immediate recurrence.

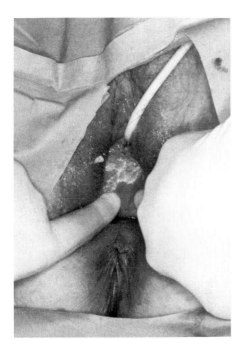

Figure 35.3. Reduction almost completed.

Careful attention to the medical condition of the patient during the operation and the convalescence will usually allow these conditions to be resolved satisfactorily.

REFERENCES

1. Chambers CB: Uterine prolapse with incarceration. *Am J Obstet Gynecol* 122:459–462, 1975.
2. Frank RT: Irreducible, strangulated, complete prolapse of the uterus, complicated by sliding hernia of the cecum and intestinal obstruction. *Am J Obstet Gynecol* 35:879–883, 1938.
3. Johnson CG: Giant calculus in the urinary bladder associated with complete uterine prolapse. *Obstet Gynecol* 11:579–580, 1958.
4. Mahran M: Vesical calculi complicating uterovaginal prolapse. *J Obstet Gynaecol Br Commonw* 79:1145–1146, 1972.
5. Molinelli EA, Porges RF: Incarcerated uterine prolapse associated with cul-de-sac abscess. *Am J Obstet Gynecol* 82:664–666, 1993.
6. Riddle PF, Lueka MH: Rupture of the small intestine as a complication of procidentia. *J Obstet Gynaecol Br Commonw* 73:685, 1966.
7. Svesko V: Total colpectomy in the treatment of a case of irreducible uterine procidentia. *Am J Obstet Gynecol* 75:213–215, 1958.

36

Genital Prolapse with Unsuspected Ventral Fixation

John H. Isaacs

Case Abstract

Vaginal hysterectomy with repair was recommended for a 68-year-old multipara with progressive genital prolapse in whom the uterine cervix, bladder, and enterocele protruded well beyond the vulva. The patient thought she underwent a partial hysterectomy because of abnormal bleeding some 35 years previously, but she did not remember the name of the doctor or the hospital. During transvaginal surgery, when the enterocele sac was opened, it was evident that the uterus extended high within the pelvis. This finding was confirmed when the anterior peritoneal cul-de-sac was opened. It was observed that traction on the cervix produced some dimpling at the lower end of an old midline abdominal scar. What was the next course of action?

DISCUSSION

Ventral fixation in modern gynecologic surgery has generally been abandoned. Various operative procedures exist, however, that use the abdominal approach to fix the uterus, cervical stump, or vaginal vault to the sacral promontory (12). Other techniques include fixation of a prolapsed uterus to the promontory with Mersilene mesh (10). In addition, the antiquated technique of transposition of the uterus between the bladder and the vagina has been resurrected (9). Two other techniques have been used in the management of uterine and/or vaginal wall prolapse. The first—fixing the uterus using an aponeurotic flap and colpoperineolevatoroplasty—is described by Krasnopol'ski et al. (6). The second consists of promontory fixation of the cervix using two Mersilene bands combined with a retropubic colpopexy (1). Although all these techniques may be quite successful, they may not give a 100% cure rate. Even in the absence of these operations, some patients who have had a classical c-section develop dense adhesions between the uterus and abdominal wall such that subsequent prolapse poses the same problems as patients with ventral fixation.

It is entirely possible that procidentia with unsuspected ventral fixation or any other than the procedures described above may defy conscientious efforts to thoroughly evaluate this patient preoperatively. However, certain precautions and considerations may serve to illuminate the situation, and the physician can then be forewarned of potential difficulties.

Mitchell (7) points out the inexperienced vaginal surgeon should not attempt a vaginal hysterectomy on patients who have a history of previous pelvic surgery or who are suspected of having other pelvic pathology. Although this advice is often given in standard textbooks, this has not been necessary in my experience nor that of others (4,5). Nonetheless, if vaginal surgery is to be performed in such cases, careful assessment of the patient's pelvis under general anesthesia prior to surgery is mandatory. Nichols and Randall (8) warn that when uterovaginal prolapse is present, the fundus may occupy a relatively normal position within the pelvis while the cervix becomes elongated and accounts for the prolapse. If significant uncertainty remains, some physicians will perform a laparoscopy prior to choosing a surgical approach rather than always using an abdominal approach.

Since the patient's previous surgical history is unknown in this case, the physician must depend entirely on the preoperative physical findings and other diagnostic techniques. The initial evaluation requires a thorough pelvic examination, keeping in mind that it is the cervix which often elongates and is the major part of the uterus contributing to the prolapse. Unless the examining physician is aware of this fact, a cursory pelvic examination may give the erroneous impression that the presenting prolapse represents the entire uterus, and the physician may fail to palpate the uterus extending high in the pelvis. Even a large leiomyoma or an adnexal mass well above the elongated cervix may not be detected unless a careful examination is carried out. One technique which may have helped preoperatively in the case presented is to insert a uterine sound into the cervix as shown in Figure 36.1. If the sound can be inserted only a short distance, this substantiates the history of a partial hysterectomy some 35 years previously. Conversely, if the uterus sounds to a depth of 8 to 12 cm, the surgeon is alerted to the possibility that the patient had a previous ventral fixation. If this precaution is taken prior to surgery, the patient can be warned of the problem and of the additional complications that can occur. A pelvic sonogram may also have been helpful in this case. With a full urinary bladder, the sonographic studies would have revealed a mass posterior to the bladder extending to the undersurface of the abdominal wall, suggesting that the uterus was still present and most likely fixed to the anterior abdominal wall.

Solution to the Problem

In this particular situation, the previous ventral fixation procedure is unsuspected and has to be resolved at the time of surgery. It is helpful if the surgeon knows about the various types of uterine suspension procedures that are and have been commonly performed so that he or she can be aware of the potential ways that the uterus can be attached to the anterior abdominal wall.

In 1924, Graves (2) described a ventral suspension wherein the fundus of the uterus and the anterior abdominal wall peritoneum was scarified and the fundus was then sutured to the anterior wall peritoneum. This type of ventral suspension was almost completely replaced later in the 1920s by another technique of ventral fixation, in which the round ligaments were used to suspend the uterus. There are a number of these suspension procedures described, including the Gilliam round ligament ventrosuspension of the uterus and the Olshausen suspension.

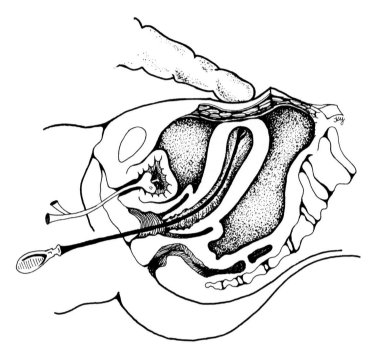

Figure 36.1. A uterine sound is inserted into the uterus. The examiner's hand, placed on the abdomen, could probably palpate the tip of the probe as it is pressed against the uterine fundus.

Basically, these operations pull the round ligaments through the anterior abdominal wall and fix them to the rectus abdominus fascia, as shown in Figure 36.2. Knowledge of these surgical procedures may give the surgeon a better idea of what is holding the uterus to the anterior abdominal wall and how these attachments may be released.

There are several possible solutions to the stated problem, and the technique employed depends a great deal on the skill and experience of the surgeon. For the less experienced vaginal surgeon, the wisest choice is to abandon the vaginal approach, open the abdomen, and remove the uterus abdominally; the large enterocele may be partially obliterated via the abdominal route through a series of purse-string sutures closing off the enterocele sac. The cystocele and/or rectocele can be repaired via the vaginal route prior to opening the abdomen.

A second option is to perform a Manchester operation and thereby leave the attached fundus in place. The reader is referred to the excellent description of the Manchester procedure in Wheeless's *Atlas of Pelvic Surgery* (11). If this technique is used, the enterocele sac is resected and the upper edge of the posterior peritoneum is attached to the posterior surface of the uterus after the cervix is amputated. The cystocele is then also repaired. The upper edges of the anterior and posterior vaginal mucosa are then sewn to the raw edge of the fundus at the point where the cervix has been removed. The result is a reconstructed vaginal canal, the prolapsed cervix is excised, and the uterine fundus remains in place.

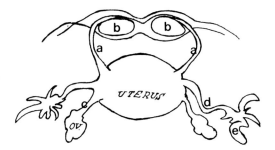

Figure 36.2. The round ligaments (*a*) are brought through the peritoneum and fixed to the fascia of the rectus abdominus muscles (*b*). The ovarian ligaments (*c*) and the fallopian tubes (*d, e*) are pulled up close to the anterior abdominal wall peritoneum but not attached to it.

Another possibility, and the one most likely to be undertaken by the more experienced vaginal surgeon, is to continue the vaginal hysterectomy and slowly work up to the round ligaments. A retractor is inserted between the bladder and the anterior surface of the uterus. A second retractor is placed between the rectum and the posterior surface of the uterus. The uterosacral ligaments, cardinal ligaments, and as much of the lower part of the broad ligaments as possible are then progressively clamped, cut, and ligated. If the top of the uterus cannot be reached, one can follow Bonney's advice (3). He suggests that a pair of volsella can be attached to the cervix on each side with one blade of each placed in the cervical canal and the other on the outside of the cervix. Gradually the uterus is then bisected moving superiorly by using a knife or a pair of strong, blunt-pointed scissors. After the uterus is bisected, a third volsellum is applied to one-half of the bisected fundus and pulled inferiorly. This will bring the upper part of the broad ligament and the round ligament into view. Clamps can be applied on the one side, and half of the uterus can be cut away.

The other half is treated in a similar fashion. The large enterocele is then excised, the neck of the sac purse-stringed, and the peritoneum closed. Additional sutures into the attenuated endopelvic fascia give support to the vaginal vault. The cystocele is also repaired.

Although the above technique may work quite well in the hands of an experienced vaginal surgeon, it is fraught with danger, which includes wounding the bladder, bowel, or ureters or the slipping of a ligature, resulting in uncontrollable bleeding. Because of this, my selection, and the one I advise for all but the most experienced vaginal surgeon, is a combined abdominal and vaginal approach. After the anterior and posterior cul-de-sacs are opened, the surgeon proceeds superiorly along the uterosacral, cardinal, and broad ligament on each side as high as possible. With such a technique the major blood supply to the uterus is clamped and ligated. When the surgeon progresses superiorly as far as is technically feasible, traction on the cervix can clearly delineate the area on the abdominal wall where the uterus is fixed. The abdomen is then prepared while the patient is still in the lithotomy position, and a small transverse incision is made over the area of fixation. The peritoneum is opened, and the round ligaments are identified close to their fundal attachments. These ligaments are then clamped and ligated, any adhesions can be lysed, and the uterus is then freed from its abdominal attachment as shown in

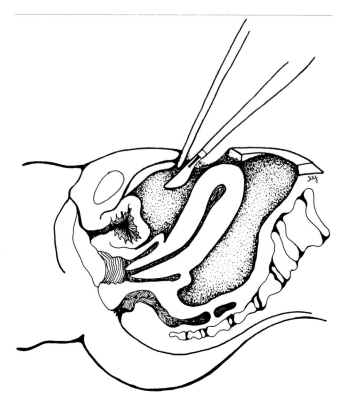

Figure 36.3.   A small transverse incision in the anterior abdominal wall over the area of the uterine fixation will expose the round ligaments. The ligaments could then be clamped, cut, and ligated, freeing the uterus from its abdominal attachments.

Figure 36.3. The ovarian ligaments and fallopian tubes are identified, clamped, cut, and ligated via this small abdominal incision, or they may be clamped and cut via the vaginal route if the uterus descends far enough for the tube and ovarian ligament to be visualized. The uterus is then delivered vaginally. The enterocele is repaired vaginally. The small abdominal incision required to accomplish the above has only minimal effect on the postoperative recovery time, and it reduces the possibility of bowel or bladder damage that may occur if all of the surgery is attempted vaginally.

If uterine prolapse occurs following a sacral promontory fixation, an aponeurotic flap, or a retropubic colpopexy, a vaginal repair may be attempted to fix the prolapse, but the patient must be forewarned that a combined abdominal and vaginal approach may be necessary. Only time will tell if the abdominal approaches to prolapse will be successful.

REFERENCES

1. Caubel P, Lefranc JP, Foulques H, Puia M, Blondon J: Treatment of recurrent genital prolapse by the abdominal approach. *J Chir (Paris)* 126(8–9):466–470, 1989.
2. Graves WP: *Gynecology*, ed. 3. Philadelphia, WB Saunders, 1924, p. 231.

3. Howkins J, Stallworthy J: *Bonney's Gynaecological Surgery.* Baltimore, Williams & Wilkins, 1974, pp. 242–246.

4. Isaacs JH: Vaginal hysterectomy. In: Sciarra J (ed): *Gynecology and Obstetrics.* New York, Harper & Row, 1984, Vol. I, Chap. 19.

5. Käser O, Iklé F, Hirsch HA: *Atlas of Gynecological Surgery*, ed. 2. New York, Thieme-Stratton, 1985.

6. Krasnopol'ski VI, Ioseliana MN, Rizhinashvili ID, Slobodianiuk AI: Current aspects of surgical treatment of prolapse of internal female genital organs. *Akush Ginekol (Mosk)* 8:58–61, 1990.

7. Mitchell GW Jr: Vaginal hysterectomy; anterior and posterior colporrhaphy; repair of enterocele; and prolapse of vaginal vault. In: Ridley JH (ed): *Gynecologic Surgery.* Baltimore, Williams & Wilkins, 1974, p. 46.

8. Nichols DH, Randall CL: *Vaginal Surgery*, ed. 3. Baltimore, Williams & Wilkins, 1989, p. 90.

9. Tescher M, Lemaire B, Michaud P: Surgical treatment of genital prolapse by vesicovaginal interposition of the myometrium. *Presse Med* 19(21):1006–1008, 1990.

10. Villet R: Treatment of prolapse using the abdominal approach. *Acta Urol Belg* 60(2):61–66, 1992.

11. Wheeless CR Jr: *Atlas of Pelvic Surgery*, ed. 2. Philadelphia, Lea & Febiger, 1987.

12. Zhiova F, Ferchiou M, Pira JM, Jedovi A, Meriah S; Uterine fixation to the promontory and the Orr-Loygue operation in associated genital and rectal prolapse. *Rev Fr Gynecol Obstet* 88(4):277–281, 1993.

37

Vaginal Hysterectomy with Intrapelvic Adhesions

J. George Moore

Case Abstract 1

A 47-year-old multipara, markedly obese and with mild urinary stress incontinence, was troubled by chronic, persistent menorrhagia which had been refractory to endocrine treatment and dilatation and curettage (D&C). She had had a Gilliam suspension of the uterus 20 years previously. The uterus, distorted by multiple leiomyomas, was estimated to be 10 to 12 weeks gestational size and minimally movable. The cervix was in first-degree prolapse. Vaginal hysterectomy was initiated. After both anterior and posterior cul-de-sacs had been opened and the cardinal ligament ligated in its entirety on each side, the corpus could not be brought into the wound. Multiple leiomyomas measuring up to 6 cm in diameter were palpable, and it became evident that the uterus was firmly attached by its round ligaments to the anterior abdominal wall. There was some rotational descent of the bladder neck.

DISCUSSION

This is not an uncommon clinical problem in which intraoperative difficulties might be anticipated. Also, postoperative pulmonary problems must be expected in a morbidly obese patient. Therefore, preoperative blood gas studies should be determined and a radial arterial line placed intraoperatively so that pulmonary problems and blood gas determinations can be monitored during and following the surgery.

The degree of prolapse of the cervix is not actually indicative of the support of the uterine corpus. Frequently, with relaxation of the lower pelvic supports, the cervix will elongate with the corpus maintaining its well-supported position (3). Also, with prior pelvic surgery (especially a uterine suspension) and with extensive postoperative adhesions, the uterine corpus may maintain its intrapelvic position and fixation.

Certainly, with this markedly obese woman, an attempt at vaginal hysterectomy and colporrhaphy was justified. Usually, following ligation and detachment of the cardinal and uterosacral ligaments together with reduction of uterine size by morcellation, sequential coring out of the myometrium, or uterine hemisection, the uterus can be brought down into the wound. Once this objective is accomplished, the uterine circulation can be secured with progressive bites up the broad ligament on either side and access thereby gained to the ovarian and/or infundibulopelvic ligaments. Hemisection of the uterus (Fig. 37.1) allows for easier access to the ovarian

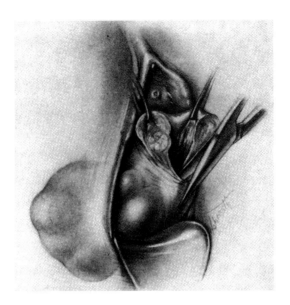

Figure 37.1. Bisection of prolapsed uterus containing multiple leiomyomata (1).

either side and access thereby gained to the ovarian and/or infundibulopelvic ligaments. Hemisection of the uterus (Fig. 37.1) allows for easier access to the ovarian ligaments and enables safer control in securing the top of the broad or infundibulopelvic ligaments (Fig. 37.2). This hysterectomy and repair were safely completed by the vaginal route.

A firm attachment of the uterine fundus to the abdominal wall (Figs. 37.2 and 37.3) would virtually preclude a safe dissection to release the attachment (3); consequently, the morcellation procedure would not allow sufficient descent of the uterus and therefore would be of little value. To solve such a patient's clinical problems (intractable menorrhagia and stress incontinence in the presence of dense fundal adhesions), the hysterectomy should be completed transabdominally along with a retropubic urethropexy (MMK or Burch procedure using a nonabsorbable suture such as no. 00 Prolene) through the space of the Retzius.

With massive obesity, a transverse lower abdominal incision (2), probably below the abdominal panniculus, should afford sufficient room for the hysterectomy and would also provide optimal access to the space of Retzius. In some instances where the pannicular apron hangs below the symphysis, the lower transverse abdominal incision may even be placed superior to the navel but just above the pubic symphysis. Jackson-Pratt suction drains should be placed laterally on either side in the space of Retzius and in the thick subcutaneous fatty tissue to decrease the chances of a seroma and/or wound disruption.

Case Abstract 2

Vaginal hysterectomy and repair were contemplated on an obese, 50-year-old multi-para with first-degree prolapse of a movable and slightly enlarged uterus, a moderate-sized cystocele and rectocele, and chronic menorrhagia. Peritonitis from an appendiceal abscess had been treated surgically by appendectomy and drainage 10 years previously, which was followed by a prolonged but gradual recovery. There had been no subsequent pregnancy. During surgery, the posterior and anterior cul-de-sacs had been opened, and the uterosacral and cardinal ligaments ligated separately, but when sustained traction was applied to the cervix, the uterus did not descend as expected. The surface of the uterus was examined digitally, disclosing dense adhesions to it of bowel, and there was a bilateral hydrosalpinx. There appeared to be a 3-cm leiomyoma in the myometrium. Aggressive traction failed to produce further uterine descent.

DISCUSSION

Prior pelvic surgery, a history of endometriosis, or a history of pelvic inflammatory disease should always suggest the possibility of intraoperative difficulty when a vaginal hysterectomy is contemplated. These features do not unequivocally preclude undertaking a vaginal hysterectomy, and the vaginal approach is still preferred, just so long as the surgeon is ready and willing to complete the procedure through a transabdominal incision if necessary. The scarring associated with postoperative endometriotic or inflammatory adhesions is associated with pelvic fixation and adherence of the

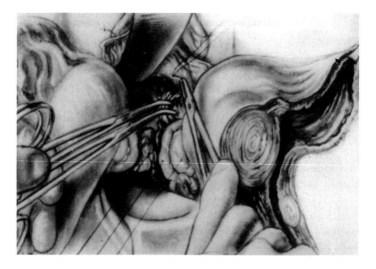

Figure 37.2.   Following bisection, the infundibulopelvic ligament of first one side and then the other is clamped and ligated (1).

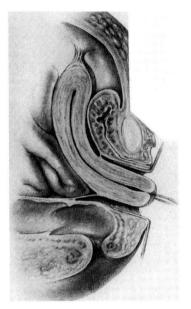

Figure 37.3.   Sagittal section of uterus after ventral fixation (1).

intraperitoneal structures (most commonly bowel) to the uterine corpus, adnexa, and broad ligaments. Under such circumstances, the possibility of injury to the urinary bladder, rectum, and intestine, inability to complete the procedure vaginally, and the necessity to complete the procedure transabdominally should always be explained to the patient when obtaining informed operative consent. Even when difficulties are not anticipated, these possibilities should always be mentioned to the patient with a planned hysterectomy, with documentation in the record.

In this patient, the history of peritonitis followed by an appendiceal abscess and surgical drainage should suggest possible operative difficulties. But other features of the preoperative evaluation might indicate that vaginal surgery could provide the best approach to correcting the clinical problems. With the uterus somewhat prolapsed and only slightly enlarged, a fractional D&C to rule out uterine cancer and a vaginal hysterectomy to correct the "chronic menorrhagia" are definitely justified. The large cystocele and moderate rectocele are certainly best (and ideally) corrected by an anterior and posterior colporrhaphy. Without extensive pelvic adhesions, fixation, and inflammatory scarring, the procedure has a good chance of proceeding without difficulty. However, in this case some problems arose.

Ligation and detachment of the uterosacral and cardinal ligaments and entry into the peritoneal cavity through both the posterior cul-de-sac and the anterior vesicouterine fold of the peritoneum went smoothly. However, at this point the uterus did not descend as anticipated, bilateral hydrosalpinx was noted, and dense adhesion of bowel to the surface of the uterus was encountered (Fig. 37.4). The 3-cm myoma was only an incidental finding and would almost certainly not create a problem. Undoubtedly, the chronic inflammatory scarring also led to fixation of the pelvic structures and prevented

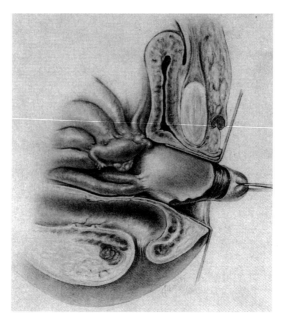

Figure 37.4.   Sagittal section during vaginal hysterectomy showing intestinal adhesions to uterine fundus (4).

descent of the corpus, although weakness of the lower uterine supports allowed elongation of the cervix and lower uterine segment (1). At this point, the operator has several decisions to make. First, should an attempt be made to persist in removing the uterus vaginally? If it were a matter of one or two filmy adhesions of bowel to the uterine fundus, they might safely be released. Often with a free space between filmy adhesions, the uterus can be hemisected (after securing the uterine circulation), and the release of adherent bowel can be carried out with better visualization (Fig. 37.1). In this instance, the scars were dense and the bilateral hydrosalpinx would have made the management of ovarian ligaments very difficult. The advisability of leaving the chronically inflamed adnexa was also a disturbing question. Hence, the decision was properly made to complete this hysterectomy and bilateral salpingo–oophorectomy through a transabdominal approach.

The second decision relates to the cystocele and rectocele. Can they be corrected through an abdominal approach? In this case, they were corrected transvaginally with an anterior and posterior colporrhaphy. In all such cases, the cardinal ligaments should also be anchored to the angle of the vagina on either side, and the detached uterosacral ligaments should be plicated. The vagina should be whipstitched for hemostasis and then the abdominal incision made for a safer approach to the hysterectomy and bilateral salpingo–oophorectomy.

As indicated earlier, contraindications to vaginal hysterectomy noted in the evaluation are only relative. Prior surgery, endometriosis, and pelvic inflammation pose the possibility of intraoperative difficulty. The experienced vaginal surgeon may be able to complete the surgery vaginally but must be prepared to back off and proceed abdominally if safety cannot be ensured.

REFERENCES

1. Benson R: Surgical complications of vaginal hysterectomy. *Surg Gynecol Obstet* 106:527–535, 1958.
2. Maylard EA: Directions of abdominal incisions. *BR J Med* 2:895, 1907.
3. Nichols DH, Randall CL: *Vaginal Surgery*, ed. 2. Baltimore, Williams & Wilkins, pp. 74–75, 189.

38

Management Challenges in Postmenopausal Bleeding

Michael P. Hopkins

Case Abstract 1

A 62-year-old gravida II, para II underwent a normal menopause at age 51. She was on hormone replacement until age 55, when she voluntarily stopped. At approximately 18 months and then 12 months previous to her visit, she noted vaginal spotting. A fractional D&C after each episode was negative. She came to the office complaining of a similar problem. Over the past week she had noticed blood in her underwear on two separate occasions.

DISCUSSION

This patient presents a vexing problem. She has not been on estrogen replacement therapy and the spotting cannot be attributable to hormone therapy. A thorough evaluation at this time must be done to evaluate other possible sources of bleeding. Although the most common cause would be related to the gynecologic system, because this patient has had negative D&C's previously, a thorough evaluation of the GI tract and the urinary system must be accomplished. The GI tract must be thoroughly investigated to eliminate a colon or rectal cancer as the source. Internal or external hemorrhoids are also a possibility. A slight amount of blood-tinged urine can present in this fashion, and an evaluation of the GU tract must also be accomplished.

My initial evaluation would be a stool guaiac. Consideration can be given for flexible sigmoidoscopy and barium enema or colonoscopy to better evaluate the large bowel. Clean-catch urinalysis should be done to evaluate for blood. This should also be repeated, and should there be any hint of blood a further urologic evaluation would be indicated. If these evaluations do not discover bleeding from the urinary or intestinal tracts, then further examination of the genital tract is warranted.

I would be concerned that the uterus had not been completely evaluated. I would review my records on the previous D&C's to ensure that I was in the cavity and a stenotic cervix had not been encountered. A transvaginal ultrasound to evaluate the uterine stripe would be useful at this point. If the patient has a uterine stripe greater than 5.0 mm, it would be more suspicious for a pathologic process in the uterus. MRI can also be utilized to further evaluate the uterus, but this is expensive and will not yield histologic information. An undiagnosed submucous fibroid or undiagnosed polyp could be the etiology. Atrophic vaginitis could be the problem. The nonestrogenized vagina is atrophic and bleeds easier with any minor trauma. An undiagnosed malignancy of either the cervix or the uterus must be considered. An adenocarcinoma of the cervix arising high in the endocervical canal can be missed on D&C, especially if a fractional D&C is not done. Rarely a cone biopsy may be necessary to diagnose the disease. Squamous cell cancer of the cervix in a postmenopausal patient will also arise high in the canal. The brush techniques for evaluating the endocervical canal have been introduced, and a very high endocervical cytologic analysis should be done.

I would recommend that this patient undergo a repeat D&C with hysteroscopic analysis of the uterine cavity. If there was any suggestion of a stenotic cervix previously, I would proceed with the D&C under ultrasound guidance. Utilizing transabdominal scanning, the sound can be identified in the uterine cavity. Although endocervical curettage is not required for staging, I still recommend that a fractional D&C be done in this situation. Occasionally, a cancer of the cervix will be diagnosed on fractional D&C done for postmenopausal bleeding.

Ultimately, I recommend that the patient undergo hysterectomy if the cause of the bleeding cannot be explained. There is a small incidence of uterine malignancy that is not diagnosed on D&C. A D&C is approximately 99% accurate for diagnosing uterine pathology. In a patient with three negative D&C's, the probability of finding pathology is small, but if the patient is otherwise healthy and continues with unexplained bleeding, a uterine source is possible.

SELECTED READINGS

Choo YC, Mak KC, Hsu C, Wong TS, Ma HK: Postmenopausal uterine bleeding of nonorganic cause. *Obstet Gynecol* 66:225–228, 1985.

Goldstein SR, Nachtigall M, Snyder JR, Nachtigall L: Endometrial assessment by vaginal ultrasonography before endometrial sampling in patients with postmenopausal bleeding. *Am J Obstet Gynecol* 163:119–123, 1990.

Stock RJ, Gallup DG: Hysterography in patients with suspected uterine cancer: Radiographic and histologic correlations and clinical implications. *Obstet Gynecol* 69:872–878, 1987.

Townsend DE, Fields G, McCausland A, Kauffman K: Diagnostic and operative hysteroscopy in the management of persistent postmenopausal bleeding. *Obstet Gynecol* 82:419, 1993.

Case Abstract 2

A 58-year-old moderately obese, gravida 0 female was recently diagnosed with complex hyperplasia on office endometrial biopsy, performed for postmenopausal spotting. She had undergone an uncomplicated total abdominal hysterectomy and bilateral salpingo–oophorectomy two days previously. The pathologist reported that he had discovered a well-differentiated superficially invasive endometrial cancer involving the left cornual region of the uterus.

DISCUSSION

The diagnosis of hyperplasia on office biopsy should alert the clinician to the possibility that endometrial cancer may be discovered in the hysterectomy specimen. When typical hyperplasia is present, a small percentage of patients will have areas of well-differentiated endometrial cancer discovered at the time of complete pathologic analysis of the uterus. An office endometrial biopsy is not as thorough as a D&C. Thus, when the only specimen available is a small biopsy, the surgeon should be aware that an unexpected endometrial cancer may be present. When operating on a patient with complex hyperplasia, I recommend that the surgeon obtain cytologic washings, carefully palpate the retroperitoneal space, and remove the ovaries. Additionally, if the surgeon is performing a vaginal hysterectomy in the presence of hyperplasia, morcellation of the uterus should never be done.

Endometrial cancer is the most common malignancy affecting the female genital tract and accounts for approximately 35,000 new cases annually. The prognosis is based on the tumor differentiation, depth of penetration into the myometrium, and lymph node status. The influence of tumor differentiation and myometrial invasion is significant in predicting the presence of metastatic disease to the lymph nodes. In a well-differentiated malignancy that is only superficially invasive or not invasive, the chance of lymph node metastases is less than 1%. Because this is a well-differentiated tumor with only superficial invasion, I would recommend that this patient not have any further surgical therapy. Pap smears of the vaginal cuff should be done every 3 months and a chest x-ray yearly. If a preoperative chest x-ray had not been done, this should be done. The CA-125 tumor antigen level has been reported to be elevated in endometrial cancer when intra-abdominal disease is present. A CA-125 tumor antigen level should be performed if the surgeon did not do a thorough inspection of the intra-abdominal contents and retroperitoneal space. A CAT scan of the pelvis and periaortic region should be obtained to evaluate for lymph node enlargement if the surgeon did not open and palpate the retroperitoneal space. In most situations, a thorough evaluation of the retroperitoneal space is not performed at the time of surgery unless the patient has a known malignancy. It is somewhat more problematic in a patient where the ovaries have not been removed. There is a small percentage of occult ovarian metastases, and if radiation is not going to be given, then reoperation for removal of the ovaries should be accomplished. If the patient is found to have a poorly differentiated tumor or deep invasion, then I usually proceed directly to pelvic radiation provided CAT scans of the pelvis and aortic region are negative.

SELECTED READINGS

Boronow RC, Morrow CP, Creasman WT, DiSaia PJ, Silverberg SG, Miller A, Blessing JA: Surgical staging in endometrial cancer: Clinical-pathologic findings of a prospective study. *Obstet Gynecol* 63:825–832, 1984.

Brinton LA, Berman ML, Mortel R, Twiggs LB, Barrett RJ, Wilbanks GD, Lannom L, Hoover RN: Reproductive, menstrual, and medical risk factors for endometrial cancer: Results from a case-control study. *Am J Obstet Gynecol* 167:1317–1325, 1992.

Prat J, Matias-Guiu X, Barreto J: Simultaneous carcinoma involving the endometrium and the ovary: A clinicopathologic, immunohistochemical, and DNA flow cytometric study of 18 cases. *Cancer* 68:2455–2459, 1991.

39

Fallopian Tube Prolapse Following Hysterectomy

W. Glenn Hurt

Case Abstract

A 31-year-old gravida III, para II, abortus I had a vaginal hysterectomy for a leiomyomatous uterus. Following removal of the uterus and inspection of the adnexa, there was concern about hemostasis, although all major bleeders had been controlled. The distal tip of a Foley catheter was placed through the vaginal cuff, and its balloon was inflated. The proximal end of the catheter was brought out through the vagina, and the cut edges of the vaginal cuff were approximated about the catheter. Postoperatively, there was minimal drainage through the catheter, which was removed on the second postoperative day.

At the time of her postoperative examination, the patient complained of a clear, watery vaginal discharge, postcoital spotting, and a pulling sensation within the pelvis. She was found to have "granulations" in the vaginal apex. These were cauterized with silver nitrate at the time of the examination, and a prescription for vaginal triple sulfa cream was provided.

The patient's symptoms persisted, and she was seen in consultation by a physician, who grasped the tissue with ring forceps, causing significant pelvic pain. The tissue was biopsied and reported to be "consistent with fimbria of fallopian tube."

DISCUSSION

Fallopian tube prolapse is an infrequent complication after hysterectomy (1,3). The surgical literature reports it as a more frequent complication of vaginal hysterectomy than of abdominal hysterectomy. In our experience, it has been seen with equal frequency following vaginal and abdominal hysterectomies, and on one occasion we saw it following a cesarean hysterectomy. In order for fallopian tube prolapse to occur, three conditions must coexist: (1) a fallopian tube of sufficient length and mobility to reach into the vagina; (2) a defect in the closure of the pelvic peritoneum; and (3) an adequate opening within the vaginal cuff (4). Contributing factors include failure to reperitonealize the pelvis; suturing of the cut ends of the adnexal pedicle into the vaginal cuff; the placement of passive or suction drainage devices through the vaginal cuff; an "open" method of cuff management; and the development of pelvic hematomas, cuff cellulitis, or pelvic abscesses that spontaneously drain into the vagina or require transvaginal surgical drainage. No single factor appears to be as important as a combination of factors in causing postoperative fallopian tube prolapse.

Patients with this condition usually complain of a clear vaginal discharge that is sometimes blood-tinged, postcoital spotting, dyspareunia, and/or lower abdominal discomfort or pain. Pelvic examination will reveal what appears to be granulation tissue at the apex of the vagina. The tissue bleeds easily when manipulated. Traction on the tissue often causes intense pelvic pain and fragmentation of the tissue. Often the patient will report that a physician has treated her vaginal cuff with silver nitrate, cryosurgery, or by trimming or avulsion of what was thought to be persistent granulation tissue.

Whenever there is a significant amount of granulation tissue about the vaginal cuff following hysterectomy, I feel that it should be biopsied and submitted for histologic evaluation. If the tissue is found to be of tubal origin, it should be excised surgically. The vaginal approach is preferred (4). Although we have not found it necessary, it is possible that in some cases laparoscopy would be of value during the dissection (3,2).

I have had to reoperate on a patient who had persistent symptoms following office removal of an intravaginal portion of their fallopian tube. Therefore, I recommend an exploratory colpotomy with total salpingectomy. Tubal remnants may be a source of persistent pelvic complaints.

Since it appears that a combination of effects causes posthysterectomy fallopian tube prolapse, the pelvic surgeon should be aware of factors that contribute to the problem. It is best not to incorporate the cut ends of the "adnexal pedicle" into the cuff closure. The adnexal pedicle usually contains the cut ends of the fallopian tube, uteroovarian ligament, and, on occasion, the round ligament. These structures are not important in supporting the vaginal apex. Incorporating them into the closure of the vaginal cuff may be counterproductive. When this procedure is used, the proximity of the cuff and adnexa provides a more direct route for ascending infection and causes the ovaries to be drawn into the cul-de-sac, where they may be a source of deep dyspareunia and possibly contribute to fallopian prolapse.

With the knowledge that the peritoneum regenerates from reserve cells, many surgeons have stopped reperitonealizing their pelvic dissections. On occasion, rough areas on the remaining pelvic organs and bowel may cause them to adhere to the retroperitoneal tissues prior to the regeneration of the pelvic peritoneum. In such instances, I feel reperitonealization may help in separating the pelvic organs from the retroperitoneal tissues and vaginal cuff. If one chooses not to reperitonealize the pelvic dissection, I feel that it is best to close the vaginal cuff.

I do not favor vaginal cuff drainage, especially when the fallopian tube remains within the pelvis and the pelvic peritoneum is not reapproximated. If the drain comes in contact with the fallopian tube, a portion of tube may be drawn into the vaginal cuff when the drain is removed.

Since the physician has very little control over manipulation of the adnexal structures during postoperative transvaginal drainage of pelvic hematomas or abscesses, the surgeon should be aware of the possibility of fallopian tube prolapse when, postoperatively, "granulation tissue" appears to be present at the vaginal apex. If transvaginal drainage of the vaginal cuff is to be performed, it seems prudent to close the peritoneum in such a way that removing the drain not pull the fallopian tube out through the vaginal cuff.

In the case presented, a transvaginal total salpingectomy was curative.

REFERENCES

1. Dao AH, Cartwright PS: Fallopian tube prolapse following abdominal hysterectomy. *J Tenn Med Assoc* 80:141–142, 1987.
2. Letterie GS, Byron J, Salminen ER, Miyazawa K: Laparoscopic management of fallopian tube prolapse. *Obstet Gynecol* 72:508–510, 1988.
3. Muntz HG, Falkenberry S, Fuller AF Jr: Fallopian tube prolapse after hysterectomy. *J Reprod Med* 33:467–469, 1988.
4. Wetchler SJ, Hurt WG: A technique for surgical correction of fallopian tube prolapse. *Obstet Gynecol* 67:747–749, 1986.

Procidentia with Adenocarcinoma of the Endometrium

William A. Cliby
Karl C. Podratz

Case Abstract

A 68-year-old woman presented for evaluation of a symptomatic protrusion from her vagina. The problem had been present for months but had recently increased in severity and was associated with symptoms of intermittent urinary outflow obstruction. The patient had long-standing hypertension and non-insulin-dependent diabetes. She had undergone menopause 14 years earlier but had noted two episodes of vaginal spotting in the past month. Examination confirmed uterine prolapse with associated cystocele and rectocele. The uterus was normal size and the adnexa were not palpable. The patient was scheduled for a preliminary dilatation and curettage (D&C) to be followed immediately by vaginal hysterectomy, bilateral oophorectomy, culdeplasty, and anterior and posterior colporrhaphies. At surgery, frozen-section examination of the D&C specimen revealed a grade 1 endometrial adenocarcinoma.

DISCUSSION

Carcinoma of the endometrium is the most common gynecologic malignancy. It is generally agreed that surgery is the mainstay of treatment, particularly for stage I disease. In 1988, FIGO modified the approach to endometrial cancer to include surgical staging. This consists of abdominal exploration with procurement of peritoneal cytology, hysterectomy, bilateral salpingo–oophorectomy, and lymph node sampling. Most gynecologic oncologists modify their surgical staging based on prognostic factors available at the time of surgery, such as histologic grade, depth of myometrial invasion on frozen section, and the presence of adnexal pathology.

A conflict arises when vaginal surgery is performed and the diagnosis of endometrial cancer is also present. Coexistent procidentia, which would best be treated vaginally, represents one such scenario. Other circumstances include morbid obesity, the presence of significant medical diseases, and occasionally the unexpected finding of cancer after postoperative pathologic exam following routine vaginal hysterectomy.

It seems logical that if lymphadenectomy for endometrial cancer is to be done selectively based on the presence of certain prognostic factors, then the ideal method of removal of the uterus can be individualized in certain cases. Several series exist which demonstrate that the 5-year disease-free survival rates for stage I patients treated vaginally are comparable to the rates of those patients treated abdominally (6,1,5,7). Particularly noteworthy are data from Scarselli et al. (7). These authors report their experience for all grades of stage I endometrial carcinoma. Treatment differed based on the institutional practice at the time of the study. Standard treatment consisted of vaginal hysterectomy for the first 2 years of study versus abdominal staging for all patients in the latter 2 years of the study. The 5-year survival rates were not statistically different, but the severe complication rate was significantly less for the vaginally operated patients.

For the patient without cancer who presents with procidentia, or significant uterine prolapse with accompanying cystocele and rectocele, treatment at the Mayo Clinic consists of preliminary D&C followed immediately by vaginal hysterectomy, removing the ovaries if possible, and the reconstruction of pelvic support by thorough culdeplasty and anterior and posterior colporrhaphies and perineorrhaphy, as described elsewhere (4). In our hands this approach provides the best chance for long-lasting repair and restoration of normal anatomy, and allows for adequate vaginal function if desired. For selected patients with endometiral cancer and procidentia, we feel this approach can safely be employed without sacrificing curability. Although there is a theoretical risk of exfoliative tumor implantation in the colporrhaphy sites, we are unaware of any such cases.

Thorough preoperative evaluation in patients presenting for vaginal hysterectomy should identify most patients with an endometrial carcinoma. In roughly 90% of patients with endometrial cancer, either vaginal bleeding or abnormal vaginal discharge will be present and office biopsy can be performed which will frequently afford a preoperative diagnosis of cancer. This thereby minimizes the chance of an unexpected diagnosis and provides adequate time for consultation and management planning. Careful preoperative evaluation will also enhance the identification of patients with obvious pelvic spread or the rare patient with distant metastasis. All patients referred to this institution for vaginal hysterectomy undergo preliminary D&C with frozen-section analysis immediately prior to hysterectomy, unless they have had recent endometrial sampling. If these guidelines are followed, it should be rare to discover an unsuspected endometrial cancer postoperatively.

Treatment options for the patient with uterine prolapse and endometrial cancer consist of the following when the diagnosis of cancer is made pre- or intraoperatively: (1) a vaginal approach, obtaining peritoneal cytology vaginally and performing bilateral salpingo–oophorectomy if feasible; (2) vaginal surgery for procidentia followed immediately by abdominal exploration and selective lymphadenectomy; and (3) abdominal hysterectomy and staging laparotomy primarily with abdominal culdeplasty, and potentially complementary vaginal repair. In all cases postoperative adjuvant treatment should be given based on analysis of available risk factors. Minor variations on these three approaches can be envisioned, and some centers may recommend preoperative radiation, although the associated anatomic distortion may compromise optimal delivery. It must also be kept in mind that these women often are morbidly obese, of advanced age, and have coexisting medical disease. These factors may sufficiently increase the operative risks of a combined approach, potentially outweighing the potential benefits. The additional risk of abdominal versus vaginal hysterectomy should also be considered (8). Although potentially attractive, the role of laparoscopy for surgical staging of endometrial cancer at present is experimental and should be confined to prospective multicenter trials.

To assess the appropriate treatment options, data from the GOG endometrial surgical pathologic studies must be considered (2,3). Although an in-depth review of these results is beyond the scope of this chapter, risk groups for nodal metastasis and distant spread can be identified. Certainly patients with disease confined to the endometrium are at very low risk of disease outside of the uterus, and hysterectomy by either route should constitute adequate therapy. In addition, approximately 80% of patients with grade 1 lesions have disease confined to the inner third of the myometrium and thus have a very low risk of metastasis. On the other hand, patients with grade 2 histology and middle third invasion or poorly differentiated lesions and any invasion are at high risk of disease spread. These patients warrant selective lymphadenectomy if they are medically suitable candidates.

Finally, certain preoperative variables should exclude a vaginal approach for therapy: (1) uterine size that would require morcellation for removal, (2) adnexal pathology, (3) grade 3 lesions on preoperative evaluation, and (4) cervical involvement. The first two criteria relate to technical difficulties that would preclude proper surgical control of the disease, and the latter two variables are associated with groups at high risk of spread outside the uterus that would best be treated with a primary abdominal procedure.

Since 1950 at our institution we have treated 52 patients having endometrial cancer and uterine prolapse solely by the vaginal approach; 6 patients received adjuvant radiation therapy. Follow-up evaluation exceeded 5 years for 47 patients and witnessed only 4 recurrences. This group includes 16 patients with grade 2 or 3 cancers, and 33 patients demonstrated some degree of myometrial invasion. This survival rate compares favorably with other reports for stage I endometrial cancers. In addition, no patient required subsequent surgery for recurrent prolapse.

Currently our recommendations for the treatment of uterine procidentia with associated adenocarcinoma of the endometrium, in the absence of the noted exclusionary factors, are described below. As previously stated, by careful attention to symptoms, pelvic exam, and preoperative sampling (either in-office or immediately preoperatively with frozen-section analysis), it should be the rare patient in whom the diagnosis of cancer is made several days postoperatively. If this does occur, and the patient is deemed medically suitable, abdominal exploration can be performed for patients with grade 1 cancers and deep invasion, grade 2 midinvasion, or grade 3 with any muscle invasion. In the absence of these factors we would not favor abdominal exploration for staging or solely to remove the ovaries if they were inaccessible at vaginal operation.

Fortunately, for the vast majority of patients, a diagnosis of cancer will be available prior to beginning the hysterectomy. If a poorly differentiated lesion is present, an abdominal approach seems most prudent, since over 90% of these patients will demonstrate some myometrial invasion and are at high risk of nodal metastasis. Abdominal culdeplasty should be performed at exploration and consideration can be given to a vaginal phase, realizing this will be more difficult after the abdominal procedure. We would avoid sacral mesh suspension, which would increase the risk of complications from postoperative radiation, if required, because of adhesions.

For patients with grade II cancers, roughly 50% have disease confined to the endometrium or inner third of the myometrium, and thus a vaginal approach seems warranted: if deeper invasion is found on frozen section we would finish the vaginal procedure and perform a midline incision to do a staging procedure. For well-differentiated cancers we would limit the operation to a vaginal approach unless deep invasion is found.

We are not advocating indiscriminate use of vaginal hysterectomy for the rare patient with procidentia and concomitant carcinoma of the endometrium. However, this approach does offer a valuable treatment alternative for certain good-prognosis patients and simultaneously provides the optimal surgical correction for procidentia. If patients are properly selected, 5-year survival should not differ from patients undergoing an abdominal operation.

In the case presented, the planned vaginal surgery was performed. After removal of the uterus, pathology confirmed the diagnosis of a grade 1 cancer that only superficially invaded the uterine fundus. The operation was completed vaginally and no postoperative adjuvant treatment given. At 7 years follow-up, the patient was without evidence of disease.

REFERENCES

1. Bloss JD, Berman ML, Bloss LP, Buller RE: Use of vaginal hysterectomy for the management of stage 1 endometrial cancer in the medically compromised patient. *Gynecol Oncol* 40:74–77, 1991.
2. Boronow RC, Morrow CP, Creasman WT, DiSaia PJ, Silverberg SG, Miller A, Blessing JA: Surgical staging in endometrial cancer: Clinical-pathologic findings of a prospective study. *Obstet Gynecol* 63:825–832, 1984.
3. Creasman WT, Morrow CP, Bundy BN, Homesley HD, Graham JE, Heller PB: Surgical pathologic spread patterns of endometrial cancer. *Cancer* 60:2035–2041, 1987.
4. Lee RA: *Atlas of Gynecologic Surgery.* Philadelphia, WB Saunders, 1992.
5. Peters WA, Andersen WA, Thornton N, Morley GW: The selective use of vaginal hysterectomy in the management of adenocarcinoma of the endometrium. *Am J Obstet Gynecol* 146:285–291, 1983.
6. Pratt JH, Symmonds RE, Welch JS: Vaginal hysterectomy for carcinoma of the fundus. *Am J Obstet Gynecol* 88:1063–1071, 1964.
7. Scarselli G, Savino L, Ceccherini R, Barciulli F, Massi GB: Role of vaginal surgery in the 1st stage endometrial cancer. *Eur J Gynaec Oncol* 13:15–19, 1992.
8. Wingo PA, Huezo CM, Rubin GL, Ory HW, Peterson HB: The mortality risk associated with hysterectomy. *Am J Obstet Gynecol* 152:803–808, 1985.

41

Injury to the Femoral Nerve During Laparotomy

Susan I. Salzberg
John O. L. DeLancey

Case Abstract

A 26-year-old gravida I, para I presented to the emergency room with 6 weeks of amenorrhea, spotting, and left lower quadrant pain. She fainted while trying to get up on the stretcher. Pulse was 142, blood pressure was 60/0, and the abdomen was distended. She was rushed to the operating room, where a left ectopic pregnancy was found at the time of emergency laparotomy. An 8-cm hydrosalpinx was present on the right side. Multiple adhesions were found bilaterally. To aid in exposure, an O'Connor-O'Sullivan retractor was placed prior to the adhesiolysis. The bowel was densely adherent to the left adnexal structures, and a lengthy lysis of adhesions was needed to define the anatomy so that hemostasis could be obtained. Meticulous dissection made it possible to preserve the tube, and an excellent reconstruction of normal ovarian-tubal anatomy was accomplished. On the first postoperative day, just after the surgeon had finished discussing the findings of the surgery with the patient and how well the reconstruction had gone, the patient stumbled as she tried to get out of bed. She had no orthostatic changes in her blood pressure and did not lose consciousness. As she was getting back in bed she complained of a weak leg and some numbness in her thigh.

DISCUSSION

Retractor-induced nerve injury is an unwelcome and devastating complication of pelvic surgery. Although it is often reversible over time, instances in which permanent nerve damage occurs are not rare. Because of the infrequency of this complication many physicians have never encountered it during their residency and know little about its prevention until after one of their patients develops the problem. In retrospect, because prevention of this type of injury is discussed in standard textbooks, explaining how this damage happens is problematic. Knowledge of the symptoms of femoral nerve injury and the closely related injury to the genitofemoral nerve can help with early recognition, and familiarity with its anatomy and the mechanism of injury helps prevent this distressing problem.

Femoral Nerve Injury

SYMPTOMS

Symptoms of femoral nerve injury include paralysis of extension of the knee, wasting of a quadriceps muscle, weakness of hip flexion, absent knee jerk reflex, and weakness in adduction and outward rotation of the thigh. These problems may be present in any degree of severity from mild paresthesias to complete numbness and loss of muscular control. With bilateral involvement the patient often fails on attempt to stand postoperatively. With less severe injury the patient is able to walk well on flat surfaces but has difficulty climbing stairs or walking uphill. Finally, sensation is lost and/or paresthesias may occur in the cutaneous distribution of the nerve, and the patient may experience pain in the anterior hip joint or lower abdomen.

ANATOMY

The femoral nerve is derived from lumbar nerves 2,3, and 4. It penetrates the psoas major muscle, and runs obliquely under it to emerge at the lower lateral border of the muscle. It then runs in the groove between the psoas major and the iliacus muscles to pass under the inguinal ligament, where it enters the thigh lateral to the femoral canal. The femoral nerve supplies the muscles of the thigh that flex the hip and extend the knee. These include the iliopsoas, quadriceps femoris, pectineus, and sartorius muscles. It provides cutaneous sensation to the anterior thigh and medial lower leg (via its saphenous branch).

CAUSE

Femoral nerve injury in association with gynecologic surgery is caused by prolonged, constant pressure by retractors. Four factors predispose to this complication: transverse incision, long operations, thin abdominal wall, and use of self-retaining retractors. A long transverse (Pfannenstiel) incision permits more lateral placement of the retractor blades and increases the likelihood of nerve injury. It should be noted, however, that femoral neuropathy has been reported with vertical incisions, so care should be taken in all pelvic laparotomies. Operative time also appears to be a factor in the pathogenesis of femoral nerve injury. Minor pressure which could be tolerated for up to 2 hours without clinical effect has produced symptoms when applied for longer periods (6). The body habitus of the patient is also a contributing factor. Patients of short stature, with thin abdominal walls, ill-developed rectus abdominus muscles, and narrow pelvises are more likely to suffer from this complication because the thin abdominal wall does not hold the retractor blades away from the nerves (1).

MECHANISM OF INJURY

Since the femoral nerve is not in the true pelvis, direct operative injury is unlikely. Stretching is also not a likely cause because it would require an extraordinary force to create such a damage injury. Studies involving retractors placed in cadavers have shown that the site of injury is 4 cm above the inguinal ligament, and that the injury is caused either by direct pressure on the nerve by retractor blades or by impingement of the psoas muscle and femoral nerve against the lateral pelvic wall by retractor blades, causing ischemic injury (1,7).

DIAGNOSIS

Diagnosis of femoral nerve injury is easily made on history and physical exam by noting the symptoms and physical findings listed above. Femoral nerve injuries can be distinguished from damage to the genitofemoral nerve because this latter nerve does not innervate any muscles. Muscular weakness of knee extension indicates the presence of femoral nerve injury. Electromyelographic studies may be confirmatory and can indicate the severity of the injury. The prognosis is excellent, with resolution of nerve function most often occurring within a few months. No treatment other than physiotherapy is usually necessary. In some instances, however, injury to the nerve can be permanent: a significant lifelong affliction.

PREVENTION

Because of the possible long-term problems from femoral nerve injury, effort should be directed toward the prevention of this complication. Retractors should be of the appropriate blade depth and should not impinge on the psoas muscle. Folded laparotomy pads should be placed between the lateral blades and the pelvic wall. Some authors recommend palpating the femoral artery after placing the retractor, with absence of pulsation indicating excessive pressure on the external iliac artery and femoral nerve. Some authors contend, however, that since the external iliac artery lies medial to the psoas muscle it could escape compression while the psoas muscle and femoral nerve are compressed. Release and reinsertion of the retractor blades for a few minutes is recommended when surgery time is greater than 2 hours (2). Finally, the length of the transverse incision should be minimized to keep the retractor blades from the vicinity of the nerve.

Genitofemoral Nerve Injury

SYMPTOMS

Symptoms of genitofemoral nerve injury include intermittent or constant pain and burning in the inguinal region with radiation of the pain to the skin of the genitalia and upper medial thigh. The pain is exacerbated by walking, stooping, and hyperextension of the hip. Recumbancy and flexion of the thigh offer some relief. There may be tenderness along the inguinal canal and hyperesthesia in the cutaneous distribution of the nerve. The pain is not reproducible by tapping over an area or point tenderness (negative Tinel's sign), which may differentiate it from ilioinguinal neuralgia.

ANATOMY

The genitofemoral nerve, which consists mainly of sensory fibers, arises from the first and second lumbar vertebral plexus. It pierces the psoas muscle near its medial border opposite the third or fourth lumbar vertebra and descends subperitoneally on the surface of the psoas major muscle. Above the inguinal ligament the nerve divides into the genital and femoral branches. The femoral branch provides sensory innervation to the femoral triangle and communicates with the intermediate cutaneous nerve of the thigh. The genital branch of the genitofemoral nerve crosses the lower end of the external iliac artery and enters the inguinal canal through the deep inguinal ring. It accompanies the round ligament of the uterus and supplies the skin of the mons pubis and labium majus.

The syndrome of genitofemoral neuralgia was first reported by Magee in 1942 (3). However, many surgeons are unaware of this entrapment neuralgia, and the syndrome is not well represented in the literature. It is thought that fibrous adhesions entrap small branches of this nerve in the region of a previous operation or blunt trauma (4).

DIAGNOSIS

Since communication between the cutaneous branches of the lumbar plexus is common and results in overlap of sensory innervation to the inguinal area, the major differential diagnosis of postoperative neuralgia in the inguinal region includes ilioinguinal, iliohypogastric, and genitofemoral nerve entrapment. Therefore, local or specific blocks should be done to determine as accurately as possible which nerve is involved (5). A local nerve block of the ilioinguinal and iliohypogastric nerves through the anterior abdominal wall as described above will alleviate the pain of ilioinguinal or iliohypogastric neuralgia. If this measure fails to alleviate symptoms, an L1/L2 plexus block (through a paravertebral route) should be performed. If this results in substantial relief of symptoms, the genitofemoral nerve should be explored. If pain is partially relieved by both blocks, one may consider staged surgical exploration of both nerves.

TREATMENT

The genitofemoral nerve is best approached through a transverse flank incision made several centimeters lateral to and above the umbilicus and extending to the anterior axillary line. The external and internal oblique and transversus abdominis muscles are divided if necessary, the retroperitoneum is exposed, and the genitofemoral nerve is identified as it penetrates the psoas muscle. A 4- to 5-cm section of the genitofemoral nerve is excised proximal to the assumed site of entrapment and proximal to the site of nerve bifurcation into the femoral and genital branches. If the bifurcation occurs within the substance of the psoas muscle, a section of both branches must be excised. The surgeon will also frequently excise a portion of the proximal ilioinguinal nerve at this time.

Hypoesthesia of the labium majus and of the skin over the femoral triangle are the most commonly reported complications of this procedure. In one study of 17 patients undergoing genitofemoral neurectomy for nerve entrapment, 12 of 17 patients experienced considerable or complete pain relief. Persistent numbness in the distribution of the nerve and loss of cremasteric reflex were the only side effects. Two patients developed subcutaneous wound infections, and a third developed a urinoma. This latter patient had had a previous ipsilateral retroperitoneal exploration with proximal ureterotomy (4). All segments of the genitofemoral nerves or proximal ilioinguinal nerves resected were normal on histologic examination.

Summation

Once aware of the potential for damage to the femoral and genitofemoral nerves, the surgeon can take steps to avoid this type of damage. Attention to the placement of self-retaining retractors and vigilance in the operating room to avoid pressure of the retractor blades on the posterior body wall will minimize the chance of nerve injury.

REFERENCES

1. Gregory F: Femoral neuropathy following abdominal hysterectomy. *Am J Obstet Gynecol* 123:819, 1975.
2. Hassen AA, Reiff RH, Fayez JA: Femoral neuropathy following microsurgical tuboplasty. *Fertil Steril* 45:889, 1986.
3. Magee RK: Genitofemoral causalgia (a new syndrome). *Can Med Assoc J* 46:326, 1942.
4. Starling JR, Harms BA: Diagnosis and treatment of genito-femoral and ilioinguinal neuralgia. *World J Surg* 13:586, 1989.
5. Stulz P, Pfeiffer KM: Peripheral nerve injuries resulting from common surgical procedures in the lower portion of the abdomen. *Arch Surg* 117:324, 1982.
6. Vanrell JA, Balasch J: Bilateral femoral neuropathy after microsurgical reversal of tubal sterilization: Case report and analysis of contributing factors. *Hum Repro* 2(4):375, 1987.
7. Vosburgh LF, Finn WF: Femoral nerve impairment subsequent to hysterectomy. *Am J Obstet Gynecol* 82(4):931, 1961.

42

Evisceration One Year After Vaginal Hysterectomy Without Colporrhaphy

David H. Nichols

Case Abstract

While lifting some heavy furniture 1 year after a vaginal hysterectomy (without repair), a 38-year-old obese multipara experienced a sudden "giving way" in the vagina accompanied by sharp pain. Thirty minutes later she noticed some intestine protruding from the vagina and went immediately to the hospital.

The patient, a mild diabetic, had been attempting over the past year to disguise a weight gain by wearing a tight girdle. She regularly had experienced several daily fits of coughing, secondary to a postnasal drip from a chronic sinusitis.

When she was seen at the hospital, several loops of very dusky bowel were found filling and protruding from the vagina through a 1-inch rent in the vault of a vertically directed vagina. A coincidental full-length rectocele was present.

DISCUSSION

The problem is that of postoperative vaginal evisceration 1 year after a vaginal hysterectomy without repair. That there was a large rectocele and a vertical axis to the vagina at the time of the present admission strongly suggests that these were present but not corrected at the time of the original surgery. In this circumstance, increases in intra-abdominal pressure as might be associated with heavy lifting, coughing, and wearing a tight girdle would be directed to the vaginal vault in an axis parallel to that of the vagina. If the tissues of the vaginal vault were poorly supported, this would over a period of time tend toward eversion of the vaginal vault or telescoping of the vagina. In the present circumstance, the full strength of these increases in pressure was directed against the site of uterine amputation. The tissue healing and qualities of scar tissue in a diabetic patient are thought to be somewhat less than those of a nondiabetic, and when the patient has a chronic cough and by habit wears a tight abdominal constricting garment, the increases in intra-abdominal pressure may be more than the integrity of the vaginal vault can withstand.

The goals of reconstructive surgery are clearly those of relieving symptoms and restoring anatomy and function to normal. Restoration to normal anatomic relationships had not been accomplished at the time of the original hysterectomy, setting the stage for the possibility of increased risk of future symptoms requiring surgical reconstruction. Had the defective vaginal axis and the rectocele been repaired at the time of the original vaginal hysterectomy, a proper upper vaginal axis now directed parallel to the levator plate and at right angles to the direction of intra-abdominal pressure should have been achieved and this surgical catastrophe likely prevented.

Adequate support of the vaginal vault at hysterectomy is clearly an important goal and accomplishment, but when there has been failure to correct a defective vaginal axis, in this case by a full-length anterior and posterior colporrhaphy and perineorrhaphy, the patient's pelvis has not been given the assurance of good postoperative equilibrium that it deserves. It is my opinion that the other anatomic abnormalities of her genital relaxation should have been corrected at the time of the original surgical treatment even though they may have been relatively asymptomatic at that time.

Emergency treatment for this patient with vaginal evisceration requires immediate laparotomy with repositioning of the bowel within the abdominal cavity, thorough inspection of the bowel to ensure its probable viability, and careful inspection of the base of the mesentery to which the prolapsed bowel had been attached to determine whether a laceration or hematoma was present that might compromise the blood supply of the bowel. This may have occurred secondary to acute traction to the intestine coincident with the evisceration. Lastly, the site of the rent through the vagina must be carefully examined, any necrotic tissue around the vaginal opening excised, the vaginal vault opening effectively closed with long-acting but absorbable suture, and the cul-de-sac of Douglas obliterated. At a future date, the anatomy of the supports of the vagina should be carefully reassessed and any abnormalities corrected by a transvaginal secondary operation, that is, colporrhaphy and perineorrhaphy when indicated.

In the case described (Fig. 42.1), the patient was taken immediately to surgery, where at pelvic laparotomy through a lower midline incision the bowel was gently drawn back into the abdominal cavity. A dusky segment of ileum measuring 13 inches in length, and located 14 inches proximal to the ileocecal valve, was noted which was without visible peristalsis or palpable pulse along the mesenteric border (Fig. 42.2). The color did not improve after a wait of several minutes. Although there was no rent in the mesentery, the involved section of bowel with its mesentery was excised, and an end-to-end anastamosis of ileum was accomplished using a two-layered technique. The edges of the defect in the vaginal vault were trimmed and closed from side to side with interrupted polyglycolic acid sutures. The deep cul-de-sac was obliterated by several purse-string sutures. A suction drain was inserted through a stab wound 3 inches lateral to the abdominal incision. Retention sutures were placed and the abdomen closed in layers. Postoperatively, the course was smooth and unexpectedly benign. There was no temperature elevation, bowel sounds returned promptly, and the patient was discharged in good condition on her sixth postoperative day. Four months later, the patient was readmitted for elective anterior and posterior colporrhaphy and perineorrhaphy, which achieved restoration of a normal vaginal axis, the upper end of which was now horizontally inclined and parallel to the levator plate. The patient had stopped smoking and had seen much improvement of her chronic cough, was no longer wearing a tight girdle, and had begun a voluntary program in weight control with appropriate weight loss. These measures greatly lessen the chance for future recurrence of the evisceration.

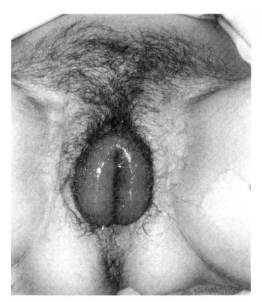

Figure 42.1.   Loops of small bowel are shown protruding from the vulva.

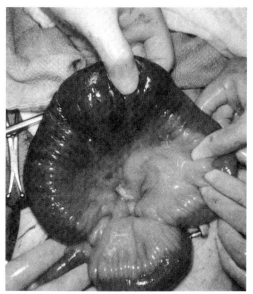

Figure 42.2.   The dusky segment of devitalized ileum is shown prior to resection.

43

Dyspareunia Following Acquired Vaginal Atresia

Tommy N. Evans

Case Abstract 1

One year following vaginal hysterectomy for uterine prolapse with repair of a cystocele and rectocele, an otherwise healthy 48-year-old multipara was unable to have satisfactory intercourse because of vaginal atresia. The introitus admitted 3 finger breadths; the vagina was only 2 inches in depth because of a stricture in the mid and upper vagina that would admit only a fingertip.

Case Abstract 2

Four years following radiation therapy for a stage II-B carcinoma of the cervix, a 43-year-old multipara complained of severe dyspareunia. Although there was no evidence of recurrent carcinoma, the vagina was virtually obliterated, with a depth of only 3 cm as a result of adherence of the vaginal walls and obliteration of the lumen by rigid cicatrix.

DISCUSSION

Case Abstract 1 describes a far too common complication of vaginoplastic surgery. Acquired vaginal atresia following colporrhaphy is a preventable and serious problem. Generally, meticulous attention to the vaginal dimensions during anterior and posterior colporrhaphy should prevent this complication. Sometimes excessive amounts of vaginal mucosa are excised. It is better to leave a little extra or redundant mucosa than to excise too much, since, after all, it is not the mucosa that is responsible for restoration of lost pelvic supports.

Endogenous and/or exogenous estrogen may be important in preventing this complication. Postmenopausal women with severe atrophic vaginitis and secondary inflammatory changes are much more likely to develop adhesive vaginitis following vaginal surgery resulting in obliteration of most, if not all, of the vagina. This may be prevented by the preoperative administration of estrogens for 2 to 3 months followed by postoperative utilization of a Milex or other suitable dilator until healing is complete. Those who have frequent coitus may require the use of a dilator for only a brief period of time or not at all. Particular attention must be devoted to those who are not sexually active during the first few months following surgery, at which time adhesive vaginitis is easily released digitally. This should be repeated monthly until healing is complete. In such situations intravaginal estrogen cream may be a useful supplement to exogenous estrogen.

Case Abstract 2 represents another example of acquired vaginal atresia which is preventable. All patients treated with radiation therapy for carcinoma of the cervix should insert a Milex or similar dilator at least two times weekly for a year or until postradiation healing is complete. Many of these patients are not sexually active for months after treatment because of decreased libido and a number of other reasons. Some husbands need to be counseled to eliminate the fear that the cancer is contagious or that intercourse would be painful for the patient. Use of estrogen cream as a lubricant when utilizing the dilator may be helpful.

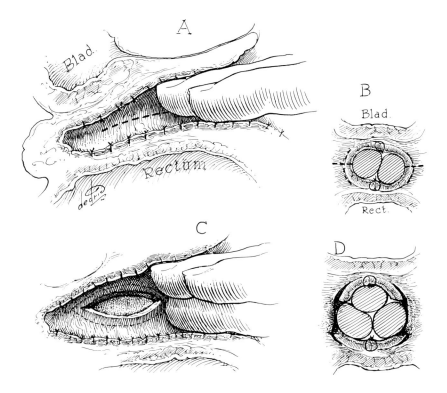

Figure 43.1.   Digital examination of the vagina immediately following colporrhaphy discloses an unexpected stenosis in the upper half that will admit but 2 finger breadths (**A**). The sites of the lateral relaxing incisions are indicated by the *dotted lines* (**B**). These incisions are made through the lateral wall of the vagina to a depth sufficient to comfortably admit 3 finger breadths (**C**). The vaginal wall is undercut for a centimeter in each direction (**D**). Any obvious bleeding vessels are clamped and tied, and a firm vaginal packing is inserted. This may be replaced in a day or so by a large vaginal obturator or mold, to keep the cut edges of the relaxing incisions apart until healing and epithelialization are well under way. This is usually by the fifth postoperative day, following which the obturator or dilator may be worn at night for an additional 2 or 3 weeks. Thus, the integrity of the colporrhaphy incisions in the anterior and posterior vaginal walls is not compromised. (From Nichols DH, Randall CL: *Vaginal Surgery*, ed. 3. Baltimore, Williams & Wilkins, 1989, with permission.)

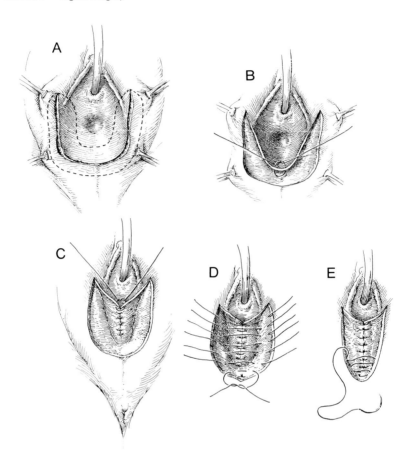

Figure 43.2.   Vulvovaginoplasty. The area of softening beneath the urethra identifies the site of the missing vagina. Following thorough infiltration with 0.5% lidocaine in 1:200,000 epinephrine solution, a U-shaped incision is made and undermined as indicated by the *broken line* (**A**). The medial margins of the incision are united by interrupted sutures (**B** and **C**) and the subcutaneous tissue by a separate layer (**D**). The lateral incisional margins are approximated separately (**E**).

Management

Management of the acquired vaginal atresia in both of these cases depends upon a number of variables. If the apex of the residual short vagina following surgery is soft and pliable, utilization of progressive dilators comparable to that described by Frank for vaginal agenesis may be adequate. More recently, Ingram has described a technique utilizing progressive dilators and a bicycle seat. When applied to highly motivated patients, these techniques may be useful in both congenital and acquired atresia. However, both the Frank and Ingram methods require many months of dedicated effort to achieve a satisfactory result.

In other instances of acquired atresia, the use of lateral transverse releasing incisions held open by an obturator or dilator until epithelialized may result in a satisfactory vaginal caliber (Fig. 43.1).

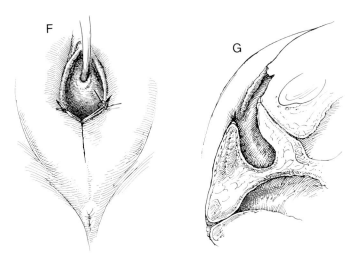

Figure 43.3. Vulvovaginoplasty at the completion of the operation is shown in frontal view (**F**) and sagittal section (**G**). (From Nichols DH, Randall CL: *Vaginal Surgery*, ed. 3. Baltimore, Williams & Wilkins, 1989, with permission.)

In most instances of acquired vaginal atresia, the best results can be achieved through utilization of the vulvoplasty technique for construction of an artificial vagina described by Arthur Williams. In Figures 43.2 and 43.3, the progressive steps utilized in performing this operation are illustrated. Following complete healing, the Williams operation should be followed by the use of a large dilator. Supplemental estrogen should be used in the estrogen-deficient patient.

In some patients with extensive cicatrix formation following previous surgery, a vaginectomy with reconstruction of a neovagina with a split-thickness skin graft may be the procedure of choice. Under these circumstances, as with congenital atresia, incision of the levator musculature bilaterally may reduce the frequency of postoperative vaginal contraction.

Acquired atresia following radiation is best treated by the Williams operation. Vaginal dissections in heavily radiated areas of devascularized tissues may result in a permanent vesicovaginal or rectovaginal fistula.

SELECTED READINGS

Evans TN, Polland ML, Boving RL: Vaginal malformations. *Am J Obstet Gynecol* 141:910, 1981.

Frank RT: The formation of an artificial vagina without operation. *Am J Obstet Gynecol* 35:1053, 1938.

Ingram JM: The bicycle stool in treatment of vaginal agenesis and stenosis: A preliminary report. *Am J Obstet Gynecol* 140:867, 1981.

Williams EA: Congenital absence of the vagina: A simple operation for its relief. *J Obstet Gynaecol Br Commonw* 71:511, 1964.

44

Genital Prolapse in a Patient with Poor Cardinal-Uterosacral Ligaments

David H. Nichols

Case Abstract

A vaginal hysterectomy and repair were being performed on a 65-year-old sexually active woman because of progression of a postmenopausal genital prolapse that recently had become virtual procidentia. The patient had been unable to retain a vaginal pessary. After the prolapsed utereus was removed, it was evident that there was practically no cardinal and uterosacral ligament strength which could be used to support the vault of the vagina to restore or maintain vaginal depth postoperatively.

DISCUSSION

When massive eversion of the vagina is the result of a general postmenopausal prolapse, atrophy of most of the endopelvic soft tissue support is often present, and there may be no strong cardinal-uterosacral ligaments to surgically develop for new support of the vault of the vagina. In most instances, the situation can be predicted by preoperative office evaluation or examination under anesthesia. This situation is probable if strong uterosacral ligaments are not palpated, and cystocele and rectocele are present; enterocele is frequently absent (Fig. 44.1). This is in sharp contrast to the more common uterovaginal or sliding prolapse, where elongated but strong and hypertrophic uterosacral ligaments can generally be identified along with a significant enterocele. The cervix and vaginal vault in the latter instance slide and descend along the anterior surface of the rectum, producing cystocele but not necessarily rectocele.

Massive posthysterectomy vaginal eversion may follow either abdominal or vaginal hysterectomy, particularly when there has been insufficient attention to the correction of defects in support of the vagina at any of several possible levels. Since a dropped uterus is the result of the genital prolapse and not the cause, a simple hysterectomy without effective repair that includes support of the vaginal vault is likely to be unsuccessful (Fig. 44.2).

There are several factors which may precipitate massive eversion. It may develop from a congenital abnormality in tissue strength, organ position, or innervation. It may also develop in response to sustained increases in intra-abdominal pressure. Obstetric damage to genital supports may be a cause. Although the condition is seen in patients of any age, it is more common among older women and appears to have some association with menopausal atrophy and involutional changes.

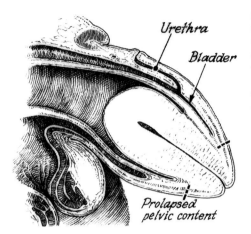

Figure 44.1. Procidentia is present with cystocele, rectocele, and descent of the cul-de-sac. There is displacement of the bladder outside of the pelvis and descent of the vesicourethral junction and proximal urethra and of the anterior rectal wall. The cul-de-sac of Douglas is displaced outside of the pelvis. (Reprinted with permission of Northern Chesapeake Publishers, Inc., from Nichols DH: Transvaginal sacrospinous fixation. *Pelvic Surg* 1:10, 1981.)

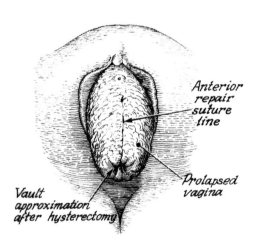

Figure 44.2. A vaginal hysterectomy has been accomplished and the attenuated cardinal and uterosacral ligaments confirmed. Any redundant peritoneum has been resected and the peritoneal cavity closed by high purse-string ligation. A full-length anterior colporrhaphy has been accomplished. (Reprinted with permission of Northern Chesapeake Publishers, Inc., from Nichols DH: Transvaginal sacrospinous fixation. *Pelvic Surg* 1:10, 1981.)

In most instances of massive vaginal eversion, however, significant uterosacral ligament strength can be identified preoperatively or intraoperatively. Shortening these hypertrophic ligaments at the time of vaginal hysterectomy is preferred (9,10) and may be combined with the New Orleans type of culdeplasty (4) or one of its modifications (9). This shortening can also be performed following abdominal hysterectomy, although appropriate transvaginal colporrhaphy should follow.

When massive vaginal eversion occurs long after total hysterectomy, cardinal and uterosacral ligaments that had been separated from the uterus but not used in support of the vagina usually will have become atrophic, so that in their weakened and attenuated condition their surgical usefulness may be less than effective in adequately supporting the vaginal vault. This should be evident at surgery, and an alternate method of support of the vaginal vault elected.

In this era of longer life span and sustained sexual activity, preservation of coital function is important to the patient, and treatment of massive eversion by surgical procedures that might obliterate the vagina or eliminate its coital function is not desirable. Colpocleisis or colpectomy may give rise to an exceedingly troublesome postoperative urinary stress incontinence (13), and enterocele or pudendal hernia may persist.

The surgical goal should be to reestablish the normal depth and axis of the vagina. The lower vagina curves cranial and posterior, and the upper vagina becomes horizontal and terminates near the hollow of the sacrum.

Victor Bonney (1) described separate primary damage in genital prolapse to either the upper suspensory system (cardinal and uterosacral ligament complex) or the lower supportive system (levator ani and pelvic diaphragm) and suggested that it is desirable, if not essential, for the surgeon to identify and overrepair the primary site of damage. In the patient with complete procidentia of vagina and uterus in which the organs are now completely outside the pelvis, the surgeon might tell which area of damage was primary by examining the patient in the lithotomy position and gently replacing the prolapse. After all instruments have been removed from contact with the patient, she is asked to bear down and the gynecologist observes that which appears first. If the cervix or vaginal vault appears first *followed* by a cystocele and rectocele, the primary site of damage has been to the upper suspensory system, and a strong cardinal uterosacral ligament complex strength cannot be expected or demonstrated. The surgeon should plan for a colpopexy to be part of the original primary operation. This might be by either transvaginal sacrospinous fixation or transabdominal sacral colpopexy following hysterectomy, the choice depending upon the operator's experience. This examining room decision will give the surgeon time to properly prepare for the operation, obtaining in advance whatever surgical assistance will be in the patient's best interest. On the other hand, if the cystocele and rectocele appear first followed by the cervix, the primary site of damage was probably to the lower supportive structures, and primary vaginal hysterectomy and appropriate colporrhaphy without colpopexy are indicated.

Various surgical approaches have been employed to treat massive eversion, some transabdominal and some transvaginal. Although ventral fixation or ventral suspension of the uterus or of the everted vagina has been described, it is not without problems. The creation of an abnormal anterior axis to the vagina may limit bladder capacity, producing a troublesome incontinence (2), and expose the unprotected cul-de-sac of Douglas to the full range of changes in intra-abdominal pressure with the significant risk of subsequent development of enterocele. Transabdominal attachment of the vault of the vagina to the promontory of the sacrum by fascia or plastic mesh through a retroperitoneal tunnel may effectively support the vault of the vagina, but effective correction of cystocele and rectocele through the same operative exposure is not possible (11). It is, however, a more physiologic and anatomically correct procedure than ventral suspension.

Transvaginal procedures include fixation of the vagina to shortened, strong cardinal-uterosacral ligaments (9,10,14), to the fascia of the pelvic diaphragm (3), or to a strong nongynecologic structure such as the sacrospinous ligament (6–9). Colpocleisis or colpectomy does not preserve a coitally useful vagina.

In the case described, appropriate colporrhaphy and transvaginal fixation of the vagina to the sacrospinous ligament is the procedure of choice. The sacrospinous ligament runs from the ischial spine to the sacrum within the substance of the coccygeus muscle. Its location is readily determined by palpation. Since the surgical anatomy describes the proximity of the pudendal vessels and sciatic nerve beneath the ischial spine, suture penetration of this ligament should occur at a preselected position 1½ to 2 finger breadths medial to the ischial spine to avoid trauma to the blood vessels and nerves.

The blunt-tipped Deschamps ligature carrier is useful, as is the Miya hook (5). The Shutt punch is remarkably easy to use (12), but with it the monofilament sutures required must be placed individually.

The choice of suture may include both absorbable (Dexon 2, or long-lasting no. 0 polyglycolic acid-type suture [PDS or Maxon]) or nonabsorbable suture such as no. 0 Prolene, Surgilene, or Novafil (10).

To expose the coccygeus muscle and ligament safely, it is desirable to proceed from an incision in the perineum that opens the rectovaginal space (Fig. 44.3) and is carried through the right rectal pillar into the right pararectal space (Fig. 44.4), exposing deep within this space the coccygeus muscle containing the sacrospinous ligament (Fig. 44.5). The muscle is grasped by a long Babcock or Allis clamp and then penetrated by the blunt tip of a Deschamps ligature carrier threaded with a full uncut length of a synthetic nonabsorbable suture or 54-inch Dexon no. 2, at a point 1½ to 2 finger breadths medial to the ischial spine, safely away from the pudendal nerve and vessels and the sciatic nerve (Fig. 44.6). The free ends of the suture are fixed to the vault of the vagina (Fig. 44.7) and, when tied, will attach the vaginal vault firmly to this area (Fig. 44.8). Appropriate anterior colporrhaphy is then completed, and after the upper 2 inches of the posterior vaginal wall have been approximated and any ballooning of the anterior rectal wall reduced by a separate running locked suture, the colpopexy stitches are tied. The knots should be snug, avoiding any suture bridges.

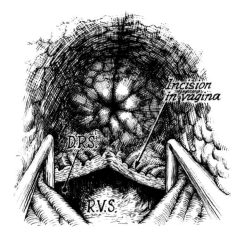

Figure 44.3. The perineum has been incised and an opening made into the rectovaginal space (RVS). The full length of the rectovaginal space has been developed to the vault of the vagina by blunt dissection and the full thickness of the posterior vaginal wall incised to a point cranial to the rectocele. The descending rectal septum (DRS), which separates the rectovaginal space from the pararectal space, is seen on the patient's right. (Reprinted with permission of Northern Chesapeake Publishers, Inc., from Nichols DH: Transvaginal sacrospinous fixation. *Pelvic Surg* 1:10, 1981.)

Figure 44.4. The right cardinal ligament and ureter have been displaced anteriorly by a Breisky-Navratil retractor in the 12 o'clock position and the rectum displaced to the patient's left by a retractor in the 4 o'clock position. An opening is made either bluntly or by using a sharp-pointed hemostat through the descending rectal septum into the right rectal space at the site of the ischial spine. This opening is enlarged by spreading the point of the hemostat or of the Mayo scissors to permit access to the coccygeus muscle, which lies in the lateral wall of the pararectal space and contains within it the sacrospinous ligament. (RVS, rectovaginal space.) (Reprinted with permission of Northern Chesapeake Publishers, Inc., from Nichols DH: Transvaginal sacrospinous fixation. *Pelvic Surg* 1:10, 1981.)

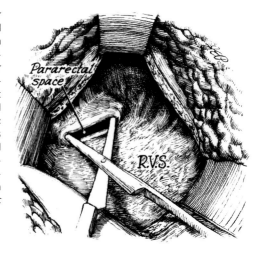

Figure 44.5. The coccygeus muscle containing the sacrospinous ligament (shown by the *dotted lines*) is visible in the depths of the right pararectal space. (Reprinted with permission of Northern Chesapeake Publishers, Inc., from Nichols DH: Transvaginal sacrospinous fixation. *Pelvic Surg* 1:10, 1981.)

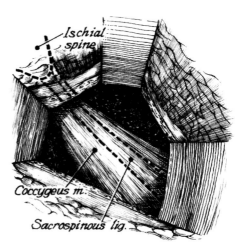

Figure 44.6. The coccygeus muscle and sacrospinous ligament have been penetrated by the blunt end of a long Deschamps ligature carrier at a point 1½ to 2 finger breadths medial to the ischial spine, safely away from the pudendal nerve and vessels and sciatic nerve. The ligature carrier had been previously threaded with a full uncut length of 52-inch no. 2 polyglycolic acid suture (Dexon). Traction to the hook exteriorizes the suture, and the Deschamps ligature carrier is removed. The end of the suture loop is cut, resulting in two strands of suture material penetrating the ligament. (Reprinted with permission of Northern Chesapeake Publishers, Inc., from Nichols DH: Transvaginal sacrospinous fixation. *Pelvic Surg* 1:10, 1981.)

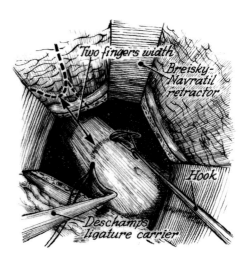

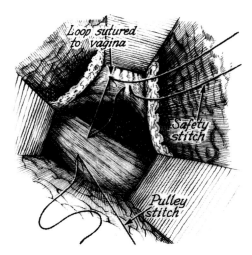

Figure 44.7.   The end of one suture is threaded on a free needle, which is sewn through the full thickness of the undersurface of the fibromuscular layer of the vaginal wall and fixed in position by a single half-hitch. The end of the second piece of suture is stitched to the undersurface of the vagina 1 cm medially. After an appropriate segment of posterior vaginal wall has been excised as part of the posterior colporrhaphy, the margins of the posterior vagina are approximated with a running subcuticular stitch of polyglycolic acid suture until the midportion of the vagina has been reached. The sacrospinous fixation stitches are tied, fixing the vagina to the surface of the coccygeus muscle–sacrospinous ligament, and the posterior colporrhaphy and perineorrhaphy are completed. (Reprinted with permission of Northern Chesapeake Publishers, Inc., from Nichols DH: Transvaginal sacrospinous fixation. *Pelvic Surg* 1:10, 1981.)

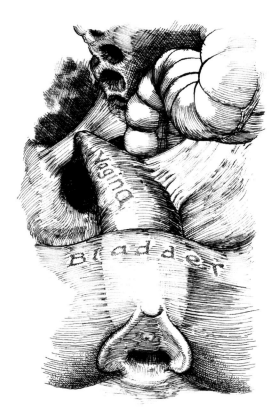

Figure 44.8.   A phantom frontal view of the sacrospinous fixation is seen, demonstrating fixation of the vagina to the surface of the right coccygeus muscle and sacrospinous ligament at a point 1½ to 2 finger breadths medial to the right ischial spine. (Reprinted with permission of Northern Chesapeake Publishers, Inc., from Nichols DH: Transvaginal sacrospinous fixation. *Pelvic Surg* 1:10, 1981.)

REFERENCES

1. Bonney V: The sustentacular apparatus of the female genital canal, the displacements from the yielding of its several components and their appropriate treatment. *J Obstet Gynaecol Br Emp* 45:328, 1914.
2. Hodgkinson CP, Kelly WT: Urinary stress incontinence in the female. III. Round-ligament technique for retropubic suspension of the urethra. *Obstet Gynecol* 10:493, 1957.
3. Inmon WB: Pelvic relaxation and repair including prolapse of vagina following hysterectomy. *South Med J* 56:577, 1963.
4. McCall ML: Posterior culdeplasty: Surgical correction of enterocele during vaginal hysterectomy: A preliminary report. *Obstet Gynecol* 10:595, 1957.
5. Miyazaki FS: Miya Hook ligature carrier for sacrospinous ligament suspension. *Obstet Gynecol* 70:286–288, 1987.
6. Morley GW, DeLancey JOL: Sacrospinous ligament fixation for eversion of the vagina. *Am J Obstet Gynecol* 158:872–881, 1988.
7. Nichols DH: Effects of pelvic relaxation on gynecologic urologic problems. *Clin Obstet Gynecol* 21:759, 1978.
8. Nichols DH: Sacrospinous fixation for massive eversion of the vagina. *Am J Obstet Gynecol* 142:901, 1982.
9. Nichols DH, Randall CL: *Vaginal surgery,* ed. 3. Baltimore, Williams & Wilkins, 1989, pp. 338–348.
10. Nichols DH (ed): *Gynecologic and Obstetric Surgery.* St. Louis, Mosby-Year Book, 1993, pp. 431–464.
11. Parsons L, Ulfelder H: *An Atlas of Operations*, ed. 2. Philadelphia, WB Saunders, 1968, pp. 280–283.
12. Sharp TR: Sacrospinous suspension made easy. *Obstet Gynecol* 82:873–875, 1993.
13. Symmonds RE, Jordan LT: Iatrogenic stress incontinence of urine. *Am J Obstet Gynecol* 81:1231, 1961.
14. Symmonds RE, Williams TJ, Lee RA, et al: Posthysterectomy enterocele and vaginal vault prolapse. *Am J Obstet Gynecol* 140:852, 1981.

45

Recurrent Genital Prolapse Following Sacrospinous Vaginal Suspension

Fred S. Miyazaki

Case Abstract

A 65-year-old multiparous female underwent a right sacrospinous vaginal vault suspension for a symptomatic grade 4 vaginal vault prolapse. Six months postoperatively, she returned with a 5-cm mass bulging through the vaginal introitus.

DISCUSSION

In symptomatic recurrent prolapse the defects usually occur in varying combinations. However, in order to simplify the discussion, they will be dealt with separately. The defects are urethrocystocele (anterior wall), enterocele (hernia from vaginal apex), and vault prolapse (descent of vault apex). The early recurrence in our hypothetical patient above suggests an error in diagnosis (missed enterocele?) or an error in corrective technique.

Postoperative cystocele is by far the most common cause of recurrence. The diagnosis is easily made by noting protrusion of the anterior vaginal wall despite a vaginal cuff apex that remains adherent to the sacrospinous ligament. A very common technical error is the insufficient narrowing of a capacious upper vault into a cylindrical tube. Patients with vaginal vault prolapse have absent apical vault support (absent cardinal and uterosacral ligaments) as well as absent lateral vaginal wall support (paravaginal defect). In these patients the preservation of a capacious upper vault allows intra-abdominal pressure to be exerted over a large area of unsupported vagina, thereby leading to the early recurrence of left anterolateral vaginal wall prolapse. This is illustrated in Fig. 45.1. This is such an important point that Nichols reiterates it six times in the one chapter on vaginal eversion in his textbook of vaginal surgery (1). In assessing vaginal caliber and redundancy, it is emphasized that intraoperative visual examination is quite misleading. With the patient under anesthesia, and in dorsolithotomy and Trendelenburg position, the overly capacious vaginal vault may appear to be grossly normal and well supported. However, traction on the anterior vaginal wall may reveal a grade 2 cystocele or a partial (L) apical prolapse. Although some experts are able to correctly "eyeball" the amount of redundant vaginal wall requiring excision, my recommended technique is as follows:

Longitudinal vaginal wall laxity is estimated by tugging on the anterior vaginal wall with a Babcock clamp. Transverse laxity is estimated by inserting two fingers into the vagina and spreading laterally. A general rule of thumb for estimating correct diameters

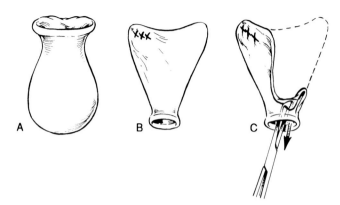

Figure 45.1.   Frontal view. **A.** Unrepaired total vault prolapse. **B.** Right sacrospinous suspension and posterior colporrhaphy. Patient is still under anesthesia and in dorsolithotomy position. Visually, the prolapse appears corrected. **C.** Traction on anterolateral vaginal wall with a Babcock clamp reveals the presence of a grade 2 anterolateral vaginal wall prolapse.

is 4 finger breadths at the introitus, 3 finger breadths in the midvagina, and 2 finger breadths at the vaginal apex. Two right-angle Allis clamps* are very helpful in making the upper and midvaginal estimation (Fig. 45.2). The clamps are applied to the midvaginal wall at approximately the 10 and 2 o'clock positions and then brought together in the midline until 3 fingers can fit in comfortably (Fig. 45.3). The clamp sites are then suture-tagged with no. 2/0 chromic suture to mark the lateral extent of the anticipated anterior wall excision. The longitudinal extent of excision is from bladder neck to the cuff apex. The excised anterior wall usually has the shape of a transverse ovoid rather than a triangle.

The three operative techniques used for correcting recurrent anterior wall prolapse appear to be equally successful; thus the choice depends mostly on the surgeon's past experience. First, a sacrospinous suspension of the opposite side and anterior col-porrhaphy could be performed. A number of experienced vaginal surgeons do bilateral suspensions which are stronger, more symmetric, and easier to perform. A bilateral suspension may have been a better choice at the time of the first prolapse surgery. Second, abdominal sacral colpopexy has also been shown to be very successful (4,5). It is mandatory to perform a prophylactic retropubic bladder neck suspension with this procedure because of the 20% to 25% incidence of stress incontinence following the procedure (4,3). Third, repair of a paravaginal defect has been efficacious as a primary procedure to correct genital prolapse (2). However, in many cases of repeat vaginal reconstructive surgery, the vaginal diameter may not be wide enough to reach from one sidewall to the other.

Recurrent enterocele is the second most common cause of recurrent prolapse following sacrospinous suspension. The most frequent type is the posterior enterocele, in which the enterocele sac lies between the posterior vaginal wall and the anterior rectal wall. The diagnosis is most easily made by simultaneous rectal and vaginal examination

*BEI Medical Systems, Chatsworth, CA 91311 (800) 223-4740.

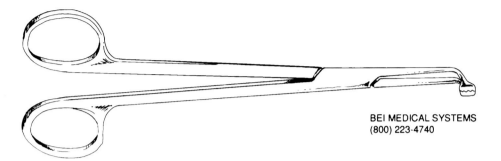

BEI MEDICAL SYSTEMS
(800) 223-4740

Figure 45.2. Right-angle (80°) Allis clamp.

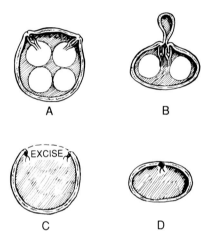

A   B

EXCISE

C   D

Figure 45.3. Estimating vaginal caliber. **A.** Capacious upper vault, a loose 4 finger breadths. Allis clamps are applied to the anterior wall at about 10 and 2 o'clock positions. **B.** Allis clamps are approximated in the midline and the vaginal caliber tested with 3 fingers. Allis clamps are readjusted until the upper vaginal canal admits 2 fingers. **C.** Allis clamps are removed and the clamp sites are suture-tagged with no. 2/0 chromic suture. The vaginal wall between the suture tags is now excised. **D.** Anterior colporrhaphy completed.

while the patient strains or coughs in the standing position. A bulge consisting of small intestines can be felt separating the two fingers. It is important to make every attempt to diagnose an enterocele preoperatively so that a thorough search for the enterocele will be made intraoperatively. Enterocele resection is fairly routine and consists of dissecting the enterocele sac off of the rectum and bladder and placing a high purse-string closure of the sac. Care should be taken laterally to take bites of only the peritoneum that has been dissected free because the ureter is usually close by.

Equally important is excision of the thinned-out posterior vaginal wall which previously covered the enterocele sac. This will bring thick, healthy vaginal wall under the peritoneum and minimize recurrence. When posterior enterocele is the predominant pathology, it is important to reduce vaginal caliber by excising attenuated posterior vaginal wall, rather than by excising healthy anterior vaginal wall at a later step.

In a central enterocele, the sac courses through the middle of the vaginal cuff and presents as a sausage-shaped mass in the middle of the vagina. The diagnosis is obvious and treatment is the same as for posterior enterocele.

In the rare anterior enterocele, the sac lies between the anterior vaginal wall and the bladder base and mimics a cystocele. However, palpation of the anterior vaginal wall may reveal gurgling small bowel. In addition, a double contour of the anterior wall prolapse may be seen when the patient valsalvas. This condition is almost always iatrogenic and follows previous vaginal surgery involving anterior colporrhaphy.

Recurrent vaginal vault prolapse is another cause of recurrent genital prolapse following sacrospinous suspension. The diagnosis is usually obvious in that the vault apex is no longer attached to the sacrospinous ligament. Pushing the cuff apex back up against the sacrospinous ligament completely relieves the prolapse. Recurrent vault prolapses are almost all due to suture bridges of various kinds which prevent good tissue-to-tissue apposition. The most common type of suture bridge results from a loosening of the knot between the first and second throws, especially with heavy monofilament sutures. This type of suture can be prevented by using a sliding granny knot for the first two throws (not a square knot). A rectal exam is then performed to rule out a suture bridge. Then four square knots are placed. Sutures twisting around each other are another form of suture bridge and can be prevented by clamping each suture end to the drapes. Finally, the vaginal cuff should be brought out between the medial and lateral sutures before placing the sutures into the vaginal wall. This prevents twisting of these sutures.

In summary, patients with vaginal vault prolapse usually have multiple defects of pelvic support, each of which needs to be correctly diagnosed and repaired. In our hypothetical patient with recurrent prolapse, the main types of prolapses, their diagnoses, and their corrections were discussed individually. If all of these diagnostic and operative procedures had been performed at the first prolapse surgery, most of these recurrences may have been prevented.

REFERENCES

1. Nichols DH, Randal CL: Massive eversion of the vagina. Ch. 16 in *Vaginal Surgery,* ed. 3. Baltimore, Williams & Wilkins, 1989.
2. Shull BL, Baden WF: A six year experience with paravaginal defect repair for stress urinary incontinence. *Am J Obstet Gynecol* 160:1432–1440, 1989.
3. Snyder SE, Krantz KE: Abdominal-retroperitoneal sacral colpopexy. *Obstet Gynecol* 77:944–949, 1991.
4. Timmons CM, Addison WA: Abdominal sacral colpopexy for management of vaginal vault prolapse. Ch. 10, p. 137, in Bayden WF, Walker T: *Vaginal Defects.* Philadelphia, JB Lippincott, 1992.
5. Timmons CM, Addison WA, Addison SB, Cavenor MG: Abdominal sacral colpopexy in 163 women with post hysterectomy vaginal vault prolapse and enterocele: Evolution of operative techniques. *J Reprod Med* 37:631–633, 1992.

46

Massive Eversion of a Shortened Vagina

George W. Morley

Case Abstract

A 45-year-old sexually active woman had had two previous operations for a troublesome symptomatic prolapse. These included a vaginal hysterectomy with colporrhaphy and a repeat colporrhaphy with excision of an enterocele. Three years following the last procedure, and over a period of several months, a recurrent vaginal eversion had developed. The vagina, though totally everted, was but 3 inches in length and could not be brought to the site of the sacrospinous ligament.

DISCUSSION

This situation poses one of the most difficult problems encountered by those interested in vaginal reconstructive surgery. Fortunately, the "short vagina" syndrome is not a frequent complication of previous hysterectomy—either vaginal or abdominal—or any other previous vaginal surgery; however, when it does occur, it is fraught with a variety of abnormal signs and symptoms and emotional frustrations. One need not discuss the etiology of this syndrome in any great detail, but certainly all who do surgery must be apprised of this possibility when performing gynecologic surgery either transvaginally or transabdominally. This is an "ounce of prevention."

The author has seen a number of these patients who have undergone transabdominal hysterectomy with removal of a portion of the upper vagina for a variety of indications; however, it is much more common in those patients who have previously undergone vaginal surgery. From a therapeutic point of view, there are a variety of ways to approach this complex problem.

A *transabdominal sacropexy* (4) certainly is an appropriate way to manage this problem; however, given a vaginal depth of only 3 inches, something more than just attaching the vaginal apex to the sacrum must be considered. One could open the apex of the vagina, after which an extension of the vagina could be fashioned from an absorbable synthetic material utilizing either a polyglycolic acid or a polyglactin 910 mesh. This newly constructed elongated "upper vagina," which can be of varying length, is then attached to the presacral ligament as performed during the more conventional transabdominal sacropexy (4). A more permanent foreign body material such as a Mersilene mesh has been used in the past, but it has the disadvantage of sometimes becoming infected or occasionally eroding through adjacent tissues or organs. Not only are these situations annoying, but the foreign body is very difficult to remove or retrieve. Currently, Gore-Tex® graft is used by some for this purpose with good results.

During the postoperative period, the absorbable synthetic material acts as a matrix or scaffolding to which fibroblastic proliferating tissue can attach. This process also stimulates the formation of granulation tissue, which carries with it an exuberant blood supply. During the healing period, an appropriately sized obturator is worn in the vagina to maintain appropriate depth and caliber. A split-thickness skin graft may or may not be required to cover the granulation bed; migratory epithelialization may occur spontaneously and quite satisfactorily. In either case, the obturator is left in place 24 hours a day for 3 months except when voiding or evacuating the lower colon or when taking a daily cleansing douche. Ultimately, the obturator can be worn for approximately 8 hours each 24-hour period—either during the day or at night.

A number of gynecologic surgeons have had considerable success with the *sacrospinous* or *sacrotuberous ligament suspension* (6) for massive eversion of the vagina; however, this simply will not work satisfactorily for this patient because this procedure will not increase the depth of the vagina and the patient will continue to experience dyspareunia. One could instruct the patient on the use of vaginal dilators in an attempt to gain more vaginal depth, and then later attach the apex of the vagina to these ligaments. However, this approach is probably of limited value.

A *vulvoplasty* (7) as described by Williams of Great Britain will certainly add depth in this area; however, this will not provide any correction for the basic problem of vaginal eversion. This technique could be used in combination with a sacrospinous ligament suspension, possibly using a synthetic nonabsorbable suture and leaving a deliberate suture bridge if the latter were thought possible in this specific case. In performing this type of vulvoplasty, one must have a sufficient amount of vulvar tissue present to fashion what is referred to as a "labioperineal pouch." Finally, the angle of inclination from this procedure is often more acute than desired. It is recommended that if one chooses to utilize this technique that the author's original description be reviewed prior to performing this unique, creative, and relatively simple operation.

In the appropriately motivated patient, the nonsurgical approach to the treatment of vaginal agenesis as described by Frank (2) certainly might benefit this patient by increasing and improving the vaginal depth and caliber over a period of time. Subsequently, it could be anticipated that a satisfactorily enlarged vagina would be developed, thus making this patient a candidate for a transvaginal sacrospinous ligament suspension as a more permanent correction of this defect. The Frank procedure is certainly simple, safe, cost-effective, and worth a try. Certainly all the hormonally depleted patients should be on estrogen replacement therapy for a protracted period of time. More recently, the Ingram "bicycle seat stool" modification (3) of the Frank procedure has been described and is worthy of review.

Some surgeons might suggest *vaginectomy followed by construction of a neovagina*. From a technical point of view this certainly can be done without any particular difficulty; however, a basic plastic surgical principle must be mentioned, which is simply that one should not "throw away" normal viable tissue. This patient's tissue can be used to some advantage and should not be discarded. If, however, one is motivated toward a total replacement of the vagina utilizing the split-thickness skin graft technique, then one can perform it without encountering any particular difficulties.

The *myocutaneous flap technique* utilizing the gracilis musculocutaneous tissues (1) is primarily used in reconstructive pelvic surgery following extensive or radical surgical procedures done primarily for gynecologic malignancy. Whereas this approach is another alternative, it appears to be more radical than that usually required to correct this defect surgically. Again, it is another option.

A combined transabdominal and transvaginal approach to the correction of this abnormality is worth mentioning. Once the vaginal apex has been located through an abdominal entry into the peritoneal cavity, the apex is opened to an ideal caliber. A split-thickness skin graft vaginoplasty of the McIndoe type is then performed. A properly fitting obturator with a split-thickness skin graft attached to the uppermost part of the obturator is inserted transvaginally to an appropriate depth and then secured externally to the vulvar tissues. The graft itself is provided with an abundant blood supply from the surrounding structures, including the surface of the small bowel. This technique has been used quite satisfactorily on pelvic exenteration patients and it provides the patient with very adequate depth.

More recently, some of these patients have been treated successfully with a full-thickness skin graft taken from the flank overlying the iliac crest (5). This type of vaginoplasty is a simple, straightforward, and effective method for treating this compromising situation. Furthermore, it has the advantage of primary closure of the donor site; familiarity with the use of the dermatome is not required and the complaint of dyspareunia is eradicated. Further, long-term observation will be needed to assess the longevity of the favorable results.

In summary, one must realize that these problems are not simple ones that can be corrected with any one of the more conventional means. These abnormalities need an individualized approach by someone familiar with these unusual findings so that these unfortunate patients can benefit from the surgeon's previous experience.

REFERENCES

1. Becker DW, Massey FM, McCraw JB: Musculocutaneous flaps in reconstructive pelvic surgery. *Obstet Gynecol* 54:178, 1979.
2. Frank RT: The formation of an artificial vagina without operation. *Am J Obstet Gynecol* 35:1053, 1938.
3. Ingram JM: The bicycle seat stool in the treatment of vaginal agenesis and stenosis: A preliminary report. *Am J Obstet Gynecol* 140:867, 1981.
4. Mattingly RF, Thompson JD (eds): *TeLinde's Operative Gynecology*, ed. 6. Philadelphia, JB Lippincott, 1985.
5. Morley GW, DeLancey JOL: Full thickness skin graft vaginoplasty for treatment of the stenotic of fore-shortened vagina. *Obstet Gynecol* 77:485–489, 1991.
6. Nichols DH, Randall CL: *Vaginal Surgery*, ed. 3. Baltimore, Williams & Wilkins, 1989.
7. Williams EA: Congenital absence of the vagina: A simple operation for its relief. *Br J Obstet Gynaecol* 4:511, 1964.

47

Enterocele, Vaginal Vault Prolapse, and Cystocele Following Vesicourethral Pin-up Operation

David H. Nichols
Kathleen Martin

Case Abstract

A 38-year-old multipara with rotational descent of the bladder neck complained of socially disabling urinary stress incontinence. Pelvic examination disclosed some multiparous relaxation with rotational descent of the bladder neck, some cystocele, an early prolapse of the uterus, and a rectocele. She was treated by the Burch modification of the Marshall-Marchetti-Krantz procedure with complete relief of her troublesome urinary incontinence.

Two years later the patient, although continent, had developed some troublesome pelvic pressure and backache, worse when on her feet. When examined, a vulvovaginal mass was identified as a large cystocele and a second-degree prolapse of the uterus with enterocele and rectocele.

DISCUSSION

This patient represents progression of some elements of genital prolapse that were present but untreated at the time of her original surgery. As Burch pointed out (1), there is a 15% incidence of enterocele subsequent to his vesicourethral pin-up operation. A change in the normally horizontal upper vaginal axis to one vertically directed exposes an unprotected cul-de-sac to the full range of changes in intra-abdominal pressure, favoring the development of enterocele.

For the patient described above, these problems now require a secondary operation, vaginal hysterectomy with colporrhaphy, which might well have been prevented had the cul-de-sac been specifically obliterated at the time of the original operation. One principle of reconstructive pelvic surgery is that if any part of the symptomatic genital prolapse is to be treated, any coincident parts, though not yet symptomatic, should be treated at the same time (10). Because there is no convincing evidence that coincident "routine" hysterectomy improves the results of the Marshall-Marchetti-Krantz or Burch operation, we would not recommend that coincident "routine" hysterectomy be a part of the original operation unless there was another reason or indication for hysterectomy, such as symptomatic leiomyomas or uterine prolapse.

The tendency toward subsequent prolapse is made worse in a patient with coincident chronic respiratory disease such as chronic bronchitis with cough, or in a patient who has the habit of regularly straining at stool to achieve an evacuation. Pregnancy itself increases intra-abdominal pressure, and is associated with an increased risk of recurrent stress incontinence when it intervenes following a surgical repair. The first operation to relieve urinary stress incontinence is the one that has the greatest likelihood of success, and the opportunity for surgical relief declines considerably with each subsequent operation. The patient is thus well advised to postpone surgical repair of the conditions causing urinary stress incontinence until after her childbearing career has been completed.

All of these factors increase intra-abdominal pressure and favor the development of subsequent symptomatic prolapse.

Since descent of the uterus is the result of a genital prolapse and not the cause, progression of prolapse is frequently seen. Prolapse of the vault of the vagina can occur independently of the presence or absence of the uterus, and not uncommonly may progress to a full vaginal vault eversion.

For the patient described above, if her childbearing career has been completed, the appropriate treatment would be vaginal hysterectomy and colporrhaphy with obliteration of the cul-de-sac (10). Had steps been taken at the time of the original surgery to obliterate the cul-de-sac, the rapid progression of subsequent events and thus the need for subsequent surgery might have been prevented.

To better elucidate the actual incidence of enterocele or rectocele formation after a retropubic urethropexy procedure such as a Marshall-Marchetti-Krantz or Burch, a review of the literature was undertaken from 1966 to the present. In Burch's review article (1) analyzing his experience from 1958 to 1968, he found a 7.6% rate of enterocele formation. Parenthetically, only 42% of the patients had been followed up longer than 20 months. Burch attributed this high enterocele incidence to the unobliterated cul-de-sac. He recommended, therefore, a dual surgical approach both from above and below, including "extensive perineorrhaphy and posterior colporrhaphy and exploration of the cul-de-sac." He further recommended obliteration of the cul-de-sac by approximating the uterosacral ligaments in the midline and by closing the pararectal gutters with interrupted sutures transabdominally. Since his paper, however, few studies have addressed the question of enterocele and/or rectocele formation after a retropubic urethropexy.

Table 47.1 summarizes the incidence of enterocele and/or rectocele after retropubic urethropexy procedures, which ranges between 7.6% and 66%. Remarkably, many of these recurrences required additional surgery. These studies confirm the vulnerable nature of the exposed cul-de-sac caused by the change of the vaginal axis created by the retropubic procedure (9). These findings also highlight the importance of finding and correcting posterior vaginal defects concomitant with the urethropexy procedure, as well as performing a cul-de-sac obliteration as, for example, by the technique of Halban (8).

In this particular case study, it is interesting that this patient developed a cystocele in addition to a rectocele and enterocele subsequent to the retropubic urethropexy. This reinforces the importance of the posterior vaginal wall as part of the support of the anterior vaginal wall and bladder. Specifically, fibers from the pubourethral ligament complex are known to interdigitate with the pubococcygeus and rectovaginal septum posteriorly, as well as to the fibromuscular wall of the vagina anteriorly (7). Therefore, disruption of one support can domino into multiple pelvic floor defects.

Table 47.1   Incidence of Enterocele and/or Rectocele After Retropubic Urethropexy

Study	Incidence of Enterocele and/or Rectocele		Defects Requiring Surgical Repair	
	Number of patients	Percentage (%)	Number of patients	Percentage (%)
Burch (1968)(1)	11/143	7.6	7/143	4.8
Stanton et al. (1976)(10)	6/40	15	1/40	2.5
Gillon et al. (1984)(3)	7/35	20	4/35	11.4
Langer et al. (1988)(5)	3/22	13.6	3/22	13.6
Eriksen et al. (1990)(2)	9/86	10.5	6/86	7
Thunedborg et al. (1990)(11)	5/19	25	Not stated	Not stated
Kiilholma et al. (1993)(4)	22/186	12	22/186	12
Wiskind et al. (1993)(12)	86/131	66	35/131	26.7

REFERENCES

1. Burch JC: Cooper's ligament urethrovesical suspension for stress incontinence. *Am J Obstet Gynecol* 100:754, 1968.
2. Eriksen BC et al: Long-term effectiveness of the Burch Colposuspension in female urinary stress incontinence. *Acta Obstet Gynecol Scand* 69:45, 1990.
3. Gillon G et al: Long-term follow-up of surgery for urinary incontinence in elderly women. *Br J Uro* 56:478, 1984.
4. Kiilholma P et al: Modified Burch Colposuspension for stress urinary incontinence in females. *Surg Gyn Obst* 176:111, 1993.
5. Langer R et al: The value of simultaneous hysterectomy during Burch colposuspension for urinary stress incontinence. *Obstet Gynecol* 72:866, 1988.
6. McGuire EJ: Abdominal procedures for stress incontinence. *Urol Clin North Am* 12:285, 1985.
7. Milley P et al: A correlative investigation of the human rectovaginal septum. *Anat Rec* 163:443–452, 1968.
8. Nichols DH: *Gynecologic and Obstetric Surgery.* St. Louis, Mosby–Year Book, 1993.
9. Nichols DH: Vaginal prolapse affecting bladder function. *Urol Clin North Am* 12:329, 1985.
10. Stanton SL et al: The colposuspension operation for urinary incontinence. *Br J Obstet Gynaecol* 83:890, 1976.
11. Thunedborg P et al: Stress urinary incontinence and posterior bladder suspension defects. *Acta Obstet Gynecol Scand* 69:55, 1990.
12. Wiskind AK et al: The incidence of genital prolapse after the Burch colposuspension. *Am J Obstet Gynecol* 167:399, 1992.

48

Vaginal Evisceration Following Pelvic Surgery

Clifford R. Wheeless, Jr.

Case Abstract 1

A vaginal hysterectomy without repair had been performed uneventfully upon an obese 35-year-old multiparous woman with second-degree prolapse, an asymptomatic cystocele and rectocele, and chronic dysfunctional uterine bleeding. The surgeon described the operation as using the "Heaney technique." The peritoneum had been closed and the vaginal vault left open for drainage, although the cut edge of the vagina had been covered with a circumferential running-locked hemostatic stitch. Chronic catgut had been used throughout. Blood loss at surgery was minimal, and no vaginal packing had been used postoperatively.

Although the patient was nauseated postoperatively, she was ambulated the evening of surgery and consumed a regular diet for supper. Nausea and sudden violent vomiting followed. The patient noted a sensation of "something giving way down below" and she returned to bed. When the perineal pad was changed an hour later (10 hours postoperatively), a loop of small intestine was found protruding from the vagina (Fig. 48.1).

Case Abstract 2

A 20-year-old primigravida, 8 weeks pregnant by dates and examination, was scheduled for therapeutic abortion by suction evacuation of the uterus. The patient was in excellent health and desired an abortion for non-medical reasons. A preoperative hemoglobin was 10.5 gm. Physical findings were unremarkable except for a uterus that was approximately 8 weeks in size. The abortion was performed under general anesthesia. The uterus was sounded to 8.5 cm. The cervical canal was progressively dilated with K-Pratt dilators to a 32 French diameter. A 10-mm straight suction cannula was introduced without difficulty, although the cervical canal was described as "tight." After the suction was turned on, the operator noted the appearance of blood-tinged amniotic fluid in the plastic curette. The curette was rotated in 180° arcs at the same time it was advanced forward and backward within the uterus. Tissue was seen in the curette. The operator advanced the curette out of the cervix and noted significant resistance. His impression was that fetal tissue was preventing the withdrawal of the suction curette. He applied additional traction on the curette and withdrew an obvious segment of small bowel through the cervix into the vagina. The vagina was intact (Fig. 48.2).

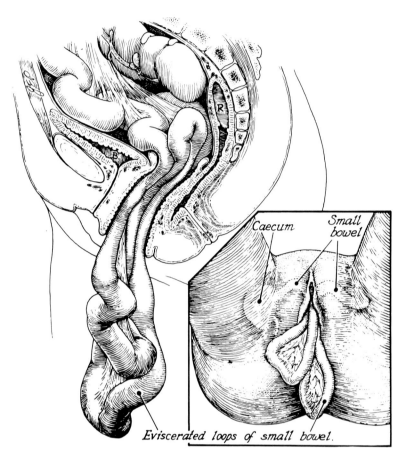

Caecum

Small bowel

Eviscerated loops of small bowel.

Figure 48.1.   A sagittal view of the lower abdomen and pelvis and a perineal view with the patient in the lithotomy position show the vaginal evisceration. The sagittal view in particular emphasizes that for complete vaginal evisceration to occur the small bowel mesentery must be mobilized in some way. Otherwise the length of small bowel mesentery is generally insufficient for the evisceration to occur. (Reprinted with permission of Northern Chesapeake Publishers, Inc., from Wheeless CR Jr: *Pelvic Surg* 2(7), 1981.)

DISCUSSION

Fortunately, vaginal evisceration of the intestine is rare (Fig. 48.1). The literature consists of individual case presentations with an occasional review article; less than 40 cases have been reported (1,2,4,5,7,8).

Evisceration usually follows vaginal hysterectomy, usually within the immediate postoperative period. However, there are cases reported years later (2,4,5). It has been reported after abdominal hysterectomy (3,5) and as a spontaneous sequel to rupture of a large enterocele with and without previous hysterectomy (2).

A contemporary source of vaginal eviscerations has been the suction curettage for termination of pregnancy during which the small intestine is sucked into the eye of a vacuum curette that has perforated the uterine wall and pulled through the perforation in the uterus and out into the vagina (Figs. 48.2 and 48.3).

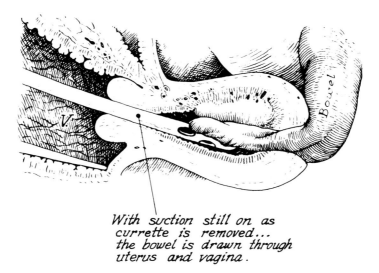

With suction still on as currette is removed... the bowel is drawn through uterus and vagina.

Figure 48.2. A sagittal drawing showing the suction curette with attached bowel being pulled through the perforated uterus during a termination of pregnancy. The gestational contents have not been removed.

The etiology of vaginal evisceration, except for that associated with suction termination of pregnancy, is confusing. There has not been one specific pattern of events that can be related in a cause-and-effect manner.

The anatomy of the small bowel and its mesentery should make vaginal evisceration difficult. Most anatomists describe the mesentery of the small bowel as being from 15 to 20 cm in length (3). Obviously, this distance is insufficient to allow the terminal ileum and/or jejunum to exit the peritoneal cavity through the vaginal cuff or a uterine perforation and eviscerate. There appear to be two possibilities. First, certain individuals could have a mesentery longer than the 15- to 20-cm average. Second, the process involved in evisceration may lengthen the small intestine mesentery by mobilizing it secondary to lacerations in the mesentery at the root of its origin. It is likely that both phenomena occur. Laceration of the small bowel mesentery threatens the continuity of blood supply to the intestine. However, the laceration could occur in such a location as to spare specific vascular arcades within the small bowel mesentery. This may explain why there are successful reports of simply replacing the small bowel into the peritoneal cavity via the vaginal route without performing a laparotomy and the patient recovering without incident. However, a procedure such as replacement of the intestine through the vaginal opening without laparotomy could be a perilous adventure. The overall mortality from vaginal evisceration has been reported at approximately 10% (8). From a review of the literature, it appears that much of this mortality is secondary to peritonitis, possibly related to intestinal necrosis. On the other hand, the morbidity from laparotomy in a modern hospital is minimal. Via laparotomy the intestine can be thoroughly inspected and suspicious areas of compromised intestine resected with primary reanastomosis.

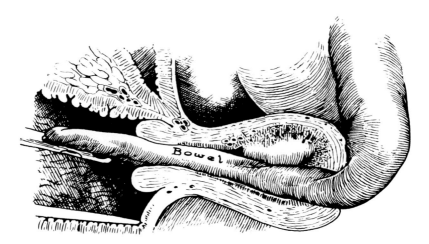

Figure 48.3. The intestine eviscerated through the cervix out into the vagina. It is at this point that one is most likely to injure the intestine by confusing it with fetal parts.

Prevention

Collective series of a significant number of patients for statistically valid results are unavailable. Therefore, the precise etiology of this problem in most cases remains unknown, except for those cases that have occurred during termination of pregnancy in which the intestine was pulled through a perforation in the uterine wall. Prevention includes considering the following: (a) whether there was failure to repair enterocele and cystocele present at the time of hysterectomy (6); (b) the pros and cons of leaving the vaginal vault open at the time of hysterectomy; and (c) choice and size of the suture material used in closing the vaginal vault, and particularly the technique of anastomosis of the stumps of the supporting ligaments of the pelvis to the angles of the vagina.

Although vaginal eviscerations have occurred from a variety of clinical and anatomic situations, most eviscerations have occurred in association with poor support of the vaginal cuff, posterior fornix, and cul-de-sac after vaginal hysterectomy (1,5,8).

The open vaginal vault is an attractive and tempting possibility for the etiology of vaginal evisceration. However, the open vaginal vault is the technique of many gynecologists, and thousands of hysterectomies have been performed leaving the vaginal vault open without the rare event of postoperative vaginal evisceration. When the vaginal vault is left open, its edge is usually sutured with a running-locked catgut suture, referred to as "reefing" the margin of the vaginal cuff. At the vaginal angles this "reefing suture" usually includes the stumps of the uterosacral and cardinal ligaments and anastomoses them to the angle of the vagina for additional support. In addition, most surgeons (but not all) peritonealize the pelvis by approximating the anterior and posterior peritoneal surfaces. This covers the open vaginal cuff. However, if one returns to the classic anatomic situation where the average length of the mesentery of the small bowel is 15 to 20 cm, evisceration would be virtually impossible unless an additional event occurred to mobilize the intestine for sufficient length to push it through an opening in the vaginal cuff. Therefore, open vaginal cuffs alone are generally insufficient to be the etiology of all vaginal eviscerations. In addition, most vaginal eviscerations reported have occurred after the vaginal cuff has been surgically closed with interrupted catgut sutures.

Choice of suture material may be a factor involved in the occurrence of posterior vaginal evisceration, but, like the open vaginal cuff, an additional factor is usually required to mobilize sufficient intestine to eviscerate out the vagina. If fine absorbable suture material is used (no. 3–0 or less), there is the attractive thesis that the anastomosis of the stumps of the cardinal and uterosacral ligaments could break down and set up the anatomic situation for evisceration. In addition, if enough pressure is acutely exerted on the mesentery of the small bowel via a Valsalva maneuver to lacerate the mesentery and thereby mobilize the intestine, evisceration could occur. However, insufficient evidence exists for placing the etiology of vaginal evisceration on choice of suture material. The author feels that absorbable suture (catgut or synthetic) in no. 2–0 to zero represents the ideal suture material for closure of the vagina and reanastomosis of the stumps of the uterosacral and cardinal ligaments to the vaginal cuff. Permanent suture used in this area would not eliminate eviscerations but would add morbidity from suture abscesses.

The method of closure of the vagina could also represent a potential threat for vaginal evisceration. All too often the vaginal cuff is closed with figure-of-eight sutures. A figure-of-eight suture, especially if tied tightly, promotes necrosis and healing by second intention. This is not the purpose of the suture in the vaginal cuff. Single sutures tied gently enough to approximate the tissue and provide hemostasis are sufficient. In addition, it is important to plicate the uterosacral ligaments behind the vaginal vault to add additional support and to reduce the tendency toward enterocele formation. The author does not feel that the classic McCall's plication of the uterosacral ligaments is necessary in all hysterectomies; in fact, it represents a threat to the ureter if the uterosacral ligaments are plicated for a distance of more than 3 cm. Although the above factors may play a role in this problem, most vaginal eviscerations are associated with significant Valsalva maneuvers, predominately vomiting, coughing, and lifting heavy objects. Severe vomiting and coughing have been reported in most cases in which evisceration has occurred after hysterectomy. Therefore, prevention must include containing these factors within moderation by eliminating overzealous oral feeding and excessive induction of postoperative coughing. Prevention of evisceration at suction abortion must include the safe utilization of techniques for performing the operation, that is, careful dilation of the cervix and repeated sounding of the uterine cavity.

Early Intervention

The key to the reduction of the severe morbidity and mortality associated with evisceration must be early recognition. Most eviscerations through the vagina are associated with lacerations of the mesentery of the small bowel, and the vascular integrity of the small bowel is at stake (Fig. 48.4A and C). When evisceration is caused by suction abortion, the additional factor of trauma by the suction curette to the surface of the bowel makes early recognition extremely important (Fig. 48.4B). Early recognition would allow surgical intervention prior to intestinal necrosis and leakage of intestinal contents into the peritoneal cavity.

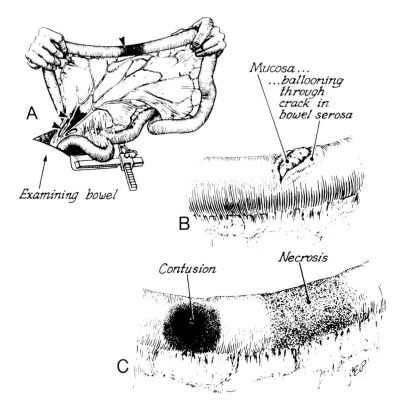

Figure 48.4.   A. This drawing demonstrates the need for complete examination of the intestine from the ligament of Treitz to the cecum. Specific areas of laceration within the mesentery should be searched for, and the relationship between the laceration and the vascular integrity of the bowel should be confirmed. **B.** Intestinal enterotomies or tears should be searched for and appropriately repaired. **C.** Areas of confusion and necrosis should be identified.

APPROPRIATE TREATMENT

Treatment for any evisceration through the vagina should start with pelvic laparotomy. Initial first aid upon discovering the evisceration should be the physiologic protection of the eviscerated loop of intestine by wrapping it in sterile saline-soaked gauze or a sterile towel. The patient should be taken to the operating room immediately, where an exploratory laparotomy through a midline incision should be done. A midline incision is emphasized because the author does not feel that the mesentery of the intestine can be inspected adequately through a Pfannenstiel incision. At the time of operation, the intestine should be carefully withdrawn through the defect, whether that be the perforated uterus or the vaginal cuff (Fig. 48.5). A complete inspection of the entire intestine and its mesentery from the ligament of Treitz to the cecum is indicated (Fig. 48.4A). The mesentery should be carefully inspected for lacerations and vascular injuries and hemostasis. Suspicious areas of intestine should be resected and reanastomosis performed (Fig. 48.6). If there have been extensive enterotomies in the large intestine with spillage of fecal material into the peritoneal cavity, primary closure should be avoided and the damaged segments of intestine should be exteriorized as the primary procedure. After

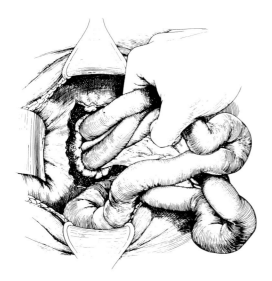

Figure 48.5. Drawing of pelvic laparotomy showing the replacement of the intestine back into the peritoneal cavity through the ruptured vaginal cuff surrounded by the torn peritoneal margins.

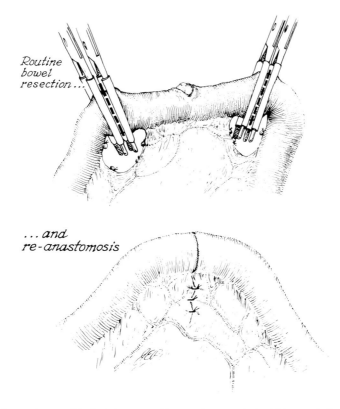

Routine bowel resection...

...and re-anastomosis

Figure 48.6. Areas of severe intestinal damage and/or vascular necrosis should be surgically resected and a reanastomosis performed.

appropriate healing has occurred, a second procedure 4 to 6 weeks later following a preoperatively prepared intestine can be performed for reconstruction of the bowel and takedown of any exteriorized intestine. There is no role for transvaginal replacement of the intestine into the abdominal cavity without laparotomy because of the possibility of lacerations in the mesentery and undetected injury to the small bowel. This is especially true when evisceration has occurred through the perforated uterus during the performance of a suction abortion. The suction curette could have damaged several pieces of small intestine other than the piece eviscerated through the uterine perforation. When the intestine has been appropriately replaced into the abdominal cavity and inspected carefully, and the damaged areas resected, the entire peritoneal cavity should be copiously lavaged with normal saline. A Salem pump nasogastric tube should be inserted into the stomach and left in place until the patient passes flatus or has a bowel movement. The hospitalization of all patients who have sustained enterotomy and probably the entire group of vaginal eviscerations should be covered with broad-spectrum antibiotics. Antimicrobial therapy should be guided by appropriate cultures taken at the time of laparotomy, but therapy should be directed toward the enteric organisms.

In those cases of evisceration associated with termination of pregnancy, it is vital to complete the termination of pregnancy as part of the repair procedure. All too often, in the panic of this unexpected and severe complication, attention is directed toward the intestinal problem and away from the potential severe complication of incomplete abortion with retained gestational contents. One solution to this problem is to have a second surgeon immediately perform laparoscopy through the umbilicus and guide the withdrawal of the suction cannula out of the peritoneal cavity and back into the endometrial cavity (Fig. 48.7), where the suction can be resumed and the termination of pregnancy completed (Fig. 48.8). Failure to do this leaves products of gestation within the endometrial cavity and creates potential for all the sequelae of incomplete abortion, that is, infection, hemorrhage, and so on.

Repair of the ruptured vagina or perforated uterus differs. The perforation site in the uterus can be closed with simple through-and-through sutures of absorbable material. However, in the case of the ruptured vagina, careful closure with a well-designed plan of ligament suspension and obliteration of the cul-de-sac should be made (Fig. 48.9). The suture material should be absorbable, and care should be made to reduce areas of necrosis to a minimum. The opening in the vagina should be excised back to fresh, healthy tissue. The vagina should then be closed with interrupted zero absorbable suture. A separate step to locate and suture the stumps of the uterosacral and cardinal ligaments to the angles of the vagina should be made (Fig. 48.9). In addition, the anterior surface of the rectosigmoid colon should be sutured to the posterior vaginal cuff to eliminate the cul-de-sac (Fig. 48.9). Complete resection should be made of all necrotic tissue along the vaginal cuff and stumps of the supporting ligaments. This is a particularly important step if fecal material has spilled into the peritoneal cavity. One should not be surprised at the development of a postoperative pelvic abscess if necrotic tissue that has been bathed in the intestinal contents is left within the pelvis postoperatively. Antibiotic therapy will not be sufficient to override this breach in surgical technique. The author advocates placing all of these patients on the "minidose" heparin schedule of 3000 to 5000 units of heparin subcutaneously twice a day. Those patients who do not have return of intestinal function within 3 to 4 days postoperatively should be given intravenous hyperalimentation. In many of the reported series in the literature, there has been prolonged ileus following

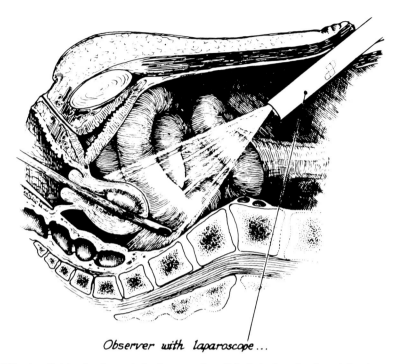

Observer with laparoscope...

Figure 48.7. A sagittal drawing demonstrating the prevention of intestinal evisceration through the uterus and vagina by performing a laparoscopy at the time of perforation of the uterus by the suction curette. The laparoscopist assists the surgeon by guiding the curette out of the peritoneal cavity and back into the endometrial cavity without sucking intestinal contents within the cannula.

vaginal evisceration. If the entire intestine has been completely explored and the surgeon is comfortable as to the vascular integrity of the intestine, prolonged ileus should be treated conservatively with nasogastric drainage and intravenous hyperalimentation. However, if the intestine has been replaced vaginally and there has not been adequate exploration of the intestine, the question of vascular integrity and necrosis of the bowel should be considered. Repeat laparotomy should be considered, and the vascular integrity of the bowel should be ensured.

Although evisceration of the small intestine through the vagina is an extremely serious event, patients have an excellent chance for recovery if intestinal necrosis and peritonitis have not occurred. Moreover, if proper closure of the vaginal vault with elimination of the cul-de-sac and careful approximation of the supporting ligaments to the angles of the vagina is made during the repair process, the likelihood of recurrence is quite small.

The average gynecologist may be in practice for a lifetime and never encounter a case of vaginal evisceration. Because of its rarity, it has been difficult for any one clinic to gain a large volume of experience in treating this phenomenon. Nevertheless, it seems logical to treat vaginal evisceration as one would treat abdominal evisceration following dehiscence of a postoperative abdominal incision. In treating evisceration of the

Figure 48.8. Sagittal drawing showing that once the suction cannula has been withdrawn into the endometrial cavity it is extremely important that the termination of pregnancy be completed. This step must be done even if intestinal contents have been pulled through the uterus and out into the vagina. It can be delayed until the intestine has been appropriately replaced into the peritoneal cavity through the laparotomy incision as shown in Figure 48.5 but must not be forgotten.

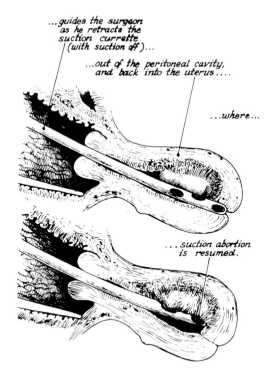

...guides the surgeon as he retracts the suction curette (with suction off)...

...out of the peritoneal cavity, and back into the uterus....

...where...

...suction abortion is resumed.

Figure 48.9. The *upper drawing* shows the repair of the ruptured vagina by suturing the vaginal cuff with a single through-and-through layer of no. 0 absorbable suture. Note that the uterosacral and cardinal ligaments have been identified and are specifically sutured to the angles of the vagina. Three separate rows of no. 0 absorbable suture are placed between the anterior surface of the rectosigmoid colon and the posterior vaginal wall and cuff to eliminate the cul-de-sac. These sutures are placed in a purse-string fashion. The *lower drawing* shows the completed repair with reperitonealization of the pelvis. A suction drain is placed adjacent to the repair.

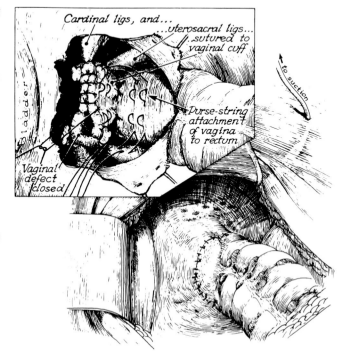

Cardinal ligs, and...

...uterosacral ligs... sutured to vaginal cuff

to suction

Bladder

Purse-string attachment of vagina to rectum

Vaginal defect closed

abdominal wall, the surgeon would never consider replacing the intestine through the traumatic abdominal opening or dehiscent wound without a thorough inspection of the peritoneal cavity. This same principle should be observed in vaginal evisceration.

REFERENCES

1. Fox WP: Vaginal evisceration. *Obstet Gynecol* 50:233, 1977.
2. Fox PF, Kowalczyk AS: Ruptured enterocele. *Am J Obstet Gynecol* 115:592, 1971.
3. Goss CM: The digestive system. In: Gray H (ed): *Anatomy of the Human Body*, ed. 28. Philadelphia, Lea & Febiger, 1972, chap. 16, p. 1230.
4. Hall BD, Phelan JP, Pruyn SC, et al: Vaginal evisceration during coitus. *Am J Obstet Gynecol* 141:115, 1978.
5. McNellis D, Torkelson L, McElin TW: Late postoperative vaginal vault disruption. *Am J Obstet Gynecol* 111:592, 1971.
6. Nichols DH, Randall CL: Complications of surgery. In: *Vaginal Surgery*, ed. 3. Baltimore, Williams & Wilkins, 1989.
7. Powell JL: Vaginal evisceration following vaginal hysterectomy. *Am J Obstet Gynecol* 115:276, 1973.
8. Rolf BB: Vaginal evisceration. *Am J Obstet Gynecol* 107:369, 1970.

49

Transvaginal Oophorectomy and Salpingo-Oophorectomy

David H. Nichols

Case Abstract

A 44-year-old multipara with a symptomatic second-degree prolapse of the uterus and coexistent cystocele and rectocele was admitted for vaginal hysterectomy and repair. Both her mother and sister had succumbed to ovarian cancer, and after some discussion, the patient requested that she receive oophorectomy simultaneously with vaginal hysterectomy. She was planning to start estrogen replacement postoperatively.

DISCUSSION

Possible oophorectomy coincident with hysterectomy should be given the same consideration whether the uterus has been just removed transabdominally or by the vaginal route (1,3–5). A decision concerning oophorectomy should be strongly influenced by the estimated risk-benefit ratio. Benefits favoring oophorectomy include potential for neoplastic ovarian disease, endometriosis, and the presumable lack of function in the postmenopausal ovary, whose very retention might increase the likelihood of subsequent ovarian cancer. Risks include the trauma of additional surgery embracing technical difficulties, intraoperative and postoperative hemorrhage, and also loss of ovarian function secondary to castration. Coincident oophorectomy through either the transvaginal or transabdominal preliminary exposure should be considered whenever the anticipated benefits outweigh the risks. An exception should be made in the case of suspected ovarian cancer, where oophorectomy should be performed only through the transabdominal exposure.

Salpingo-oophorectomy should be considered when the infundibulopelvic ligament is long. This is often the case when the uterus prior to hysterectomy has been prolapsed or retroverted. Salpingo-oophorectomy does, however, leave a raw intraperitoneal surface after ligation with the small risk of subsequent bowel adhesion to the raw area. This might precipitate a future volvulus or intestinal obstruction. Oophorectomy alone may be considered when the infundibulopelvic ligament is short, as transvaginal exposure of such an infundibulopelvic ligament may be difficult (6).

The ovary may be grasped with a sponge forceps and brought into the operative field, where the mesovarium can be clamped only under direct vision. Oophorectomy alone permits the tube and its mesosalpinx to fall over the raw area of the ligated mesosalpinx, lessening the chance of subsequent bowel adhesion in this area. When a benign neoplastic ovarian cyst is encountered, freely movable and without adhesions, the ovary should be removed intact, providing that the tumor is of such a size that it can pass unruptured through the vagina. When space is cramped, the mesovarium may be clamped between two forceps and cut and the forceps attached to the ovary used as a gentle handle to deliver the most narrow diameter of the ovary into the vagina. A larger neoplasm requires pelvic laparotomy. Trocar aspiration through the cyst wall to reduce the size should be used rarely and only when the cyst is unilocular, the wall nonpapillary, and the content serous-like. Spilling of cyst contents may soil the peritoneal cavity, risking possible implantation of even benign tumor cells, especially those of the mucinous cystadenoma.

The infundibulopelvic ligament or mesovarium should be securely ligated and under direct vision. Proximity of the ureter should be noted when transfixation ligatures are applied to the infundibulopelvic ligament (2). Ideally, the ligament or mesovarium should be penetrated only once to minimize the risk of slippage or hematoma (3). A useful stitch is shown in Figure 49.1. Polyglycolic acid suture, no. 0 or 00, is ideal (Dexon or Vicryl). When salpingo-oophorectomy is being contemplated, a stitch can be placed in the infundibulopelvic ligament by penetration with the Deschamps ligature carrier and tied. This provides penetration of the infundibulopelvic ligament by a blunt needle, lessening the chance of laceration of the ovarian artery. When the clamp or forceps is eliminated, the suture is placed farther away from the nearby ureter, lessening the chances of ligating or compromising its integrity. The suture may be tied in the same fashion illustrated in Figure 49.1, which minimizes slippage. The ovary and tube may then be cut free and removed from the operative field and a separate free tie applied to the infundibulopelvic ligament distal to the fixation stitch. Alternately, the infundibulopelvic ligament may be clamped as shown in Figure 49.2, the adnexa removed, and a fixation stitch placed as shown, which may be followed by a free tie to the ligament stump. Postoperative care should include careful observation for unexpected and concealed intraperitoneal bleeding, which, if significant, should make itself known by unexplained tachycardia or a postoperative fall in hemoglobin/hematocrit. Severe, steady suprapubic or lumbar pain or a palpable intra-abdominal mass is strongly suggestive of retroperitoneal hematoma, and prompt exploratory laparotomy should be anticipated. Estrogen supplementation may be considered, especially if the patient is sexually active and the hormone not medically contraindicated.

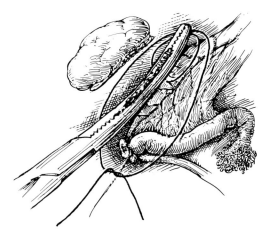

Figure 49.1. The entire mesovarium has been clamped by a Heaney-type forceps and the ovary cut free. The mesovarium is penetrated once through its midportion. Each end of the suture is passed around the tip of the forceps as shown and tied at the heel of the forceps, while the latter is being unlocked and slowly removed.

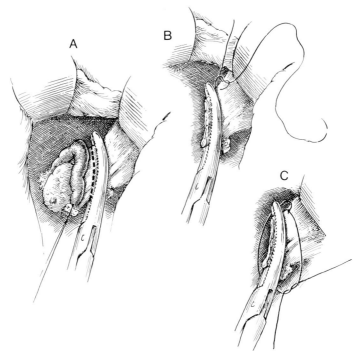

Figure 49.2.   A. The infundibulopelvic ligament is clamped. **B.** The adnexa are removed and a transfixion stitch anchored. **C.** The stitch is tied. (Reprinted with permission from Nichols DH, Randall CL: *Vaginal Surgery*, ed. 3. Baltimore, Williams & Wilkins, 1989.)

If one is preoperatively contemplating oophorectomy, it is well to obtain the patient's permission for this ahead of time; always disclose to the patient postoperatively what was done during surgery.

When considering coincidental elective oophorectomy, one should ask whether it appears that the patient will likely benefit from this procedure or whether circumstances exist under which the need and desirability of subsequent oophorectomy are likely. If the decision has been made to consider oophorectomy or salpingo-oophorectomy, one should assess the technical aspect of the particular problem and determine its feasibility and safety.

Laparoscopically Assisted Vaginal Hysterectomy (LAVH)

Coincident translaparoscopic oophorectomy or salpingo-oophorectomy may be performed by the experienced endoscopic surgeon using endoscopic coagulation, the endoloop, or endoscopically applied staples. Translaparoscopic transection of the infundibulopelvic ligament can precede vaginal hysterectomy and the adnexa removed with the surgical specimen. Because of the extra-operative time involved, this adds to the expense and imposes the risks of the extra procedure, often scheduled as a LAVH.

If there has been a uterine retroversion, the infundibulopelvic ligament has probably elongated, bringing the ovary closer to the vaginal operative field and making transvaginal oophorectomy technically easy. If no uterine retroversion preceded surgery, the surgeon should anticipate no elongation of the infundibulopelvic ligament and expect to find the ovaries higher within the pelvis.

In the interest of cost containment and effectiveness the surgeon has the option of doing the vaginal hysterectomy first and seeing if at that time the ovaries can be safely removed transvaginally (as will be demonstrated in the majority of patients), avoiding the expense and risk of laparoscopy. If they cannot safely be removed transvaginally, and the patient strongly desires that they be extirpated, this can be accomplished by transabdominal laparoscopy at the conclusion of the hysterectomy, after the peritoneal cavity has been closed or the vagina obturated (vaginal hysterectomy laparoscopically assisted (VHLA)).

One must remember that although bilateral oophorectomy reduces the likelihood of developing subsequent ovarian carcinoma, it does not eliminate completely the chance of future development of this disease. There are a number of instances in which following oophorectomy the patient developed an abdominal malignant disease histologically indistinguishable from ovarian carcinoma, the tumor having possibly arisen in some ovarian rest tissue not occupying the exact position of the ovary. For this reason the surgeon should assure a patient that ovarian cancer is much less likely to develop following oophorectomy, but one should never promise or guarantee that the patient will never in the future develop postoophorectomy "ovarian" cancer, for if the patient does, the surgeon might be held liable for breach of contract should litigation arise.

If it appears that transvaginal oophorectomy or salpingo-oophorectomy can be performed safely and under direct vision, it should be done. Should surgical exposure present a serious problem, there is no place for risky surgical acrobatics.

REFERENCES

1. Funt MI, Benigno BB, Thompson JD: The residual adnexa: Asset or liability? *Am J Obstet Gynecol* 129:251, 1977.
2. Hofmeister FJ, Wolfgram RC: Methods of demonstrating measurement relationships between vaginal hysterectomy ligatures and the ureters. *Am J Obstet Gynecol* 83:938, 1962.
3. Nichols DH: A technique for vaginal oophorectomy. *Surg Gynecol Obstet* 147:765, 1978.
4. Nichols DH, Randall CL: *Vaginal Surgery*, ed. 3. Baltimore, Williams & Wilkins, 1989.
5. Ramney B, Abu-Ghazaleh S: The future function and fortune of ovarian tissue which is retained in vivo during hysterectomy. *Am J Obstet Gynecol* 128:626, 1977.
6. Wright RC: Vaginal oophorectomy. *Am J Obstet Gynecol* 120:759, 1974.

50

Anterior Vaginal Wall Prolapse After Cystectomy

William J. Hoskins

Case Abstract

A female infant born with exstrophy of the bladder underwent bilateral ureterosigmoid-ostomy for urinary diversion at age 1 year. This was later followed by transvaginal cystourethrectomy. At age 22 years, the patient delivered a normal infant vaginally after an uncomplicated antepartum course. One month postpartum there was a marked prolapse of the anterior vaginal wall. This progressed, and at examination 1 month later, a mass including the uterus protruded beyond the vulva and was a source of discomfort to the patient.

DISCUSSION

When the cloaca fails to close anteriorly in the developing embryo the resulting defect is called exstrophy of the bladder (from Greek meaning "to turn out"). The occurrence of bladder exstrophy is reported to be 1 in 30,000 to 40,000 live births and is five times more common in males than in females (3,7). The anterior wall of the bladder, the urinary sphincter, urethra, pubic arch, and lower abdominal wall are absent to varying degrees. In the female, there is often abnormally wide separation of the labia and a cleft clitoris. The separation of the pubic bones often leads to a waddling gait when the child begins to walk. This instability of gait rarely persists into adult life. With early involvement of expert urologic, orthopedic, and plastic surgical treatment, approximately one-third of these patients may have surgical closure of the defect and retain urinary continence. Closure is usually effected in stages, including osteotomy to provide firm pubic apposition, bladder closure, reconstruction of the external genitalia, and bladder neck reconstruction.

When closure is not possible, urinary diversion and excision of the bladder and urethra are carried out. Although abdominal closure can usually be accomplished without osteotomy, this procedure will usually result in a better anatomic result. Genital reconstruction is performed as a later procedure. Historically, direct ureterocolonic anastomosis was the method of choice in urinary diversion for bladder exstrophy; but ascending infections, colonic stenosis, and acidosis are frequent complications. Ideal conduit diversion in the young child is also associated with many long-term complications. One good alternative appears to be formation of a nonrefluxing sigmoid conduit with external drainage for 4 to 5 years followed by colosigmoid anastomosis of the conduit to the rectosigmoid.

Modern surgical techniques in the management of bladder exstrophy have resulted in females reaching adulthood with intact reproductive organs. Gynecologic problems that such patients are prone to develop are (1) uterine descensus with procidentia and (b) anterior vaginal wall defects. Although reports are rare, Damm (1) reported a case of uterine prolapse following a vaginal cesarean section in a patient with a dead fetus and 50 hours of obstructed labor. This patient had undergone excision of the bladder exstrophy at age 2 years. DeCarle, in a discussion of a case presentation by Overstreet and Hinman (5), presented two additional cases of uterine prolapse following vaginal delivery in patients who had undergone excision of bladder exstrophy and recommended that these patients be delivered by classical cesarean section to prevent postpartum genital prolapse.

When considering how to effect surgical repair of a patient as described in the abstract, three factors must be considered: (a) Does the patient desire to retain childbearing capacity? (b) Should repair be accomplished via an abdominal or a vaginal approach? (c) Should one suspend the genitalia anteriorly or posteriorly? Factors a and b are closely related because the applicability of a vaginal approach would be dependent on the patient not wanting to preserve childbearing. If such was the case, vaginal hysterectomy with sacrospinous suspension of the vaginal vault according to the method of Randall and Nichols (6) would be the procedure of choice. The anterior vaginal defect could then be excised and closed. If the perineal body (as is often the case in these patients) is particularly broad, a relaxing perineoplasty might be helpful. This method of repair has the distinct advantage of avoiding an abdominal operation in a patient who probably has extensive scarring and where extensive pelvic dissection might disrupt function of the ureterosigmoid anastomosis.

If the patient desires to retain childbearing function, it is unlikely that repair can be effected by the vaginal approach alone. In this case, one must decide whether to perform an anterior suspension of the vagina and uterus or to choose some form of sacropexy (2). An anterior approach has the advantage of avoiding the ureterosigmoid anastomotic sites and, in addition, would place the suspended uterus between the weak anterior vagina and the direction of intra-abdominal pressure. The author recommends a Pfannenstiel incision with mobilization of an inferior strip of aponeurotic fascia 1 to 2 cm in width and as long as the incision (Fig. 50.1). These fascial strips could then be tunneled through the internal inguinal ring beside the ligament and retroperitoneally to the lower uterine segment and upper portion of the cervix. These should be sutured under tension anteriorly with interrupted nonabsorbable sutures so as to elevate and bring forward the cervix and uterus (Fig. 50.2). Excess anterior vaginal tissue should be excised approximately in the midline, or this portion of the operation could be performed by a vaginal approach. Anterior suspension of the uterus could be accomplished in a variety of ways. If the round ligaments are normal in size and not attenuated (as is often the case in patients with exstrophy), a modified Gilliam suspension should be performed (Fig. 50.2).

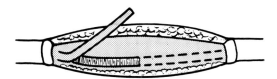

Figure 50.1. A Pfannenstiel incision has been made and a strip of aponeurotic fascia 1.5 cm wide and 8 cm long has been mobilized.

Figure 50.2.   A. A modified Gilliam suspension has been performed to support the fundus of the uterus. **B.** Aponeurotic fascial strips have been utilized to support the lower uterine segment.

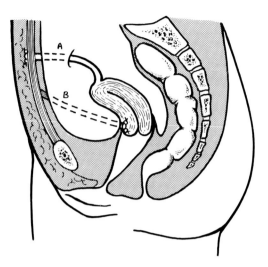

If the round ligaments are attenuated, a separate fascial strip from the upper portion of the aponeurotic fascia can be used to suspend the fundus of the uterus anteriorly, or one can suture the fundus directly to the anterior abdominal wall. Of the above methods of suspending the fundus of the uterus, the modified Gilliam suspension would be the least likely to be disrupted by pregnancy because the round ligaments will stretch when the uterus enlarges.

The second option for suspension of the genitalia involves some type of sacropexy (2,4). This operation is performed by suturing a strip of nonabsorbable material to the posterior vagina and lower uterine segment. The supporting strip is then tunneled retroperitoneally on the right side of the rectum and sutured to the periosteum of the sacrum. A variety of synthetic mesh materials as well as fascial strips can be utilized to suspend the genitalia. The advantage of this type of suspension is that the normal axis of the vagina is maintained and the resulting suspension is very durable. Two major disadvantages in this patient would be the danger of disrupting the ureterosigmoid anastomoses and the absence of the uterus anteriorly, which would predispose the patient to recurrence of the anterior vaginal prolapse secondary to the force of intra-abdominal vaginal pressure. In addition, the fixation of the uterus posteriorly might result in compromise of the urinary diversion when the uterus enlarges in pregnancy.

When all options are considered, the best procedures are vaginal hysterectomy and sacrospinous ligament suspension in the patient who does not desire childbearing, and anterior abdominal suspension in those patients who desire to retain childbearing capacity. In any case, a relaxing perineoplasty should be performed, if necessary, to retain or improve coital function. Should the patient become pregnant, cesarean section at term is the preferable method of delivery to avoid disruption of the surgical repair.

REFERENCES

1. Damm PN: Geburt bei spathecken. *Zentralb J Gynok* 61:440, 1937.
2. Hendee AI, Berry CM: Abdominal sacropexy for vaginal vault prolapse. *Clin Obstet Gynecol* 24:217, 1942.

3. Jeffs RD: Exstrophy and clinical exstrophy. In: Whitehead ED, Leiter I (eds): *Current Operative Urology*. Philadelphia, Harper & Row, 1984.
4. Käser O, Iklé FA, Hirsch HA: *Atlas of Gynecological Surgery*, ed. 2. New York, Thieme-Stratton, 1985.
5. Overstreet EW, Hinman P Jr: Some gynecologic aspects of bladder exstrophy. *West J Surg* 64:131, 1956.
6. Randall CL, Nichols DH: Surgical treatment of vaginal inversion. *Obstet Gynecol* 38:327, 1971.
7. Winter CC, Goodwin WE: Malformation of the urinary bladder. In Karafin L, Kindall AR (eds): *Urology*. Hagerstown, MD, Harper & Row, 1974.

51

Posterior Colporrhaphy — Lost Needle

Robert F. Porges

Case Abstract

A posterior colporrhaphy and perineorrhaphy were being accomplished following vaginal hysterectomy and anterior colporrhaphy upon a married 52-year-old multipara. The technique being used included "levator" stitches intended to bring the medial bellies of the pubococcygei together between the vagina and the rectum. As a deep levator stitch was placed, an audible "snap" was heard, and it was discovered that the swaged-on needle had been broken at its midpoint, and the missing needle segment was no longer visible. Although the fractured end of the missing segment could be initially felt but not visualized, additional palpation pushed it deeper within the substance of the muscles to a point where it could no longer be palpated.

DISCUSSION

Every effort must be made to retrieve the end of the broken needle, the length of which can easily be determined by comparison with a similar needle to the one having been passed.

Anatomy

In Figure 51.1, the relationship of the medial border of the levator muscle to the rectum is shown clearly. The posterior aspect of the medial border of the levator muscle hugs the wall of the rectum several centimeters above the anal sphincter. The levator muscle and the vagina intersect obliquely, rather than perpendicularly, resulting in a more distal intersection between the anterior wall of the vagina and the levator muscle.

The rationale for the placement of sutures into the levator muscle is to bring the muscle bundles anterior to the rectum, thereby reducing the dimensions of the genital hiatus both anteroposteriorly and laterally. Usually one does not see as much of the muscle within the operative field as is shown in Fig. 51.1. In those elderly women who stand to gain the most from posterior repair, the fibers of the levator muscle often will be attenuated and set far laterally, resulting in a very wide genital hiatus.

Technique of Posterior Colporrhaphy

Although individual surgical preferences may vary, usually, following triangular denudation of the distal portion of the posterior wall of the vagina and portion of the

222

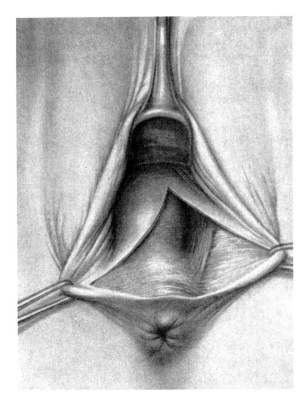

Figure 51.1. The relationship of the medial border of the levator muscle to the levator is shown. (Reproduced with permission from Halban J: *Gynäkologische Operationslehre.* Vienna, Urban & Schwarzenberg, 1932.)

perineum (Fig. 51.2), the pelvic urogenital diaphragm is incised on each side to provide access to the levator muscle. The levator muscle may be identified by its tone and the direction of the muscle fibers, which span in an anteroposterior direction and may be palpated readily from the inferior border of the pubic ramus medially to the arcus tendineus more posteriorly. Some surgeons grasp the levator muscle with an Allis clamp, pulling it into the operative field and making it more accessible for placement of the suture. The disadvantage of the Allis clamp is that it traumatizes the delicate muscle fibers and often results in some bleeding from the border of the muscle. Other surgeons dig the needle directly into the depth of the muscle and pull the muscle medially and more superficially into the operative field. It is just this maneuver that may cause the needle to snap if the traction on the muscle is not exactly along the course of the curve of the needle. One or two, seldom three, sutures are usually sufficient for the levator muscle.

PREVENTION

The operator should use a large, fairly thick needle with swaged-on no. 0 Dexon or an equivalent suture. Instead of pulling the bulk of the muscle medially with the needle, he or she should push the index finger against the rectal wall medial to the

Figure 51.2. Triangular denudation of the distal posterior vaginal wall and postion of the perineum. (Levator muscle to the levator is shown.) (Reproduced with permission from Halban J: *Gynäkologische Operationslehre.* Vienna, Urban & Schwarzenberg, 1932.)

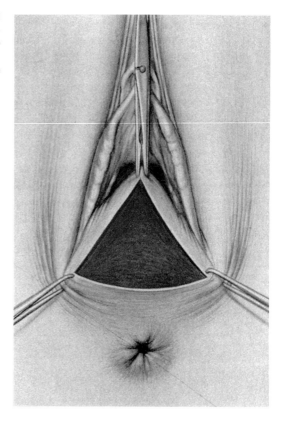

levator muscle so that the needle will be passed into a free space, only deeper in the operative field. The needle should always be passed in a path corresponding to its own curve. One must not invent a new curve for the needle with one's own wrist. The cervix is another area in gynecologic surgery where, if the needle is not passed exactly in its own curve, it may snap.

How to Find the Needle

Normally, the needle holder will grasp the needle at the three-quarter:one-quarter junction so that if the needle does break it will be likely to do so halfway between the needle tip and the needle holder, leaving a substantial length of needle fragment within the tissues.

Many operating rooms have some form of metal detector, and ophthalmologists occasionally use powerful magnets to retrieve metal from the eye. If these instruments are available they may be found useful. The most practical way to retrieve the needle is to probe for it with a tonsil clamp, using the digit of the other hand in back of the levator muscle as a baffle.

Occasionally, a clue to the location of the needle may be obtained by placing a finger into the rectum. If this fails, then sutures should be placed above and below the site of needle passage for traction and hemostasis. The portion of the muscle between these sutures may even be excised. In unusual circumstances, a Schuchardt incision may provide better access to the levator muscle directly and assist in the retrieval of the broken needle.

SELECTED READINGS

Halban J: *Gynäkologische Operationslehre*. Vienna, Urban & Schwarzenberg, 1932.

52

Mass in the Lateral Wall of the Vagina

Winfred L. Wiser

Case Abstract

A 16-year-old nulligravid patient who had been regularly menstruating for 3 years was troubled by increasing dysmenorrhea and a persistent intermenstrual dark bloody discharge. Although the uterus appeared to be of normal size, pelvic examination was somewhat difficult to perform. It was determined that there was a mass distending the full lateral wall of the left side of the vagina. The mass measured approximately 3 cm in diameter and appeared to be cystic, although the mass was tense. Careful examination revealed a pin-hole-size opening in the lateral vaginal wall about 3 cm cranial to the hymenal ring, and pressure on the mass expressed some dark mahogany discharge through the opening.

DISCUSSION

There are a few cases of lateral vaginal wall masses. A differential diagnosis must include the following:

1. Obstructed hemivagina
2. Mesonephric, paramesonephric, and urogenital sinus cysts
3. Leiomyoma
4. Vaginal adenosis
5. Vaginal hematoma
6. Advanced vaginal malignancy

The patient described above demonstrates the diagnostic dilemma of the lateral vaginal mass. Her history and physical findings are highly suggestive of failure of lateral fusion and central canalization of müllerian ducts, which results in a double uterus, a patent vagina, and an obstructed hemivagina. If this diagnosis is correct, she will likely have ipsilateral absence of the kidney (Fig. 52.1).

Mesonephric cysts are found along the route of the Gartner's ducts. Paramesonephric cysts occur at any point in the vaginal wall; urogenital sinus cysts arise in the vestibule. These embryonic cysts are seldom symptomatic.

Leiomyomas most frequently occur in the anterior wall of the vagina but may be found along the lateral vaginal wall. They may extend cephalad into the hollow of the sacrum and vary in consistency from firm to semicystic. The predominant symptom is the sensation of partial vaginal obstruction.

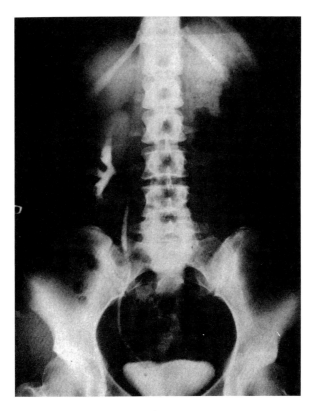

Figure 52.1.   IVP — unilateral absence of kidney and collecting system.

The woman with a traumatic vaginal hematoma will give a history of recent trauma or vaginal delivery.

Lateral vaginal fusion defects are associated most frequently with a uterus didelphys. However, they may be associated with a bicornuate or septate uterus. The hemivagina may be completely or partially obstructed. The point of obstruction may vary from low in the vagina to near the corpus of the uterus (Fig. 52.2). With incomplete obstruction, a fistula may occur at any point in the vaginal septum, or there may be lateral communication with the double uterus usually at the cervix.

Symptoms and physical findings correlate with the degree of obstruction (i.e., complete or incomplete obstruction), the location of the obstruction, and the presence or absence of a communicating fistula.

Symptoms in women with complete obstruction are progressive, severe dysmenorrhea with intermittent episodes of intermenstrual, lower abdominal aching pain; this pain usually begins 1 to 2 years following menarche. These women have a normal menarche, regular menstrual cycles, and occasional premenstrual spotting. They always present with a bulging lateral mass (Fig. 52.3). Women who have incomplete vaginal obstruction present with lower abdominal pain and moderate-to-severe dysmenorrhea. In addition, they have an intermittent, foul-smelling, mucopurulent discharge, and a

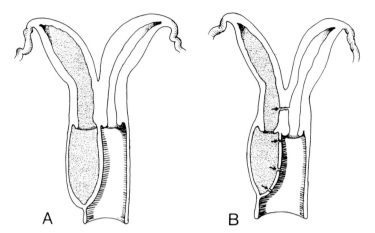

Figure 52.2.   **A.** Double uterus, double vagina with complete obstruction, hematocolpos, hematometra on one side. **B.** Double uterus, double vagina with incomplete obstruction of hemivagina.

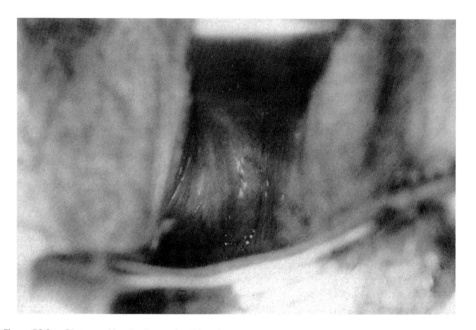

Figure 52.3.   Obstructed hemivagina on the right side with bulging hematocolpos.

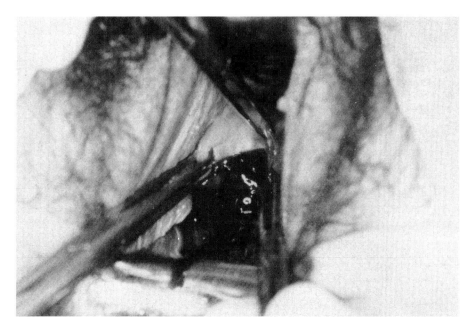

Figure 52.4.   Incision through wall of obstructed hemivagina. Old blood from hematocolpos.

history of polymenorrhea with irregular staining between menses. An ill-defined or recurring mass may be found on physical examination. A pelvic abscess in the obstructed
vagina may be the presenting sign in some women, but it is more common in those women
with a very small connecting fistula where a previous attempt at dilatation of the fistula has
been made.

The diagnosis of this problem requires a high degree of suspicion. Palpation
of a cystic mass in the lateral vaginal wall, a tender pelvic mass, and/or visualization of old
blood coming from the lateral vaginal wall should increase suspicion of an obstructed
hemivagina. A hysterosalpinogram is helpful if there is a lateral communication at the
level of the cervix. In the completely obstructed hemivagina, a hysterosalpingogram may
be useful to define what appears to be a normal unicornuate uterus on the side opposite
the mass. An intravenous pyelogram (IVP) revealing ipsilateral absence of the kidney
increases the likelihood of diagnosis. Aspiration of old blood from the mass in complete
obstruction completes the diagnosis.

Treatment is simple. A large window is made between the two vaginas by
excising a portion of the thick-walled septum. Because the septum is thick, the surgeon
may be somewhat apprehensive in making the initial entry into the blind pouch. When the
obstruction is complete, manifested by a bulging mass, an incision can be easily made over
the mass. Placing a needle into the hematocolpos is helpful in establishing the optimal site
of the incision. When a fistula is present between the two vaginal canals, a small probe
with a hook can be passed through the fistula and traction applied toward the midline. An
incision can then be made in the septum with relative ease (Fig. 52.4). The mucosa of the

blind vaginal pouch is velvety smooth and glistening in appearance. The vaginal cavity and uterus should not be irrigated since irrigation increases the chance of pelvic infection. Once a window—which is large enough to prevent stricture—has been made, interrupted hemostatic sutures of no. 3–0 chromic catgut are placed in its circumference (Fig. 52.5).

The most common error in management of the obstructed hemivagina is failure to make the correct diagnosis before initiating a treatment regimen. The patient is frequently subjected to an abdominal exploration. The surgeon finds a double uterus with one side enlarged with a hematometra. The mass below the uterus extends to the pelvic floor. The hematometra should not be drained through the uterine fundus. The abdomen should be closed and a vaginal window made from below.

In the completely obstructed hemivagina, the epithelium is always composed of cuboidal cells, whereas the incomplete obstructed canal will be lined with squamous cells. When the canal is lined with cuboidal cells, a period of 2 to 3 years may be required for the metaplastic process to produce a squamous cell lining. Therefore, following creation of a vaginal window, these patients are likely to have a profuse, water-like discharge for months, until a squamous epithelium has replaced the cuboidal epithelium.

Reproduction, following treatment of unneglected cases, appears to be approximately the same as that in women with the equivalent uterine deformity but without an obstructed vagina. Pelvic endometriosis may result if the obstruction is not recognized and treated early. The incidence of endometriosis, however, is more common in the duplicated uterus without vaginal obstruction.

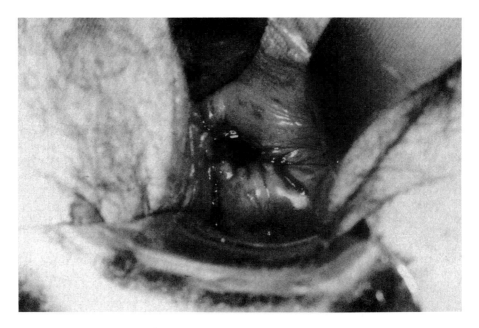

Figure 52.5.   Window completed between obstructed vagina and normal vagina.

SELECTED READINGS

Jones HW Jr: Reproductive impairment and malformed uterus. *Fertil Steril* 36:137, 1981.

Jones HW Jr, Wheeless CR: Salvage of the reproductive potential of women with anomalous development of the müllerian ducts: 1868–1968–2068. *Am J Obstet Gynecol* 104:348, 1968.

Rock JA, Jones HW Jr: The double uterus associated with an obstructed hemivagina and ipsilateral renal agenesis. *Am J Obstet Gynecol* 138:339, 1980.

Yoder IC, Pfister RC: Unilateral hematocolpos and ipsilateral renal agenesis: Report of two cases and review of the literature. *AJR* 127:303, 1976.

53

Wolffian Duct Cyst at the Vaginal Vault

Ricardo M. Azziz
Lisa A. Peacock
John A. Rock

Case Abstract

A 3-cm cyst on the right side of the vaginal vault of a 23-year-old patient had become a source of dyspareunia. The cyst with its lining was surgically excised by sharp dissection. Because of some troublesome oozing at the base of the cavity from which the cyst had been removed, several figure-of-eight sutures using no. 0 chromic were placed, effectively controlling the bleeding. On the morning of the second postoperative day, the patient called complaining of severe backache. By that afternoon, the pain appeared to be concentrated in the right costovertebral angle. The patient felt anorexic and nauseated. The following morning the abdomen was distended with minimal bowel sounds. The temperature rose to 38.7°C. A urinalysis revealed 1+ hematuria, with occasional WBCs and bacteria. The blood count revealed a WBC of 12,300 per ml with a left shift and a hematocrit of 36%.

DISCUSSION

The differential diagnosis in this case should include unilateral ureteral obstruction with superimposed pyelonephritis, simple pyelonephritis, acute appendicitis, or intrapelvic abscess. Physical examination findings may be similar in all four diagnoses. With appendicitis, however, there may be greater rebound and tenderness to palpation over McBurney's point, although this is not always true with a displaced or retrocecal appendix. Urinalysis will be negative in 90% of surgical injuries to the ureter; however, hematuria may be present secondary to bladder manipulation and catheterization.

Postoperative ureteral obstruction is usually secondary to ligation or to acute angulation from a suture placed in the periureteral tissue. Rarely, it may also be the result of transection or resection of a segment of ureter. In addition, progressive ureteral edema and inflammation can convert a partial occlusion to a complete obstruction. Alternatively, a stitch placed directly through the ureter will not commonly produce obstruction, but may result in fistula formation.

An intravenous pyelogram (IVP) should be performed as soon as a ureteral obstruction is suspected. With complete occlusion, the kidney will continue to excrete urine for days to months, albeit at a decreased rate. The ureter will become distended, and renal blood flow and glomerular filtration will decrease. Since iodinated contrast medium is heavier than urine, the most dependent portion of the obstruction will opacify first. In the event of nonvisualization, higher doses of radio-opaque medium and repeat films taken up to 24 hours later should be employed. Approximately 10 days after complete ureteral obstruction, the kidney ceases to filter enough contrast material to produce a urogram. Nevertheless, in these cases, a tubular nephrogram may still be seen. If the IVP is not diagnostic, real-time ultrasonography will usually reveal the dilated and tortuous obstructed renal tract. Injection of iodinated contrast dye can then be achieved either percutaneously (antegrade pyelography) or through cystoscopically placed ureteral stents (retrograde pyelography), thereby precisely locating the site of obstruction.

Management

Once the diagnosis of ureteral obstruction is made, the operator must (a) assess bilateral renal function, (b) treat any infectious process, (c) drain the affected kidney, and (d) restore normal urinary flow.

Because of the high iodine concentration in contrast material used to illuminate the renal tract, the sole presence of a tubular nephrogram does not necessarily reflect adequate parenchymal function. In this situation, a radionucleotide scan can provide important prognostic information relating to cortical blood flow and subsequent renal function. Experimental evidence in dogs indicates that irreversible vascular damage to the kidneys occurs 30 to 40 days after complete ureteral ligation. Nevertheless, there are isolated reports in humans of full renal recovery up to 12 weeks after occlusion. In the present case good return of renal function can be expected if the obstruction is promptly relieved. The serum creatinine, blood urea nitrogen, and electrolytes should be carefully followed.

Concurrent pyelonephritis places the patient at risk for septic shock and can aggravate existing renal damage. In addition, surgical repair of the obstructed ureter can become more technically difficult with a higher risk of failure and fistula formation. Pending urine culture and sensitivity results, either a second-generation cephalosporin or a broad-spectrum semisynthetic penicillin administered intravenously will provide appropriate coverage with minimal side effects. Although 70% of the antibiotics mentioned are excreted unchanged into the urine, the dosage requires adjustment for impaired renal clearance, as demonstrated by the serum creatinine. Patients with unilateral obstruction will usually have a normal creatinine clearance if the unobstructed kidney is healthy. In addition to antibiotic therapy, drainage of the affected kidney will dramatically aid the resolution of infection.

Alternative methods for drainage of the obstruction and restoration of urinary flow include (a) simple deligation, (b) ureteral or nephrostomy stent placement, with or without deligation (and possible later repair), and (c) immediate surgical intervention.

A cystoscopically placed ureteral stent (size 5 or 6 French, silastic) permits drainage of the infected urine if the stent can be passed into the renal pelvis beyond the obstruction. In a small number of patients, the ureteral occlusion will resolve spontaneously and without sequelae as the misguided suture dissolves. The stent should remain in place for a minimum of 10 to 14 days, secured to a transurethral Foley catheter. In the majority of cases in which the offending suture remains in situ, a ureteral stricture will form independent of the type of suture or stent used. Later surgical repair or transureteral dilation may be required. Unfortunately, because of the associated edema and inflammation of the bladder mucosa, visualization of the ureteral stent is sometimes impossible. Attempts to cannulate the obstructed ureter should therefore be performed judiciously, since the risk of ureteral perforation in these circumstances may be high, and perforation can result in the formation of a retroperitoneal urinoma and abscess.

If the ureter cannot be cannulized beyond the obstruction, percutaneous nephrostomy should be performed under radiographic or sonographic guidance. Under no circumstances should the kidney remain obstructed. Drainage should be continued for 6 weeks to 3 months while the patient unfortunately carries with her a constant reminder of the complication. As stated before, the ureteral occlusion will sometimes resolve spontaneously, although a residual stricture usually will persist.

In view of the high incidence of ureteral stricture when the stitch is left in situ, deligation should be attempted. In dogs, if the suture is removed within the first week of obstruction, the majority of cases resolve without sequelae. With removal between 7 and 14 days, full recovery occurs in 50%. If the deligation occurs after 2 weeks of occlusion, most ureters demonstrate a persistent mild to moderate pyelocaliectasis. In the present case, a deligation attempt should be attempted transvaginally. Removal of the sutures 48 hours after surgery will not usually disrupt the hemostasis achieved; nevertheless, exposure will be difficult and the tissues will be very friable. Concomitant cystoscopic stenting of the ureter may assist in identification and repair of the obstruction. Finally, great care must be taken not to induce further damage to the ureter during attempts at deligation or repair.

After successful deligation, follow-up IVP studies should be performed at regular intervals, because the development of a stricture or fistula has been observed up to 1 year later. If a fistula develops or a stricture is unresponsive to transureteral dilation, delayed surgical repair of the ureter is required. Surgical repair should be performed no earlier than 6 weeks, and preferably at 3 months, from the original operative procedure. In the case presented, with the occlusion so near to the ureterovesical junction, the preferred method of repair would be a ureteroneocystotomy, with or without a bladder flap or psoas hitch procedure.

As previously noted, convention has dictated that surgical reconstruction of the injured ureter be delayed for several weeks to allow resolution of the edema and inflammation, which may make repair both technically difficult and prone to failure and fistulization. Alternatively, several reports have indicated that early repair may be technically easier because of the lack of dense fibrosis, resulting in good repairs with minimal failures or residual sequelae. Therefore, in the young, healthy patient without extensive induration or infection, immediate repair may be considered as early as 10 to 14 days after obstruction. In general, early aggressive reconstruction with resection of the damaged segment is indicated if the obstruction is recognized within 72 hours of surgery. Because the patient presented with acute pyelonephritis, however, such an approach would not be advisable.

Prevention

As the ureter passes underneath the uterine artery and through the cardinal ligament, it curves caudally, anteriorly, and medially, forming what is known as the ureteral "knee." The portion of ureter caudad to the uterine artery averages 1.9 cm in length, of which the majority is transvesical in location. The ureteral knee is located from

0.8 to 2.5 cm lateral to the cervix, approximately 1.2 cm cephalad to the lateral vaginal vault, and 1.8 cm medial to the ischial spine. As the ureter enters the base of the bladder, it lies approximately 1 cm above the anterior vaginal fornix.

In this patient, the anatomy was distorted by a Wolffian duct cyst present in the vaginal vault. Gartner duct cysts are dilations of Wolffian remnants composed of a single layer of cuboidal or columnar cells overlying a thin smooth muscle coat. They may be multiple and are generally found lateral to the uterus, cervix, and vagina. They may be found within the broad ligament, extending downward and anteriorly between the bladder, cervix, and vagina, or they may appear in the lateral vaginal vault as asymptomatic submucosal cysts.

When removing these cysts, the operator must remember that Gartner duct cysts, unless very superficial, are extremely difficult to excise completely. Their close proximity to the cervical and vaginal branches of the uterine and vesical arteries and their possible extension deep into the parametria can create a situation in which hemorrhage is difficult to control. Partial resection with marsupialization to the vaginal mucosa will usually be sufficient to alleviate symptoms. Bleeding during this procedure arises from the cut surfaces of the vaginal mucosa and may be controlled with a continuous running-lock suture or interrupted sutures which include only the mucosa and underlying fascia.

A cyst at the base of the broad ligament and upper vaginal vault may displace the ureter medially toward the cervix. Downward and lateral traction on the cervix during the procedure may further displace the ureter medially and downward toward the vaginal vault, where it can be readily ligated by a misplaced suture. In order to identify the course of the ureter preoperatively, an IVP may illuminate any medial displacement due to the mass effect of the cyst. In addition, at the conclusion of the operative procedure ureteral patency can be readily confirmed by the intravenous administration of 3 to 5 cc of a chromogen (e.g., indigo-carmine or methylene blue) and cystoscopy some 5 to 10 minutes later. Cystoscopic visualization of the efflux of dye from both ureteral orifices, after instillation of 100 to 200 cc of sterile saline into the bladder, confirms bilateral ureteral patency. Ultimately, prevention of a ureteral injury is best achieved by a heightened awareness of the presence of the ureter, thorough knowledge of the anatomy involved, and careful assessment of any concurrent distortions.

SELECTED READINGS

Bright TC, Peters PC: Ureteral injuries secondary to operative procedures. *Urology* 9:22, 1977.

Brubaker LT, Wilbanks GD: Urinary tract injuries in pelvic surgery. *Surg Clin North Am* 71:963, 1991.

Gurin JI, Garcia RL, Melman A, Leiter E: The pathologic effect of ureteral ligation, with clinical implications. *J Urol* 128:1404, 1982.

Hoch WH, Kursh ED, Persky L: Early, aggressive management of intraoperative ureteral injuries. *J Urol* 114:530, 1975.

Pearse HD, Barry JM, Fuchs E: Intraoperative consultation for the ureter. *Urol Clin North Am* 12:423, 1985.

Raney AM: Ureteral trauma: Effects of ureteral ligation with and without deligation-experimental studies and case reports. *J Urol* 119:326, 1978.

Reisman DD, Kamholz JH, Kantor HI: Early deligation of the ureter. *J Urol* 78:363, 1957.

St. Lezin MA, Stoller ML: Surgical ureteral injuries. *Urology* 38:497, 1991.

Smith AD: Percutaneous nephrostomy and insertion of nephrostomy tubes and ureteral stents. In: Kaye KW (ed): *Outpatient Urologic Surgery.* Philadelphia, Lea & Febiger, 1985, pp. 131–144.

Stanhope CR, Wilson TO, Utz WJ, Smith LH, O'Brien PC: Suture entrapment and secondary ureteral obstruction. *Am J Obstet Gynecol* 164:1513, 1991.

Tarkington MA, Dejter SW, Bresette JF: Early surgical management of extensive gynecologic ureteral injuries. *Surg Gynecol Obstet* 173:17, 1991.

Thompson JD: Operative injuries to the ureter: Prevention, recognition, and management. In: Thompson JD, Rock JA (eds): *TeLinde's Operative Gynecology,* ed. 7. Philadelphia, JB Lippincott, 1992, pp. 749–783.

Toporoff B, Sclafani S, Scalea T, Vieux E, Atweh N, Duncan A, Trooskin S: Percutaneous antegrade ureteral stenting as an adjunct for treatment of complicated ureteral injuries. *J Trauma* 32:534, 1992.

54

Retroperitoneal Postoperative Hemorrhage

R. Clay Burchell

Case Abstract

A vaginal hysterectomy and repair had been accomplished on a 38-year-old para VII. The patient was not anemic at the onset of surgery, and blood loss was estimated at 500 cc during the operative procedure. The vagina was lightly packed at the conclusion of surgery.

On the first postoperative day the patient was reasonably comfortable but somewhat restless. The blood pressure was recorded as 100/70 and the pulse rate 110, at rest. A routine hemoglobin and hematocrit were reported as 8 gm and 24%, respectively. Palpation of the abdomen disclosed some lower abdominal tenderness but without discrete masses. Bowel sounds were active, and the patient was not particularly nauseated.

DISCUSSION

The abstract presents a typical history of a patient with severe postoperative hemorrhage after vaginal surgery. Unfortunately, this complication occurs more commonly than it should and is often unrecognized. When there is severe internal hemorrhage, particularly if it is retroperitoneal, adequate treatment may not be instituted, and a significant number of patients have died without effective therapy.

Obviously, the first problem in the history presented is to make a diagnosis. The blood counts should be repeated, but, in my experience, a marked reduction in hematocrit and hemoglobin postoperatively always means blood loss which must be explained. There is virtually never any benefit in praying, denying, or hoping that something is amiss with the laboratory determinations. What is amiss is that there has been unrecognized operative or postoperative hemorrhage and the patient needs treatment.

In this situation, it is unlikely that all the bleeding occurred at operation and was unrecognized. It is common to underestimate the operative bleeding by some factor (even half), but in this patient there is an unexplained loss of 3 or more units of blood. Thus, the most likely diagnosis is postoperative hemorrhage and this is probably retroperitoneal, since the gastrointestinal tract does not seem to be disturbed.

A rapid pulse either at rest or upon having the patient sit up suddenly would help to confirm the diagnosis. Absence of shifting dullness with abdominal and flank percussion would tend to support retroperitoneal rather than intraperitoneal hemorrhage. With a large retroperitoneal hemorrhage, hematomas may have dissected laterally and anteriorly so that there may be flank dullness, but this will not shift when the patient is moved. At times, hematomas have extended superiorly to the diaphragm and interfered with diaphragmatic excursion. Ultrasound examination might demonstrate a retroperitoneal mass and support the diagnosis.

From the abstract one could assume that the active bleeding had stopped because there should be a marked change in vital signs in 24 hours with continued hemorrhage of this severity; the change in blood count shows that the bleeding has been severe. Assuming that the active bleeding has stopped, there are basically two options for subsequent care.

One approach is to transfuse the patient, use all supportive measures as necessary based upon the clinical course, and attempt to avoid an operation. The other option is to operate immediately after transfusion, evacuate the hematoma, and ensure hemostasis. There are pros and cons with each option.

A useful approach to the decision-making process is to consider the worst and best outcomes with each option and subsequently balance the conflicting forces. The significant danger with not operating is that the hematoma may become infected. An infected retroperitoneal hematoma is a most serious complication of pelvic surgery and, at best, results in prolonged morbidity; at worst, death ensues. A large hematoma is difficult to drain without operating transabdominally, and there is the certainty of total peritoneal infection with a celiotomy. A common sequela of an infected retroperitoneal hematoma is septic pelvic thrombophlebitis because the great veins of the pelvis and abdomen are surrounded by the abscess. If thrombophlebitis ensues and an anticoagulant-antibiotic regime is not effective, the vena cava must be ligated or death is virtually certain.

On the other hand, with the best possible outcome for the nonoperative course, the bleeding may not recur, the hematoma may not become infected, and there may be very little subsequent morbidity. In time, the hematoma will resorb without permanent sequelae. The key question is based on the risk of the hematoma becoming infected.

The other approach is to operate when the patient is in good condition. This approach necessitates a major operation, evacuation of a large hematoma, and probably dissection of a large retroperitoneal area. The operation demands anatomic familiarity with the operative area, and not all gynecologists will feel comfortable with the operation. This, however, should not preclude the operative option from being considered. The advantages to the operative approach are that any pelvic bleeding can be stopped with certainty and the hematoma can be evacuated so that there will not be a large culture media for abscess formation. Even if the retroperitoneal space does become infected, a large abscess should not form and antibiotics should be effective. Again, one is balancing the odds of an infected hematoma against the morbidity of a major operation to prevent a disaster that may not occur.

There are several other considerations that may assist in making the decision. Prior to the days of antibiotics, it was known that a postoperative patient could be reoperated upon within the first 24 to 36 postoperative hours without serious danger of infection. If the abdomen was reopened after the first day and within a week, peritonitis was virtually certain. Although antibiotics enable the surgeon to operate when necessary, this old rule of thumb is of some help. When postoperative hemorrhage is discovered within the first day, there are significant advantages to operating. If the hemorrhage is discovered after several days, there may be advantages to waiting unless there are any signs of infection. When an abscess develops, it must be drained. In addition, if a patient with a hematoma is several days postoperative and there is no sign of infection, this may provide some assurance that an infection will not ensue.

In the patient presented, with the internal bleeding discovered on the first postoperative day, the best treatment would be early operation with evacuation of the clots. It is also important that any bleeding points be ligated. A very effective procedure is bilateral internal iliac artery ligation. This operation will prevent the necessity of religating all the pedicles and has been found effective in second operation for postoperative hemorrhage. Since iliac ligation has no effect on the hemodynamics of ovarian artery flow, the ovarian arteries should be surveyed and religated if they are a source of bleeding. In my personal experience, there have been several deaths when the patients were observed without reoperation, but no serious morbidity from early reoperation.

In a situation of this type, there is naturally a good deal of retrospective critique. Is hemorrhage inevitable in some patients, or should it always be preventable? What steps can be taken to prevent postoperative bleeding? Suffice it to say that the surgeon is always subject to some self-censure when there is a serious complication, even if the objective view is that it could not have been prevented.

In a series reporting the clinical use of internal iliac ligation, the author found that the procedure was utilized for postoperative hemorrhage twice as often after vaginal as after abdominal hysterectomy (4). There are several reasons why postoperative hemorrhage is more common after vaginal than abdominal procedures. The operator has only one good opportunity to ligate vessels with the vaginal operation—the first time the pedicle is sutured. If tags are not left on the pedicle, it retracts upward; if tags are present, there is likelihood of traction causing bleeding. A total survey of the field at the end of the operation is not available with vaginal hysterectomy. The procedure must be done correctly at each step.

An additional factor is that many gynecologic surgeons are not thoroughly familiar with tissue planes in the vaginal approach and thus are unable to stay out of trouble. One of the commonest mistakes is to circumcise the cervix too low, with the result that the vaginal cuff is too small for the subsequent operation. Pedicles are poorly ligated from inadequate exposure, and hemorrhage is likely.

Postoperative hemorrhage of significance is virtually always arterial in origin. Small veins tend to cease bleeding because there is no pulse pressure to prevent clotting. A small artery, however, will continue to bleed for hours and often will not stop spontaneously. The prevention of postoperative hemorrhage is based upon understanding the arterial anatomy, careful suturing of pedicles the *first time*, and gentle handling of tissues so that, once placed, pedicle sutures are not dislodged or loosened. Postoperative hemorrhage should be rare and might always be preventable in a theoretical sense for a specific patient. Unfortunately, statistics do catch up, and any surgeon will have a small incidence of postoperative hemorrhage.

When this complication occurs, a good clinician will not deny the change in vital signs hoping that there is no hemorrhage but will make a prompt diagnosis and institute early treatment. There are more options for therapy before than after the patient has gone into shock.

Internal iliac artery ligation certainly has a place in the treatment of pelvic hemorrhage. Understanding how and why the operation results in hemostasis will enable the surgeon to decide when to utilize the procedure. Understanding is hampered by a number of misconceptions about the pelvic blood supply and internal iliac ligation, and these should be corrected.

First, the blood supply to the human female pelvis is unbelievably abundant. After ligation of the main arteries (internal iliac), there is no deprivation of blood supply. There is an interlacing network of collateral anastomosis which functions immediately. Since the collateral network is already present, the concept that collateral channels develop over a period of time after ischemia is untrue for the human female pelvis. The second major point is that iliac ligation always promotes clotting, even though it may not always, by itself, stop the bleeding. As the blood flows through the small-diameter anastomosis after internal iliac ligation, the high arterial pulse pressure is "damped out" so that clots are not dislodged from vessels once they form.

Bilateral ligation affects the pulse pressure in the entire pelvis. Unilateral ligation has primarily a unilateral effect, so that ligation of one vessel will suffice if the bleeding is arising from a unilateral source. When the bleeding site is unknown or in the middle of the pelvis, both vessels should be ligated. Understanding the physiology of iliac ligation leads to several other obvious conclusions (1,2). The operation will be effective with hemorrhage from uterine atony and certainly should be employed prior to a decision to perform cesarean hysterectomy with patients who desire more children. With uterine atony the ovarian arteries should also be ligated because they supply large amounts of blood to the upper portion of the fundus. The uterine blood supply is sufficient to support a term pregnancy after ligation of all four vessels—both internal iliac and both ovarian arteries (6).

The operation is technically simple and not difficult for the experienced gynecologic surgeon to learn. Nevertheless, it is too infrequently used, and some women have unnecessary hysterectomy simply because it is not in the surgeon's experience at the crucial time. All gynecologists should not only be competent but confident of their competency to perform internal iliac ligation when indicated.

The ability to perform the operation only requires a knowledge of the retroperitoneal anatomy and the patience to dissect carefully. The actual ligation of the vessel is unimportant in the learning process. Anatomy of the iliac vessels and of the ureter should be learned from fresh dissection by any gynecologist in training if he or she is to be capable of preventing accidents in subsequent practice.

When iliac ligation alone does not stop the bleeding, pelvic packing will be an additional help. The so-called umbrella pack has been found to be particularly useful because, with this ingenious concept of Logothetopulos as adopted from Mikulicz, positive pressure of any desired amount can be applied to pelvic bleeding sites (3,5,7,8). Obviously, in the most critical situations, there are two hemostatic agents to reinforce each other, and together they should control any pelvic bleeding.

References

1. Burchell RC: Arterial physiology of the human female pelvis. *Obstet Gynecol* 31:855, 1968.
2. Burchell RC: Physiology of internal iliac artery ligation. *J Obstet Gynaecol Br Commonw* 75:642, 1968.
3. Burchell RC: The umbrella pack to control pelvic hemorrhage. *Comm Med* 32:734, 1968.
4. Burchell RC, Mengert WF: Internal iliac artery ligation: A series of 200 patients. *Int J Gynecol Obstet* 7:85, 1969.
5. Logothetopulos K: Eine absolut sichere Blutstillungs methode bei vaginalen und abdominalen gynakologischen operationen. *Zentralbl Gynaekol* 50:3202, 1926.

6. Mengert WF, Burchell RC, Blumstein RW, et al: Pregnancy after bilateral ligation of the internal iliac and ovarian arteries. *Obstet Gynecol* 34:664, 1969.
7. Mikulicz J: Ueber die Anwendung der Antisepsis bei Laporatomieen, mit besonderer Rucksicht auf die Drainage der Peritoneal hohle. *Arch Klin Chir* 26:111, 1881.
8. Parente JT, Dlugi H, Weingold AB: Pelvic hemostasis: A new technique and pack. *Obstet Gynecol* 19:218, 1962.

55

Bleeding Three Hours Following Vaginal Hysterectomy

George W. Mitchell, Jr.
Fred M. Massey

Case Abstract

A vaginal hysterectomy and repair had been performed on a 42-year-old woman because of troublesome menorrhagia unrelieved by previous curettage, with mildly symptomatic cystocele and rectocele. Although the surgery proceeded swiftly, the blood loss throughout the procedure was greater than usual, and at the conclusion of the procedure, a Foley catheter was placed in the bladder and a pack placed in the vagina. Three hours from the conclusion of the operation the surgeon was notified that the postoperative vaginal bleeding was persistent and excessive and the packing was saturated with blood, which was slowly soaking some sanitary napkins that had been placed.

DISCUSSION

A small amount of bleeding may be expected after every vaginal hysterectomy and repair, and the nursing service on the surgical floor must be alerted to this fact in order to avoid unnecessary calls. The decision to intervene depends upon both quantitative and qualitative factors. Usually a sponge or light pack has been placed in the vagina immediately following the conclusion of the surgical procedure, and this sponge is ordinarily saturated with a serosanguineous discharge, which may be profuse enough to soil the perineal pad and the immediately adjacent bedclothes. If the discharge is red rather than serosanguineous and if it is definitively progressive, so that the spot outside the packing continues to increase in size, there is a strong likelihood that the bleeding will not stop spontaneously, and a look at the operative site is indicated. More objective confirmation of blood loss can be obtained by the postoperative hematocrit, which should be routinely ascertained when the patient is in the recovery room, or shortly thereafter, and should be repeated when there is any suspicion that bleeding persists. The time factor is also important, in that most small bleeding points which would be likely to be sealed by clotting should be dry within an hour of the operation. Persistent bleeding 3 hours after the operation strongly suggests that hemostasis has not been secured. A patient who has bled excessively during the procedure should be kept under particularly close observation postoperatively because of the possibility that normal clotting will not have taken place.

Gynecologists often tend to forget that abnormal uterine bleeding may not be a manifestation of uterine disease or simple ovarian dysfunction. A history of menorrhagia unrelieved by conservative treatment should indicate a good bleeding history and complete preoperative blood studies, including prothrombin time, partial thromboplastin time, and bleeding time, to rule out a bleeding tendency; if abnormal values are found, a consultation with the hematology service is essential. Often such a consultation will permit elective surgery to go forward but will recommend that such adjuncts as platelet transfusions or fresh-frozen plasma be immediately available.

Intraoperative control of bleeding is of the utmost importance in vaginal surgery, as in other types of surgery. Some surgeons believe erroneously that bleeding from the broad tissue planes that have been opened is to be expected and that this bleeding can be left uncontrolled until the conclusion of the operation, when it may be eliminated by closing the vaginal mucosa, and by using packing. In addition to careful ligature of the major vascular pedicles, small bleeding points on the vaginal mucosa and the bladder and rectal muscle should be clamped and either tied or coagulated. Many surgeons find it simpler and quicker to use the electrocoagulation unit to seal these small vessels. Abnormal bleeding during the operation suggests the possibility of a bleeding diathesis, as previously noted, or the possibility that the wrong tissue planes have been dissected.

At the conclusion of the operation, the uterosacral, cardinal, and ovarian ligaments which had been previously ligated should be carefully inspected for further bleeding. This is most easily done by leaving the second suture on each of these ligaments long and using that suture for traction to pull the stump back into the field. The uterine vessels, which should not be directly placed on traction, will usually be exposed by this maneuver. When the vaginal mucosa has been closed over the cystocele and rectocele repair, there should be a short delay before packing to make certain there is no persistent bleeding. If there is, it is essential to reopen the vaginal mucosa at this time and search for the source of the bleeding. Not infrequently, this will be far superior and lateral to the vesical neck, where the rich venous plexuses of the urogenital diaphragm may have been ruptured during the dissection. This area is difficult to expose, but it is necessary to place one or two mattress or figure-of-eight catgut sutures in the area to bring this bleeding under control.

There are varying opinions about whether to close the vaginal mucosa completely following vaginal hysterectomy and repair, to leave the cuff open, to insert a small drain, or to place the dissected area and the peritoneum immediately above the vaginal cuff under constant drainage. Each has its own supporters, but if the operative field is dry, the vaginal cuff can safely be closed without drainage. If there is some concern about hemostasis and some slight drainage persists, it is well to leave the vaginal cuff open. Drains are seldom necessary and if left in too long postoperatively, may constitute a hazard because of the introduction of infection.

The amount of packing to be placed in the vagina after surgery is also the subject of some debate. Common sense dictates that, if very heavy packing of the type associated with radium applications must be inserted, the surgeon does not feel very secure about hemostasis. This type of packing is most uncomfortable to the patient and may cause damage to the bladder or rectum or gangrene of the vaginal flaps. A loose packing of gauze soaked with some medication, such as iodoform, to reduce unpleasant odor is introduced to assist with hemostasis, obliterate dead space, and prevent the soiling of bedclothes and linen, which can be objectionable to the patient and her family. Such a pack should never be left in longer than 24 hours.

When the call comes from the floor that a patient is bleeding progressively and/or the hematocrit is falling after vaginal hysterectomy and repair, the surgeon must order the patient to the examining room, where, with the patient in lithotomy position and in a good light, he or she can remove the first pack and carefully inspect the operative site. If the bleeding is not excessive and seems to be coming from the vaginal closure anteriorly or posteriorly, one or two superficial sutures at the bleeding site may serve to control it. Otherwise, heavier packing is indicated. This should be done using gauze rolls 2 to 3 inches in width and a long dressing forceps. At the time of this examination, the patient should also be examined for the possibility of intraperitoneal bleeding. The signs one ordinarily associates with this may be masked by the effect of recent surgery, and the hematocrit is the best check of the situation. A culdocentesis may be attempted if the issue remains in doubt. The secondary pack should not be left in longer than 24 hours, even if it is effective, and should again be removed in the treatment room under good conditions for another examination. If the secondary pack is unsuccessful and the bleeding continues, other steps are necessary.

If, at the time of first examination, removal of the pack reveals large clots, if the bleeding is excessive, or if the location of the bleeding seems to be at the vaginal apex, it is unlikely that a secondary pack will prove effective. The surgeon has a choice of trying this, of course, so long as the patient's general condition remains stable, but he or she should be thinking about reexploration in the operating room.

When transferred to the operating room, the patient should be given general anesthesia and again inspected vaginally. Any obvious bleeding points may be ligated at this time, but brisk bleeding strongly suggests the likelihood that a large vessel has escaped its ligature. This is particularly true if the bleeding is arterial. At this point, the vagina should be packed to make its identification easier suprapubically, and an abdominal incision, either vertical or transverse, made through the peritoneum. Good exposure of the pelvic floor is often difficult to obtain because of the presence of hematomas and the disruption of tissues by surgery. Both ovarian pedicles should be identified and, if necessary, religated and an attempt made to localize the uterine artery and vein. If this is impossible, consideration must be given to ligating the uterine artery and vein on either side, at their origin from the hypogastric vessels. If the clotting has progressed to the lateral pelvic walls, making identification of these vessels difficult, it may be necessary to ligate the hypogastric artery close to its origin from the common iliac. Under these serious circumstances, ligation of both arteries is indicated, even if the bleeding seems to be from only one side. If bleeding is coming from an unsecured ovarian artery, it should be ligated. How rapidly the surgeon must proceed from simple nonoperative bleeding to hypogastric artery ligation depends, of course, upon the magnitude of the bleeding and the patient's general condition. Serious complications require serious measures.

56

Unanticipated Spontaneous Vaginal Hemorrhage Following Straining at Stool on Tenth Postoperative Day

David H. Nichols

Case Abstract

A vaginal hysterectomy with repair and bilateral salpingo–oophorectomy had been performed on a 42-year-old patient because of troublesome, persistent menometrorrhagia and some mild degree of genital prolapse. The postoperative convalescence was smooth and unremarkable. But on the tenth postoperative day (3 days after discharge from the hospital), the patient called her surgeon to report that, following some straining at stool, the postoperative vaginal bleeding, which had almost stopped, had suddenly increased and was now flowing so freely that it ran down her leg and she was unable to contain it.

DISCUSSION

This is an uncommon but potentially serious problem, and the source of bleeding may be either venous or arterial, most likely the latter. The major vessels from which hemorrhage can arise in the patient described are a uterine artery, a vaginal artery, or an ovarian artery. Another source of bleeding is from spontaneous transvaginal evacuation of an old postoperative hematoma. The character of the blood is significant in identifying the etiology. Bright red blood which readily clots is generally of arterial origin and may occur from either "scab" disruption secondary to prematurely increased physical activity or prematurely timed coitus, or consequent to increased intra-abdominal pressure from straining at stool. A profusion of dark unclotted blood suggests evacuation of a hematoma, which, although dramatic by its volume, is usually self-limited.

Sanguinopurulent discharge may indicate spontaneous evacuation of an infected hematoma or of an abscess cavity. In the latter instance there will generally have been antecedent fever, and if there was coincident fresh bleeding it may have resulted from premature absorption of a vascular pedicle ligature or an erosion by the abscess into a nearby blood vessel. An additional source of hematoma might be that which is secondary to a previously undiagnosed blood dyscrasia or coagulopathy, but in most instances there will be a history of a previous bleeding tendency and ease of bruising.

For the complication described in the abstract, the vagina should be examined in either the office, the hospital emergency room, or the hospital operating room, depending upon the amount of hemorrhage, either with or without anesthesia. An examination must be accompanied by an examination light from an adequate source. The immediate treatment depends upon what is found at the examination.

A bleeding artery should be clamped and ligated. At the site of the colporrhaphy, this will generally be a branch of the vaginal artery; at the vault of the vagina, it may be either uterine or ovarian.

If a specific site of bleeding cannot be identified, microfibrillar collagen (Avitene) may be applied (carefully avoiding any region near the ureter, lest it initiate periureteral fibrosis with future obstruction) and the vagina packed for 24 to 48 hours. A transurethral Foley catheter may or may not be necessary, depending upon the extent of vaginal distention from the packing. At the end of 24 to 48 hours, the pack is gently removed and the patient observed for an additional 24 hours.

Complete blood count, hematocrit, and bleeding and clotting time determinations are made and appropriately treated if abnormal. Ascorbic acid (vitamin C) 500 mg two to three times daily may be administered and stool softeners and laxatives prescribed to eliminate straining at stool in the immediate future. The patient should remain at rest until a new clot has formed and has begun to be organized at the site of the bleeding. The protocol for postoperative convalescence is then restarted.

If the above measures are not successful, bilateral hypogastric artery ligation may be performed through either a transperitoneal or extraperitoneal exposure. If this procedure does not promptly stop the hemorrhage and the services of a skilled radiologist are available, selective embolization through a vascular catheter may be employed.

The prevention of delayed postoperative hemorrhage begins with a careful preoperative workup to diagnose and treat any possible coagulopathy. Postoperative care should include a comparison of the postsurgical with the preoperative hemoglobin and hematocrit, and instructions to the patient on going home should include adequate rest, the prescription of stool softeners and laxatives to avoid straining at stool, the avoidance of excessive exertion, and postoperative prohibition of coitus for 4 to 6 weeks.

Adequate hemostasis at surgery is essential, and postoperative supplementation by vitamin C may be desirable, especially if the patient is a smoker, to diminish the effect of nicotine-induced oxidation of ascorbic acid.

Careful examination of the patient described above disclosed some "scab disruption" in the vault of the vagina, the cause uncertain but possibly from some straining at stool or from unreported coitus. There was generalized ooze with no single site of bleeding. A vaginal pack was inserted and the patient placed on bedrest. The packing was removed 24 hours later, and the patient was observed for an additional 24 hours, then ambulated and sent home with prescriptions for vitamin C and stool softeners. The remainder of the convalescence was uneventful.

Recurrent Protrusion of the Anterior Vaginal Wall with Vault Eversion, Paravaginal Defects, and Thin Vaginal Epithelium

Bobby L. Shull

Case Abstract

A 45-year-old woman with uterine procidentia, cystocele, and rectocele was treated by transvaginal hysterectomy and anterior and posterior colporrhaphy. A few months following surgery, she experienced a recurrence of pelvic pressure and began to observe tissue protruding from the vaginal opening.

The physical examination was performed with the patient in lithotomy position and bearing down. The urethrovesical junction prolapsed to the hymen, the Q-tip deviated 60° from the horizontal, the bladder prolapsed halfway outside the hymen with lateral, midline, and superior loss of support, the cuff prolapsed 2 cm outside the hymen, the cul-de-sac and rectum had adequate support, and the introitus admitted 4 finger breadths easily. The perineal body measured 1.5 cm. The anal sphincter was intact. (See Figure 57.1.)

DISCUSSION

Persistence or recurrence of pelvic support defects following reconstructive surgery is a problem frequently described in the gynecologic literature. The specific sites of support defects, however, are not always clearly defined. This particular patient had support defects for the urethra, the urethrovesical junction, the bladder, and the vaginal cuff, and in addition had a perineal body which was small and an introitus which was abnormally large.

A clear understanding of normal pelvic support is essential before one can prevent or treat this surgical problem. The urethra and bladder normally rest on the pubocervical fascia. The pubocervical fascia is trapezoidal in shape, fused with the perineal membrane distally, attached to the arcus tendineus fasciae pelvis laterally, and attached to the cervix or cuff, broad ligament, and ligaments superiorly (Figure 57.2). In addition, the pubocervical fascia may be weak centrally, allowing formation of a midline cystocele. Paravaginal, or lateral, support defects are frequently associated with hypermobility of the urethra and loss of the lateral sulci of the vagina, allowing the urethrovesical junction and lateral vaginal supports to sag with straining. Midline support defects are

Figure 57.1. A patient with loss of support laterally, centrally, and superiorly. A few rugae can be seen in the upper third of the pubocervical fascia closest to the urethrovesical junction. The remainder of the anterior segment is elongated and has lost its rugae. The apices prolapse < 2 cm past the hymen. (From *Issues in Clinical Obstetrics and Gynecology.* Philadelphia, JB Lippincottt, 1993, with permission.)

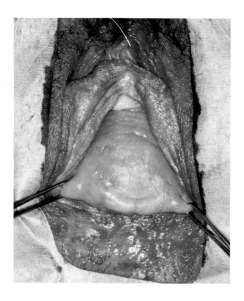

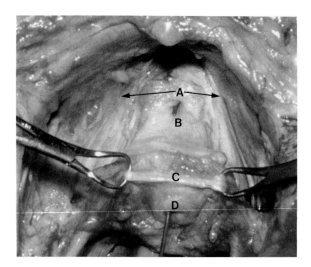

Figure 57.2. An autopsy dissection of the pubocervical fascia. (**A.** Arcus tendineus fasciae pelvis. **B.** Silver wire through the urethra. **C.** Towel clamps on the superior portion of the pubocervical fascia. **D.** Silver wire through the cervix.) (From *Issues in Clinical Obstetrics and Gynecology.* Philadelphia, JB Lippincott, 1993, with permission.)

seen with a cystocele which may protrude to or through the hymen, but with normal vaginal sulci. Superior (transverse) defects occur with elongation of the anterior vagina, loss of rugation of the epithelium, and the appearance of thin, shiny vaginal epithelium, particularly at a point near the junction of the bladder and vaginal cuff. These lateral, midline, and superior defects may occur individually or in combination. The vaginal cuff is normally suspended from the cardinal uterosacral ligament complex (3). Prolapse of the vaginal cuff outside the hymen indicates that either the cuff is not suspended to the cardinal uterosacral ligament complex or that those ligaments cannot provide their proper suspensory function.

The perineal body is formed by transverse perineal muscles, the bulbocavernosus muscles, and the perirectal fascia and anal sphincter. Usually the length of the perineal body is greater than the distance from the inferior margin of the urethral meatus to the posterior edge of the hymen. When the introitus admits 3 to 4 finger breadths with ease, one can presume the perineal body is not intact or there is poor levator muscle tone.

Prevention

The ideal therapy would have been to use techniques in the original operation designed to reduce the likelihood of persistence or recurrence of the support defects. The patient's preoperative examination did not document the specifics of each support defect. Review of the operative note indicated that she had midline plication of the pubocervical fascia using synthetic absorbable suture material. The superior portion of the pubocervical fascia was not incorporated into the closure of the vaginal cuff. No mention was made of shortening the cardinal uterosacral ligament complexes and no perineorrhaphy was performed. It is imperative to identify each support defect preoperatively and to confirm the findings intraoperatively. There are three sites in the pubocervical fascia which must be repaired to offer the patient an opportunity for cure: midline, lateral, and superior. The vaginal angles must be suspended to a point of fixation at or above the level of the ischial spines. A perineorrhaphy with incorporation of the perirectal fascia and bulbocavernosus muscles to the perineal muscles and anal sphincter must be performed.

Treatment Options

There are several management options. It is important to document the presence or absence of genuine urinary incontinence, constipation, or fecal incontinence, and to record the patient's desires for preservation or enhancement of vaginal size for intravaginal sexual intercourse. When the subpubic arch admits 3 to 4 finger breadths and the primary complaint is not genuine incontinence, surgery can be approached by the vaginal route exclusively. The author performs a vertical midline incision from the urethrovesicle junction to the apex of the vagina, reflecting the vaginal epithelium away from the bladder and pubocervical fascia. One should look for an enterocele and, if one is identified, enter the sac and perform high ligation of the enterocele using nonabsorbable suture. One continues the anterior dissection into the space of Retzius bilaterally, identifies the arcus tendineus fasciae pelvis from the ischial spine to the back of the pubic bone, and places a series of interrupted permanent sutures through the white line from its origin near the ischial spine to the back of the pubic bone. The suture nearest the ischial spine is placed in the most superior portion of the pubocervical fascia and the underlying vaginal epithelium at the apex. The sutures in the white line are individually sewn into the pubocervical fascia perivesically and periurethrally in a progressive fashion. When the sutures on one side have all been placed, one should tie them individually and repeat the same procedure on the opposite side. Next, any midline defect in pubocervical fascia is plicated using a series of interrupted nonabsorbable sutures. The superior portion of the pubocervical fascia is attached to the apex of the vagina using a series of interrupted nonabsorbable sutures. In most cases, it is unnecessary to excise any vaginal epithelium. The epithelium is approximated using absorbable suture. This approach allows correction of the midline, superior, and lateral support defects in the pubocervical fascia. A perineorrhaphy and posterior colporrhaphy should be performed next. The repair begins with excision of a diamond-shaped wedge of tissue from the perineum and introitus. The dissection continues to the vaginal apex. The perirectal fascia is approximated using polyglycolic acid sutures beginning at the cuff. The perirectal repair is completed by attaching the fascia to the perineal body. The bulbocavernosus muscles are used in the perineal reconstruction leaving the introitus 2 finger breadths wide.

In the patient with significant genuine urinary incontinence and with poor pubococcygeal muscle tone, or in the patient with a narrow subpubic arch, the author performs the midline plication of the pubocervical fascia and the reattachment of the superior portion of the pubocervical fascia to the vaginal cuff transvaginally. The dissection for the posterior colporrhaphy is carried to the apex of the vagina and the angles of the vagina are suspended to the iliococcygeus fascia near the ischial spine (8). After completion of the posterior colporrhaphy, the perineal body is reconstructed incorporating perirectal fascia and bulbocavernosus muscles. The goal would be to have the axis of the vagina posterior and the introitus accept 2 finger breadths. Next, one repositions the patient and performs a transabdominal paravaginal repair (or retropubic repair), reattaching the pubocervical fascia to the arcus tendineus using a series of interrupted nonabsorbable sutures.

There are other options for surgical management of the patient with anterior vaginal anatomic defects and stress urinary incontinence. Benson reported a small series of patients treated with minimal incision needle endoscopic suspension of the urethrovesicle junction as an adjunct to other pelvic reconstructive procedures (1). His short-term results were excellent, 91% were cured of stress incontinence, but he cautions that follow-up for 5 to 10 years is required before this approach can be fully evaluated. Gardy reported a group of 62 women with cystocele, 45 of whom had stress incontinence (4). Fifty-eight had urodynamic evidence of urethral dysfunction. They were treated one of several ways, including needle suspension only, needle suspension plus cystocele repair, pubovaginal sling plus cystocele repair, or cystocele repair only. Functional results were excellent; however, persistent or recurrent support defects occurred in 12% of patients who had cystoceles prolapsing through the hymen.

Nichols advocates the use of the Kelly plication to correct urethral funneling and pubourethral ligament plication to elevate and stabilize the hypermobile urethra (5).

What about the role of anterior repair and sacrospinous ligament suspension in this particular patient? The author would not choose that option because the major support defect is for the pubocervical fascia. Suspension of the apex of the vagina to the sacrospinous ligament offers the patient an excellent opportunity for suspension of the vaginal apex, but may predispose her to persistence or recurrence of the anterior segment defects (9,2). Sacrospinous ligament suspension may be incorporated with vaginal paravaginal repair, although the author has found that it may be unnecessary to perform sacrospinous ligament suspension if the vaginal paravaginal repair extends to the origin of the white line near the ischial spine (6). In some patients attachment of the cuff to the iliococcygeus fascia adds depth to the vagina and enhances the posterior axis of the vagina when performed in association with vaginal paravaginal repair.

The author's preference is treatment by an exclusively transvaginal approach unless there is a significant concern about genuine urinary incontinence. The advantages of the vaginal approach are the reduced recovery time and decreased morbidity. Many of these patients who are older recover more easily with surgery than with abdominal surgery. Ina woman with significant genuine incontinence, it is uncertain that the cure rate for vaginal paravaginal repair is equal to the cure rate for transabdominal vaginal paravaginal repair (7). It is the author's clinical impression that women with urethral hypermobility and good pubococcygeal muscle tone have better bladder control after vaginal paravaginal repair than do women with urethral hypermobility and poor or absent pubococcygeal muscle tone.

REFERENCES

1. Benson JT, Agosta A, McClellan E: Evaluation of a minimal-incision pubovaginal suspension as an adjunct to other pelvic-floor surgery. *Obstet Gynecol* 75:844, 1990.
2. Bonney V: The principles that should underlie all operations for prolapse. *J. Obstet Gynaecol Br Emp* 41:669–683, 1934.
3. DeLancey JOL: Anatomic aspects of vaginal eversion after hysterectomy. *Am J Obstet Gynecol* 166:1717–1728, 1992.
4. Gardy M, Kozminski M, DeLancey J, Elkins T, McGuire E: Stress incontinence and cystoceles. *J Urol* 145:1211, 1991.
5. Nichols DH, Randall CL: *Vaginal Surgery,* ed. 3. Baltimore, Williams & Wilkins, 1989.
6. Shull BL: Unpublished data.
7. Shull BL, Baden WB: A six-year experience with paravaginal defect repair for stress urinary incontinence. *Am J Obstet Gynecol* 160:1432–1440, 1989.
8. Shull BL, Capen CV, Riggs MW, Kuchl TJ: Bilateral attachment of the vaginal cuff to iliococcygeus fascia: An effective method of cuff suspension. *Am J Obstet Gynecol* 168:1669–1677, 1993.
9. Shull BL, Capen CV, Riggs MW, Kuchl TJ: Preoperative and postoperative analysis of site-specific pelvic support defects in 81 women treated with sacrospinous ligament suspension and pelvic reconstruction. *Am J Obstet Gynecol* 166:1764–1771, 1992.

SECTION VI

URINARY TRACT PROBLEMS AND INJURIES

58

Accidental Cystotomy During Vaginal Hysterectomy

John D. Thompson

Case Abstract

A vaginal hysterectomy and repair were being performed on a 35-year-old multipara because of recurrent dysfunctional uterine bleeding (unrelieved by repeated curettage and hormonal therapy) and some pelvic floor relaxation. The uterus was in first-degree prolapse, with a modest cystocele and rectocele. Traction to the cervix brought the latter down to the vaginal outlet.

A posterior colpotomy was made without difficulty, but a problem was encountered in finding the anterior peritoneal fold. The more the operator dissected in this area, the less his visibility, and the more troublesome the bleeding became. Suddenly there was a free flow of clear fluid, and it was evident that the dissection had encroached upon and lacerated the bladder.

DISCUSSION

When a complication is encountered during a gynecologic operation, the question of whether there were proper indications for the operation will likely be asked. Details regarding the magnitude of this patient's dysfunctional uterine bleeding are not given in the case abstract. Also, details regarding her conservative management are not given. However, heavy, frequent, and, possibly, prolonged bleeding must have been the main indication for the hysterectomy. Although the degree of uterovaginal prolapse was modest at best, there were no symptoms. Asymptomatic uterovaginal prolapse of a "modest" degree does not require surgery for relief. It is difficult to make an asymptomatic patient feel better with an operation. Therefore one must assume that the recurrent dysfunctional uterine bleeding was the major reason for the decision to perform a vaginal hysterectomy.

There is nothing in the case abstract to suggest that the vaginal approach for removing the uterus was contraindicated. Indeed, one might assume that this multiparous patient with modest relaxation had normal anatomy. Under these circumstances, a vaginal hysterectomy and repair should have been accomplished without difficulty. The fact

(Author's Note: This chapter was originally written by the late Dr. Richard F. Mattingly, a distinguished pelvic surgeon. Although it has been revised and updated by the current author, many of the thoughts in the chapter were originally expressed by Dr. Mattingly and are preserved.)

that a laceration of the bladder occurred is another example of how the sword of Damocles can fall unexpectedly even during the simplest operations.

General Discussion

The close anatomic relationships of the bladder, uterus, and upper vagina cause the bladder to be the most vulnerable and frequently injured organ of the lower urinary tract during pelvic surgery. The bladder and lower genital tract are so intimately approximated in their embryologic development and later in adult life that they have been characterized as the "uroreproductive unit." It is understandable, therefore, that bladder injury may occur during dissection of the cervix and lower uterine segment. Bladder injury occurs in approximately 0.5% to 1.0% of all major pelvic operations. The incidence of bladder injury with vaginal hysterectomy is lower than the incidence of bladder injury with abdominal hysterectomy. This is due to the fact that there is little deformity of the uterus and intrapelvic pathology is usually absent when the vaginal approach is selected for hysterectomy. With the recent trend toward vaginal hysterectomy to remove large uterine leiomyomas with morcellation, there could be an increase in the incidence of bladder injury with vaginal hysterectomy. Dissection of the bladder base from the cervix and lower uterine segment and identification and opening of the anterior peritoneal fold during vaginal hysterectomy can be the most difficult technical steps of this operation. Bladder injury during vaginal hysterectomy occurs more frequently than injury to the terminal ureter or rectum.

Factors Related to Bladder Injury

Alterations of anatomy from previous pelvic surgery may increase the risk of bladder injury during vaginal hysterectomy. Previous operative procedures such as cesarean section, abdominal myomectomy, or other procedures which might produce advancement of the bladder peritoneum on the anterior wall of the uterine corpus render a patient at risk for potential bladder injury. When there is a history of previous pelvic surgery, a vaginal hysterectomy has a greater potential for associated injury to the bladder than when the procedure is done by the abdominal route. Many skilled surgeons do not consider previous pelvic operations to totally contraindicate the performance of a vaginal hysterectomy. Yet, only extensive surgical experience can surmount the adhesive scars and advancement of the bladder base from a previous low cervical cesarean section. In such cases, the surgeon would be well advised to make certain that the patient has been informed of this small, but important, risk of bladder injury during vaginal hysterectomy.

The present author does not believe that a history of previous low cervical cesarean sections is a contraindication to vaginal hysterectomy. Indeed, in such cases the dissection of the bladder base from the cervix is usually easier to do vaginally than abdominally.

Uterine enlargement due to small leiomyomas may cause distortion of the anterior cul-de-sac and bladder base. Occult pelvic endometriosis may also involve the bladder peritoneum, produce coincidential scarring and bleeding, and make entry into the peritoneal cavity difficult. The bladder may have been advanced on the anterior uterine surface at the time of cesarean section or uterine suspension. Such advancement of the bladder can cause technical difficulties.

Lack of operator experience must be included as one of the important risk factors associated with bladder injury at the time of vaginal hysterectomy. Dissection beneath the bladder base in search of an elusive peritoneal fold is one of the most difficult parts of this operative procedure. Extensive operative experience is required for the surgeon to feel totally secure and technically precise in the dissection of this troublesome area. Individual gynecologic surgeons can recall vividly the period in their early operative experiences when difficulties with this dissection were encountered. As experience increases, dissection of the fascial plane between the bladder and lower uterine segment is done with greater ease and facility while inadvertent injury to the bladder wall becomes an infrequent and unusual event.

Operative Technique

A variety of vaginal hysterectomy techniques that are equally effective and technically sound have been described. However, there are certain points that are common to all. Exposure and illumination of the operative field must be optimum. If exposure is limited by a narrow subpubic arch or a tight vaginal introitus, a median episiotomy or Schuchardt's incision will be required. Retractors and cervical tenacula can be moved around during the operation to provide optimum exposure. The proper use of these instruments for traction and countertraction is essential. Breisky-Navratil retractors of different sizes are preferred. Deaver retractors are not used in vaginal hysterectomy. The sharp edge of a Deaver retractor may cause trauma and may become a weapon when used improperly, especially beneath the bladder. Dissection in the proper plane can be facilitated by injecting sterile saline beneath the vaginal mucosa around the cervix (Fig. 58.1). A vasopressor is not added to this saline solution since host tissue defense mechanisms against infection may be adversely affected by using vasoconstrictors in the tissue. With the cervix pulled forward, an incision is first made posterior to the cervix in the

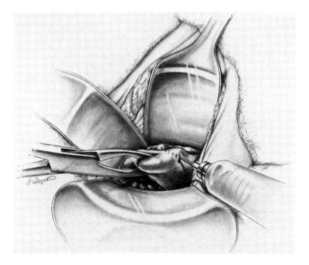

Figure 58.1. The anterior cervix is grasped with a tenaculum and sterile saline is injected beneath the vaginal mucosa around the cervix. (Reprinted with permission from Thompson JD, Rock JR: *Te Linde's Operative Gynecology*, ed. 7. Philadelphia, JB Lippincott, 1992.)

posterior vaginal fornix. Although this dissection may be done with the scissors or scalpel, the electrocautery (Bovie) unit is preferred. The blade tip is bent approximately 45 degrees and the dissection is made with brief strokes through the tissue in much the same manner as an artist strokes a canvas with a brush. With proper traction on the cervical tenaculum and countertraction with a retractor, the tissue will fall away when only lightly touched with a Bovie blade. Small bleeders may be quickly cauterized as they are encountered. Entry into the posterior cul-de-sac is followed by clamping and ligating the uterosacral ligaments bilaterally. After bleeding from the posterior vaginal cuff is controlled, saline is injected submucosally at the point of attachment of the vaginal mucosa to the cervix anteriorly. It is critical to find the correct plane of dissection between the bladder and the lower uterine segment. By moving the cervix in and out several times one can demonstrate the point of attachment of the vaginal mucosa to the cervix. The incision should be made 2 to 3 mm above the border between the smooth cervical mucosa and the vaginal rugae (Fig. 58.2). Then with strong traction on the cervical tenaculum downward and countertraction with a retractor lifting up on the anterior vaginal wall, the incision is made with the blade tip of the Bovie unit. The tissues will separate more easily when the proper plane of dissection between the bladder and cervix is found. Scissors dissection also may be used if the handle is elevated and the points directed downward against the uterus (Figs. 58.3 and 58.4). Pushing upward between the bladder and the cervix with a gauze-covered index finger may cause too much tissue trauma, but gentle finger dissection without gauze may be helpful. However, the surgeon should avoid pushing the peritoneum away with the finger. After the fascial attachment between the bladder and the cervix has been incised, the peritoneal reflection of the anterior cul-de-sac can usually be easily seen as two transparent layers sliding back and forth against one another

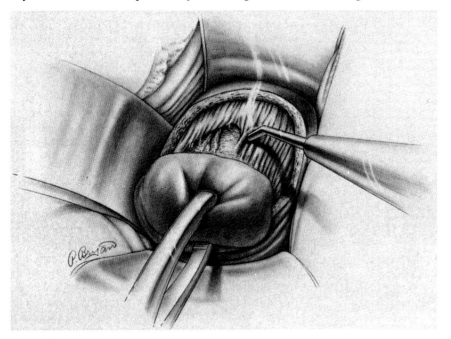

Figure 58.2.   The incision in the vaginal mucosa is extended anterior to the cervix. The blade tip of the Bovie unit is used to dissect the bladder away from the cervix and lower anterior uterine segment.

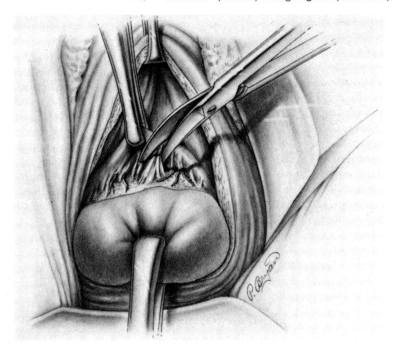

Figure 58.3. Scissors dissection also may be used to find the proper plane. (Reprinted with permission from Thompson JD, Rock JR: *Te Linde's Operative Gynecology,* ed. 7. Philadelphia, JB Lippincott, 1992.)

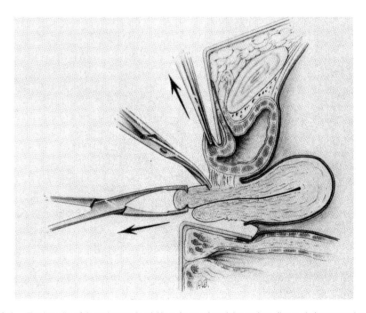

Figure 58.4. The handle of the scissors should be elevated and the points directed downward against the uterus. Strong traction and countertraction will facilitate the dissection. (Reprinted with permission from Thompson JD, Rock JR: *Te Linde's Operative Gynecology,* ed. 7. Philadelphia, JB Lippincott, 1992.)

(Figs. 58.5 and 58.6). At this point, a small incision can be made in the peritoneum. A retractor is placed through this incision in order to identify loops of small intestine or omentum to confirm that the peritoneal cavity rather than the bladder has been entered. Only after this is confirmed is the incision in the peritoneum extended laterally on each side.

Difficulty in finding the proper plane of dissection between the bladder above and the cervix and lower uterine segment below may be the result of making the incision between the cervix and the vaginal mucosa improperly. If the incision is made too low in the cervix, the plane of dissection may go deep in the cervix and anterior lower uterine segment, thus causing unnecessary bleeding. If the incision in the vaginal mucosa is too high, the wall of the bladder might be injured. Too frequently, the impatient surgeon attempts to separate the bladder from the uterus bluntly without first having incised and released the dense areas of adherence which are always present in the midline. This is one of the most frequent causes of bleeding from the wall of the adherent bladder which, if great pressure is vigorously applied, may cause a tear in the musculature or frank disruption of the full thickness of the bladder wall. In some cases of difficult dissection, a uterine sound or Kelly clamp may be passed through the urethra to demonstrate how low the bladder base is attached to the cervix. This will help to locate the bladder in relation to the plane of dissection. Instilling a few milliliters of methylene blue in the bladder will stain the bladder mucosa. The blue color will assist in identifying a more correct plane of dissection and may prevent an entry into the bladder.

In some instances, the operative field is too obscured with bleeding to make an accurate visual determination of the boundaries of the bladder wall. When the operator has reached this point of surgical frustration, the following steps are proven to be exceedingly helpful:

1. Obtain adequate but gentle exposure and illumination of the surgical field.
2. Avoid trauma to the bladder wall caused by firm pressure from an angulated, narrow, sharp bladder retractor.
3. Identify carefully all bleeding vessels and control each with individual suture ligatures.
4. Distend the bladder with 200 cc sterile saline lightly stained with methylene blue.
5. Follow the wall of the bladder from the anterior vaginal margin to the apex of the surgical field. The wall of the bladder should be carefully inspected to determine if there is a defect in the muscularis or mucosa from which there may be significant bleeding.
6. Facilitate exposure by clamping and securely ligating the uterosacral ligaments, cardinal ligaments, and uterine vessels bilaterally. This usually will allow greater descent of the cervix to gain better visibility of the plane of dissection.
7. If, in spite of these measures there is still difficulty in identification of the anterior peritoneum, the index and middle fingers of one hand can be inserted through the cul-de-sac of Douglas, passed over the uterine fundus, and used to distend the boundaries of the anterior peritoneal fold, which can then be safely incised (Fig. 58.7).

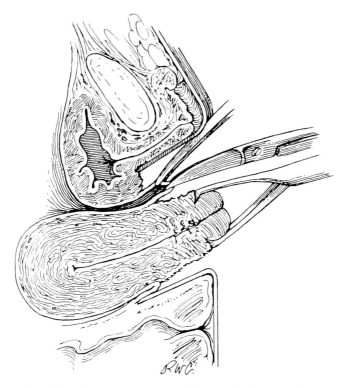

Figure 58.5. A small incision is made in the peritoneal reflection between the bladder and the uterus. (Reprinted with permission from Thompson JD, Rock JR: *Te Linde's Operative Gynecology,* ed. 7. Philadelphia, JB Lippincott, 1992.)

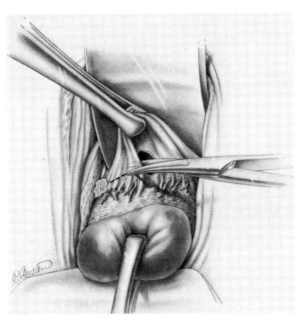

Figure 58.6. If the surgeon is certain that the peritoneal cavity has been entered, then the incision in the peritoneum can be extended laterally. If entering the peritoneal cavity anteriorly is difficult, then it can be delayed until later but should be done before the uterine vessels are clamped and ligated. (Reprinted with permission from Thompson JD, Rock JR: *Te Linde's Operative Gynecology,* ed. 7. Philadelphia, JB Lippincott, 1992.)

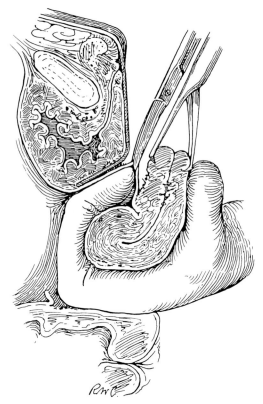

Figure 58.7. Lateral view of posterior cul-de-sac approach for identification and incision of bladder peritoneum between index and middle fingers. In difficult cases, this approach is sometimes helpful. (Reprinted with permission from Thompson JD, Rock JR: *Te Linde's Operative Gynecology,* ed. 7. Philadelphia, JB Lippincott, 1992.)

Should inadvertent entry into the bladder occur during the dissection, it will usually be identified by the sudden gush of clear or blood-tinged fluid that follows the scissors incision of the fold of tissue that was thought to be the anterior peritoneum. This may also occur following vigorous, blunt finger dissection of the bladder base from the uterine wall. To have this complication occur and to fail to recognize it could prove to be a serious medical-legal liability. If there is the slightest suspicion, a defect in the bladder can be recognized simply by instilling sterile saline which has been slightly tinged with methylene blue in the bladder. Although it is not necessary to do this in every case, it should be done without hesitation in those cases where there has been even the slightest concern about possible injury to the bladder wall.

Surgical Repair of Bladder Laceration

If an injury to the bladder can be recognized at the operation of injury and repaired properly, a vesicovaginal fistula is not likely to occur. However, since the bladder base is the most dependent portion, injuries in this location are especially likely to result in fistula formation if they are not recognized and repaired correctly at the operation of injury.

It must be clearly understood that the surgical injury to the bladder during a vaginal hysterectomy will occur almost exclusively in an area of the bladder base that is above and separate from the trigone and lower ureters (Fig. 58.8). These anatomic facts are important in undertaking the surgical repair of the bladder defect. One should recall that the female urethra measures approximately 4 cm from its origin at the vaginal introitus to the urethrovesical junction. The urethrovesical junction is located at the level of the junction of the middle and upper third of the anterior vaginal wall. The trigone and ureteral orifices are contiguous with the upper one-third of the vagina and the anterior vaginal fornix. The remainder of the bladder base rests intimately on the cervix and the lower portion of the lower uterine segment. Injury to the bladder during the dissection of the tissue plane that separates the cervix and lower uterine segment from the bladder base will involve only that portion of the bladder wall that is above the trigone. In other words, cystoscopy will reveal that the bladder laceration is above the interureteric ridge and does not involve the intramural portion of the ureters unless the laceration is very extensive and lateral to the midline. Of course, if the bladder laceration occurs during the dissection for an anterior colporrhaphy, the trigone of the bladder may be involved. If there is any question of ureteral involvement, cystoscopy can be done. If the ureteral orifices cannot be located easily, 5 ml of indigo-carmine given intravenously will cause blue urine to spurt from the orifices in only a few minutes, facilitating their identification through the cystoscope.

It is our experience that immediate repair of the bladder defect is advisable rather than deferring the repair until completion of the hysterectomy. The peritoneal cavity should be opened prior to the repair in order to facilitate exposure and to relieve tension on the suture line. The immediate bladder repair avoids loss of identification of the anatomic landmarks and the extent of the bladder injury. Therefore, it is preferable to repair the bladder wall as soon as the injured area has been clearly outlined. On the other hand, there are two circumstances under which it might be preferable to proceed with the hysterectomy first. Sometimes the presence of the

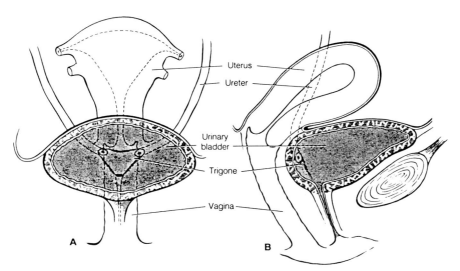

Figure 58.8. **A.** Anterior view of the normal anatomy of the ureter and bladder. The terminal end of the ureter passes medially from the lateral pelvic wall and crosses over the anterior fornix, where it enters the trigone of the bladder, which rests on the upper one-third of the anterior vaginal wall. **B.** Sagittal view of anatomical relationship of ureter and bladder base. Note that the ureter enters the trigone in the area of the upper one-third of the vagina. (Reprinted with permission from Mattingly RF, Thompson JD: *Te Linde's Operative Gynecology*, ed. 6. Philadelphia, JB Lippincott, 1985.)

uterus will interfere with exposure of the margins of the bladder laceration and thus interfere with the repair. Also, sometimes significant bleeding will be present which can be best controlled by completing the hysterectomy part of the operation. Under these circumstances, judgment may dictate that the hysterectomy be completed before the bladder laceration is repaired.

Once the bladder opening has been identified, the lateral boundaries of the laceration wall should be marked by traction sutures or Allis clamps. The defect should be closed in three layers (Fig. 58.9). A continuous suture of no. 3-0 delayed absorbable suture is used for the initial layer of closure to invert and close the bladder mucosa, making certain that the entire defect is securely closed. Formerly, a major concern was the inadvertent placement of sutures through the bladder mucosa during the repair of a bladder laceration. Today, this is no longer a matter for concern. The initial suture line should be placed without undue traction on the delicate and fragile bladder mucosa. However, it is important that the repair be watertight. Therefore, the integrity of the initial suture layer should be tested with instillation of weakly stained solution of saline into the bladder. If there are sites of obvious leakage through the initial suture layer, these sites should be reinforced with additional interrupted, inverting horizontal mattress sutures placed in the same plane as the bladder defect. The first layer of closure should be reinforced with a second layer of continuous or interrupted no. 3-0 delayed absorbable sutures placed in the muscular-fascial tissue imbricating and supporting the initial suture line broad surface to broad surface without tension. Finally, a third layer of interrupted no. 3-0 delayed absorbable sutures may be necessary to reinforce the previous suture layers. A final test of the security of the closure may be done at this point. Any point of leakage should be identified and reinforced. The final step in the repair is an important one. The anterior peritoneal edge behind the bladder should be sutured to the anterior vaginal cuff or to the bladder wall below the defect to interpose another layer between the site of bladder repair and the vaginal vault and to relieve tension on the suture line. This is a very useful maneuver and should be done to reinforce any suspected area of trauma to bladder muscle even if the bladder has not actually been entered. In any case of suspected weakness of the bladder wall, the bladder muscle must not be left approximated and over the vaginal apex.

It should be understood that primary healing after intraoperative bladder injury is not dependent on placement of a large number of sutures in the bladder wall. Rather, tissue healing is enhanced by the accurate placement of the correct number of sutures that will repair the bladder wall correctly and not interfere with its blood supply.

After injecting 5 cc of indigo-carmine intravenously, cystoscopy should be performed to be certain that dye spurts from both ureteral orifices.

Postoperative Care

Bladder drainage should be achieved by means of a transurethral or suprapubic catheter. Regardless of the technique of bladder drainage, it is critical to proper healing that the bladder remain empty and the bladder undistended for at least 7 days. The patient may be allowed to ambulate. She is carefully observed so that bladder distention does not occur. When the catheter is finally removed, careful observation is necessary to be certain that adequate voiding occurs without a high residual urine volume.

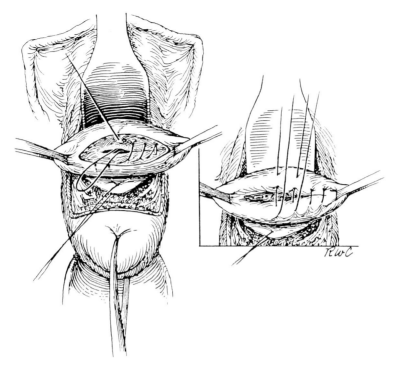

Figure 58.9. Closure of accidental laceration of bladder in two layers; continuous 3–0 chromic or delayed-absorbable suture includes bladder mucosa and intermuscularis in first layer; interrupted inverting 2–0 sutures in muscularis form the second layer. Free margin of bladder peritoneum held with suture may be advanced over the suture line for additional support to watertight closure. (Reprinted with permission from Mattingly RF, Thompson JD: *Te Linde's Operative Gynecology,* ed. 6. Philadelphia, JB Lippincott, 1985.)

Conclusion

It is the author's position that the gynecologic surgeon should be technically capable of closing a bladder defect once he or she has created it. It is important for the gynecologist to understand that the primary responsibility for the bladder injury falls on the shoulders of the surgeon who caused it and cannot be transferred to another specialist who might be summoned to perform the repair. It is comforting to know that the bladder has a rich collateral blood supply and will heal rapidly when closed correctly.

SELECTED READINGS

Everett HS, Mattingly RF: Urinary tract injuries resulting from pelvic surgery. *Am J Obstet Gynecol* 71:502, 1956.

Heaney NS: Techniques of vaginal hysterectomy. *Surg Clin North Am* 22:73, 1942.

Jaszczak SE, Evans TN: Intrafascial abdominal and vaginal hysterectomy: A reappraisal. *Obstet Gynecol* 59:435, 1982.

Mattingly RF, Borkowf HI: Lower urinary tract injuries in pregnancy. In: Barber HK, Graber EA (eds): *Surgical Disease in Pregnancy.* Philadelphia, WB Saunders, 1974.

Mattingly RF, Moore DE, Clark DO: Bacteriologic study of suprapubic bladder drainage. *Am J Obstet Gynecol* 114:732, 1972.

Thompson JD, Rock JR: *Te Linde's Operative Gynecology,* ed. 7. Philadelphia, JB Lippincott, 1992.

Williams TJ: Urologic injuries. In: Wynn RD (ed): *Obstetrics and Gynecology. Annual 1975.* Vol. 4. New York, Appleton-Century-Crofts, 1975, pp. 347–368.

59

Urine Leakage Through Vagina After Vaginal Hysterectomy and Anterior Colporrhaphy

Richard E. Symmonds

Case Abstract

A vaginal hysterectomy and anterior colporrhaphy had been performed on a 37-year-old multiparous patient with symptomatic genital prolapse. On the third postoperative day, the Foley catheter was removed and the patient was found to be leaking urine through the vagina.

DISCUSSION

Regardless of the surgeon's experience and ability, an occasional bladder perforation will occur with vaginal hysterectomy and anterior colporrhaphy; if fistula formation is to be prevented, the bladder injury must be recognized and repaired. The recognized injury that is repaired immediately will almost never lead to fistula formation. Leaving a retention catheter in the bladder for 7 to 10 days after all difficult vaginal hysterectomies that may have been traumatic to the bladder provides additional "insurance." For instance, with a vaginal hysterectomy that is done after a low cervical cesarean section or a previous anterior uterovaginal surgery of another type, some bladder "demuscularization" may occur without actual perforation. In such patients, prolonged catheter decompression of the bladder may obviate the development of a fistula.

With a patient leaking urine 3 days after vaginal hysterectomy and anterior colporrhaphy, the bladder distention associated with a cystoscopic evaluation should be avoided and a more simple effort should be made to determine the nature of the fistula. With the insertion of a tampon in the vagina and the instillation of methylene blue into the bladder, leakage of urine (rather than peritoneal fluid) often can be confirmed by the presence of dye on the vaginal tampon; this finding suggests that a vesicovaginal fistula is present. If, after a time, the methylene blue has failed to stain the vaginal tampon, another tampon is inserted, followed by the intravenous administration of indigo-carmine. If this dye stains the vaginal tampon, whereas the methylene blue in the bladder had failed to do so, the patient can be considered as having a ureterovaginal fistula.

With confirmation of a vesicovaginal fistula by the dye test, cystoscopic evaluation need not be done merely to determine the size or location of the fistula. It is much too soon to consider surgical intervention to correct the fistula; generally, cystoscopic overdistention of the bladder will not be beneficial and could be detrimental. A large-caliber transurethral catheter should be inserted to maintain bladder drainage and decompression; on occasion, even fistulas of rather large size can heal spontaneously. This is particularly true for the high fistula that is leaking urine through the vaginal vault by a relatively long and perhaps circuitous tract where fibrotic obliteration of the tract (rather than epithelialization) can occur. During catheterization, the patient can be up and about and even dismissed from the hospital; rest in bed or assuming the prone position usually does not promote healing of the fistula. If the fistulous tract fails to heal with catheter drainage within 4 to 6 weeks, it is unlikely to do so.

If the patient continues to leak urine after the catheter has been removed, the catheter should be left out to allow the irritation and infection that has occurred from prolonged catheterization to subside. Any consideration of surgical correction of the fistula should be deferred for approximately 3 months. During this time, the suture material from the hysterectomy should have been absorbed or expelled, edema and infection will have subsided, and the tissues will become soft, pliable, and "workable." The use of cortisone does not significantly speed up this process. The first surgical effort to correct the fistula has the best possibility of success; thus, one should be certain that the tissues are in absolutely optimal condition before repair is attempted.

When the "two-dye test" has reliably excluded the presence of a vesicovaginal fistula and suggests that the urinary leakage is from a ureterovaginal fistula, cystoscopic investigation of its location should be promptly done. An effort should be made to insert a ureteral catheter well above the level of the ureterovaginal fistula; when this can be accomplished and the catheter has been left in place for 2 to 3 weeks, approximately 30% of the fistulas subsequently will heal spontaneously. The fortunate patient who obtains spontaneous healing of the ureterovaginal fistula must be observed most carefully by the use of excretory urography after intervals of 3, 6, and 12 months to be sure that a stricture of the ureter does not occur. A delayed stricture of the ureter can severely impair or even totally destroy renal function; such a stricture can be occult and completely "silent" clinically.

Occasionally, a ureteral catheter cannot be inserted because of its kinking or distortion at the level of the fistula; in this instance, additional action is not urgent, provided the kidney is not being jeopardized by high-grade obstruction and infection. If the kidney is being drained well by the fistula and there is no infection, one can procrastinate and allow the patient sufficient time to recover from the operation. After 10 to 15 days, another effort can be made to insert a ureteral catheter; on occasion, due to the subsidence of edema, suture relaxation or dissolution, or other changes, a ureteral catheter can be inserted, and this may promote spontaneous healing of the fistula.

The situation becomes urgent when the patient has significant pyeloureterectasis, poor drainage, and upper urinary tract infection; permanent impairment of function or even loss of the kidney can result. Depending on the patient's condition, the surgeon must consider either a prompt nephrostomy or an abdominal approach to repair the ureterovaginal fistula. When the patient is critically ill and toxic, a nephrostomy (open or percutaneous) is the safer approach.

If 3 days after vaginal hysterectomy and repair the patient has no evidence of vault infection and is in reasonably good condition, immediate repair of a ureterovaginal fistula frequently is the treatment of choice. This soon after a vaginal hysterectomy there may be relatively little edema or tissue reaction to the surgery involving the higher pelvic portion of the ureter and the broad ligament; abdominal exploration and a ureteroneo-cystostomy frequently can be accomplished utilizing relatively normal tissues. This is in decided contrast to the quality of the tissues that usually will be found in the patient in whom a ureterovaginal fistula has developed several days after total abdominal hyster-ectomy for conditions such as endometriosis, pelvic inflammatory disease, and malig-nancy. Any consideration of accomplishing an immediate repair of a ureteral injury after abdominal hysterectomy for such problems is to be definitely deplored.

When the condition of the patient has indicated the need for a temporizing nephrostomy, definitive repair of the ureterovaginal fistula should be deferred for 2 or 3 months. Depending on the degree of urinary extravasation and infection that has oc-curred, an earlier approach may reveal significant edema, inflammatory reaction, and suture material that can make the dissection difficult and the repair less than satisfactory.

In summary, bladder-ureteral injuries must be recognized and repaired at surgery. When doubt exists at the time of surgery, the instillation of dye (or milk) into the bladder may disclose an otherwise unrecognizable perforation. Even when an actual bladder perforation has not occurred, prolonged catheterization after operation is advis-able whenever the surgeon considers the degree of bladder trauma to be unusual and excessive.

Once the fistula has occurred, the surgeon should not be coerced into early surgical intervention by the anxious patient and her family. In a series of 600 patients referred to the author's clinic with fistulas, more than half had had an unsuccessful fistula repair. The most prevalent cause of the unsuccessful repairs appeared to have been premature surgical efforts to correct the fistula. The initial repair should be deferred until the tissues are in optimal condition.

SUGGESTED READINGS

O'Connor VJ Jr, Sokol JK, Bulkley GJ, et al: Suprapubic closure of vesicovaginal fistula. *J Urol* 109:51, 1973.
Symmonds RE: Prevention and management of genitourinary fistula. *J Cont Educ Obstet Gynecol* 21:13, 1979.
Symmonds RE: Ureteral injuries associated with gynecologic surgery: Prevention and management. *Clin Obstet Gynecol* 19:623, 1976.
Symmonds RE, Hill LM: Loss of the urethra: A report on 50 patients. *Am J Obstet Gynecol* 130:130, 1978.

Vesicovaginal Fistula Following Total Abdominal Hysterectomy

John D. Thompson

Case Abstract

Because of annoying, dysfunctional uterine bleeding unresponsive to hormonal manipulation and dilatation and curettage (D&C), a total abdominal hysterectomy was performed on a 36-year-old woman whose two children had both been delivered previously by an uncomplicated low cervical cesarean section.

During the performance of the hysterectomy, there was dense adherence between the posterior surface of the bladder and the cervix at the site of the cesarean section scars. Considerable difficulty was encountered in establishing a proper plane using both blunt and sharp dissection. Much oozing from the posterior surface of the bladder was controlled by several interrupted mattress stitches of no. 3-0 chromic catgut.

Although the urine was blood-tinged, the Foley catheter was removed the morning of the second postoperative day. Slight hematuria, dysuria, and fever continued for several more days. On the eighth postoperative day, the patient noted partial urinary incontinence and was totally incontinent of urine on the ninth postoperative day. No diagnostic studies were performed, and the patient was sent home with an indwelling transurethral Foley catheter connected to a leg bag. She was reassured that "the leakage from the vagina will surely stop spontaneously in a few more days." However, urine was still leaking through the vagina 8 weeks later whenever the catheter was clamped. The patient and her husband became increasingly upset and began asking direct questions of the surgeon about the cause of this problem and its potential for solution.

DISCUSSION

When a major complication is encountered in the surgical treatment of gynecologic disease, the patient's clinical history and physical findings should be carefully reviewed to determine if the operation was indicated in the first place. From the clinical history given, it does seem that this patient's operation was appropriate, although information about the amount of bleeding, the presence or absence of anemia, the number of D&C's performed, and so on is not provided in the abstract. Hysteroscopy with endometrial ablation might have been considered as an alternative management option.

After determining that the operation was indicated, one might then ask if the operation was performed correctly. Here there may be some room for discussion:

1. Certainly in the absence of pelvic pathology (such as tumors or indurated adnexal tissue) a vaginal hysterectomy can usually be performed with ease even though the patient has had no previous vaginal deliveries. In the author's opinion, the vaginal approach is preferable when hysterectomy is indicated in a patient who has had previous low cervical cesarean section(s). The dissection of the bladder from the lower uterine segment is usually easier when done vaginally, especially since it is always possible to put an instrument in the bladder through the urethra to help locate the proper plane of dissection. If there are no contraindications to vaginal hysterectomy, then a history of previous low cervical cesarean section should be considered an indication rather than a contraindication to the vaginal approach.

2. In the presence of normal anatomy and healthy tissues, dissection of the bladder away from the anterior lower uterine isthmus and upper vagina can usually be done without difficulty or abnormal bleeding, and in a proper plane. The dissection must displace the bladder inferiorly and laterally for a distance sufficient to allow removal of the cervix without injury to the bladder. Sharp dissection with the scissors is preferred rather than tearing the tissues apart by pushing down vigorously with a sponge forceps or gauze-covered finger. When the dissection is adequately done, it should be possible to approximate the anterior and posterior vaginal walls together below the cervix in the midline and laterally (Fig. 60.1). The pubovesicocervical fascia covers the cervix

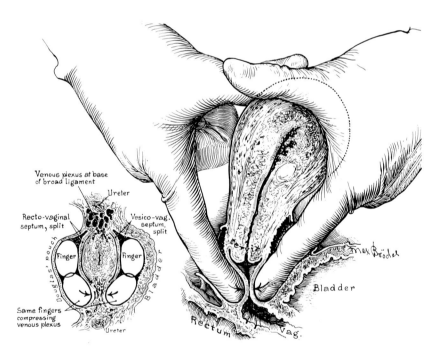

Figure 60.1.   Total abdominal hysterectomy. Testing the depth of the anterior and posterior dissections. The *inset* shows the method of segregating the vascular plexus on each side into a narrow zone adjacent to the basal segment of the broad ligament. (Reprinted from Richardson EH: A simplified technique for abdominal panhysterectomy. *Surg Gynecol Obstet* 48:248, 1929, with permission.)

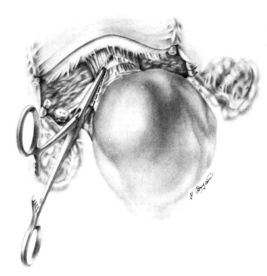

Figure 60.2. Total abdominal hysterectomy. A T-shaped or V-shaped incision is made in the pubo-vesicocervical fascia anterior to the cervix. Straight Ochsner's clamps are placed across the cardinal ligaments lateral to the cervix and inside the fascia in such a way that the fascia is actually peeled off the cervix. An incision is made at the dotted line and the clamp is replaced with a no. 0 delayed-absorbable suture. Several bites may be needed in each cardinal ligament.

anteriorly. An incision can be made in this fascia and the dissection between the bladder and cervix accomplished using an intrafascial technique. With this method of removing the cervix, the bladder is less likely to be injured (Fig. 60. 2).

3. When difficulty with the dissection is encountered (as in this case), the surgeon must decide whether the benefits of removing the cervix are worth the risk of bladder injury and possible postoperative vesicovaginal fistula formation. It should be possible to remove the cervix safely in almost every case, but not necessarily in every case. In those rare instances when the danger of removing the cervix exceeds the danger of leaving it in, the surgeon should leave it in. The incidence of postoperative vesicovaginal fistula is almost zero when a subtotal hysterectomy is done.

    If a decision is made to leave the cervix in place, the endocervical canal can still be removed as recommended and illustrated by Noble in 1928 (Fig. 60. 3). If it is not possible to remove the entire canal all the way to the external cervical os from above, the remainder of the canal can be extensively cauterized transvaginally or a conization of the remaining cervix can be done at the end of the operation or later if necessary. It is worthwhile to consider this alternative course of management when the cervix is difficult to remove for any reason.

4. "Much oozing from the posterior surface of the bladder was controlled by several interrupted mattress stitches of no. 3–0 chromic catgut." Several comments about this statement in the case abstract must be made. Although one cannot be certain, it seems that the bladder wall may have been seriously damaged during the dissection. If so, it would be prudent to test the integrity of the bladder wall before sutures are placed. This can be done by instilling 200 to 300 cc of sterile saline into the bladder and observing the traumatized area for weakness, thinning, or an actual entry into the bladder through which saline will be seen to extravasate. By doing this the surgeon can make a better decision about what suture and suture

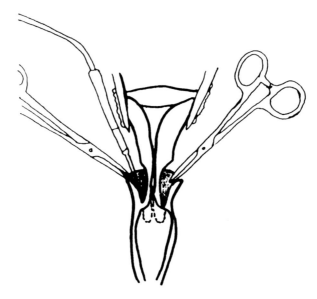

Figure 60.3.   Diagrammatic sketch showing removal of core of cervix with endotherm needle. (From Noble GH: *SMJ* 21:832, 1928.)

technique to use. "Several interrupted mattress stitches of no. 3–0 chromic cat-gut" can cause ischemic necrosis of an already traumatized posterior bladder wall and actually interfere with the healing process if not placed correctly.

    When the bladder is injured during total abdominal or vaginal hysterectomy, meticulous closure of the defect should be followed by another important step. The peritoneal edge behind the bladder should be sutured securely to the anterior vaginal incision with interrupted no. 3–0 delayed-absorbable sutures. This will separate the closure of the bladder defect from the vaginal apex and interpose another layer of tissue between the two (Fig. 60.4). Thus the bladder is more likely to heal and a vesicovaginal fistula is less likely to form.

5. At the end of each gynecologic operation, abdominal and vaginal, indigo-carmine should be injected intravenously and cystoscopy performed to observe efflux of the dye from each ureteral orifice. This will confirm integrity of the ureters. At the same time, the bladder can be inspected for evidence of injury. If sutures have been used to control bleeding from the posterior bladder wall, one should examine this area inside the bladder with the cystoscope, looking for sutures that may have been placed through the bladder mucosa.

6. When there has been trauma to the posterior bladder wall and urine is still "blood-tinged" on the second postoperative day, one must suspect that a postoperative vesicovaginal fistula may develop and must therefore leave the Foley catheter in place for 10 to 14 days postoperatively. This will give the injured bladder wall the best possibility of healing spontaneously without a fistula forming. If grossly bloody urine continues for several days and

the patient complains of dysuria and is febrile, the possibility of a vesico-vaginal fistula forming is even greater. In this situation, the inside of the bladder should be examined cystoscopically for evidence of trauma that was not recognized during the operation.

7. When a patient becomes incontinent of urine on the eighth postoperative day following a difficult total abdominal hysterectomy, diagnostic studies should be done to determine the reason for the incontinence. Circumstances in this case would point to a vesicovaginal fistula as the most likely diagnosis. However, this diagnosis must not be assumed until proven. Postoperative urinary incontinence may also be transurethral and may be from a unilateral or bilateral ureterovaginal fistula. Proper management depends on a correct diagnosis. Diagnostic studies that should be done include transurethral instillation of methylene blue dye, excretory urography, and cystoscopy. The patient should

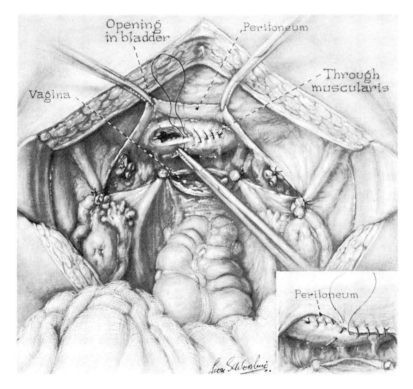

Figure 60.4.   Closure of accidental opening of bladder during total abdominal hysterectomy. The bladder is closed with a continuous no. 3-0 delayed-absorbable suture inverting mucosa into the bladder. A second muscular layer of interrupted sutures should support the initial layer. The suture line is then reinforced by bringing the peritoneum over the operative defect and suturing it in place. Advancement of the bladder peritoneum over the suture line will protect it from postoperative pelvic cellulitis and make certain that no leakage occurs into the vagina. The edge of the bladder peritoneum may also be sutured to the anterior vaginal cuff.

not simply be discharged from the hospital with reassurance "that the leakage from the vagina will surely stop spontaneously in a few more days." Spontaneous healing of a posthysterectomy vesicovaginal fistula is unusual.

Management of Simple Vesicovaginal Fistula Following Hysterectomy

It was formerly taught that one must wait at least 6 months after the operation of injury before attempting a vesicovaginal fistula repair. It was believed that this much time was required for the tissues to become sufficiently healthy to hold sutures and to heal. Recent experience indicates that most simple postoperative vesicovaginal fistulas may be repaired successfully without delay. Certainly, this is the opinion of this author. More complicated fistulas may require a waiting period for tissues to improve.

With a small vesicovaginal fistula, the urinary leakage will be slight and in some instances will depend on the position of the patient. Women with such a small fistula may void a good quantity of urine, whereas in those with large fistulas sufficient urine does not collect in the bladder to permit voiding. Most often patients are totally or almost totally incontinent of urine, require rubber sheets to protect the mattress, and need diapers or rubber pants to protect their clothing. With marked incontinence, the vulva usually becomes reddened, tender, and excoriated over time. The odor of urea may be so offensive as to be disgusting and embarrassing to the patient and repulsive to others. Social and sexual activity are markedly restricted or nonexistent. Such patients often become reclusive and depressed. Frank psychotic depression may result from prolonged incontinence if repair is delayed too long.

After a fistula is diagnosed, one can offer the patient the option of wearing or not wearing an indwelling transurethral bladder catheter. The urine loss through the fistula can be controlled better if a large-caliber Foley catheter is used. However, some patients will have so much discomfort from the catheter that they will prefer instead to wear rubber pants and/or disposable diapers until a repair can be done.

Those surgeons who prefer to wait 3 to 4 months to repair a simple posthysterectomy vesicovaginal fistula are especially concerned that the tissues be completely normal and without edema and infection so that a proper dissection, proper suturing, and proper healing will result in a successful closure. Meanwhile, the patient is terribly uncomfortable. Collection devices and indwelling catheters usually do not keep her dry and may aggravate the perineal irritation. Since she is embarrassed, depressed, and restricted in her social and marital activities, she is not easily convinced that she should remain in this unpleasant state for several more months before anything is done to close the fistula. The patient is likely to become impatient and seek other advice.

Patients with simple, uncomplicated posthysterectomy vesicovaginal fistulas can be offered an earlier repair with reasonable chance of success, and much unpleasantness can be avoided. Although it is always important to think in terms of doing a successful repair, it is also important to consider reducing the total number of patient wet days as much as possible. If given a choice, most patients will opt for early repair.

A careful preoperative evaluation is carried out with particular reference to the proximity of the ureteral orifice to the fistula margin, the presence of more than one fistula, coexisting ureteral stenosis, urinary tract infection, and especially the degree of induration of the tissues. Preoperative steroids are of questionable value and are no longer used by this author.

The transvaginal partial colpocleisis described originally by Latzko is the preferred operation to repair simple posthysterectomy vesicovaginal fistulas (Fig. 60.5). The operation is rapid and simple to perform, and the recovery is prompt. Debridement of all indurated tissue is essential. Bleeding vessels are secured. The tract of the fistula is excised completely and in such a way as to allow exact identification of the freshened edge of the bladder mucosa. When the vesicovaginal fistula tract is mature and completely epithelialized, it may not be necessary to excise the tract. However, when the fistula is fresh and includes indurated tissue, the entire tract must be excised even though this may result in a larger hole in the bladder. For a successful result, sutures must be placed in healthy tissue so that the repair can be done in several layers. The vaginal mucosa should be mobilized widely in all directions around the fistula.

The choice of sutures is important. The author's present preference is for no. 3–0 delayed-absorbable sutures throughout the repair. The first layer of interrupted vertical mattress sutures includes the bladder mucosa and adjacent bladder muscle. The bladder side of the fistula must be closed securely. The adequacy of the closure is tested by instilling 200 cc of a weak solution of methylene blue into the bladder through a catheter. If there is any point of leakage through this initial suture line, reinforcement is required. The first layer closing the bladder mucosa must be watertight. Following this, several more layers (two or three) of horizontal mattress sutures are placed in such a way that the bladder base is approximated "broad surface to broad surface without tension" over the first layer of sutures. Further dissection and mobilization must be carried out if there is tension on the suture line. Finally, the excess vaginal mucosa is trimmed away and the vaginal edges are approximated transversely. When the repair is completed, 5 cc of indigo-carmine are injected intravenously. The bladder is emptied and 200 cc of clear sterile saline are instilled. A cystoscope is inserted to watch for efflux of dye from the ureteral orifices. This is necessary to prove ureteral integrity at the end of the operation even if ureteral catheters were in place during the operation.

Postoperatively, adequate bladder drainage must be provided. Although a suprapubic catheter may be needed for complicated fistulas, a transurethral Foley catheter can be used for simple fistulas that are easily and securely repaired. Usually the catheter is left in place about 10 days. However, this time may be shorter or longer depending on the size of the fistula and the security of the closure. If the fistula is very small and the repair is very secure, the patient may be discharged early without a catheter with instructions to void frequently. Early ambulation is allowed in patients with simple fistulas. Maintenance of an adequate urine output is more important in preventing urinary tract infection postoperatively than is the use of urinary antiseptics.

It should be understood that this discussion has been written with the above case abstract in mind. Very special operative techniques and postoperative care will be needed for patients with complicated fistulas. Complicated fistulas are those that are large; those that have had previous unsuccessful attempts at repair; those that involve the urethra, vesical neck, or ureters; those that are associated with intestinal fistulas; and those that result from radiation or surgery for gynecologic malignancies. Although the standard principles for fistula repair still apply, and perhaps should be applied more strictly, other special techniques may be necessary to achieve continence. A longer period of time may be required before the tissue around the fistula is mature or healed and ready

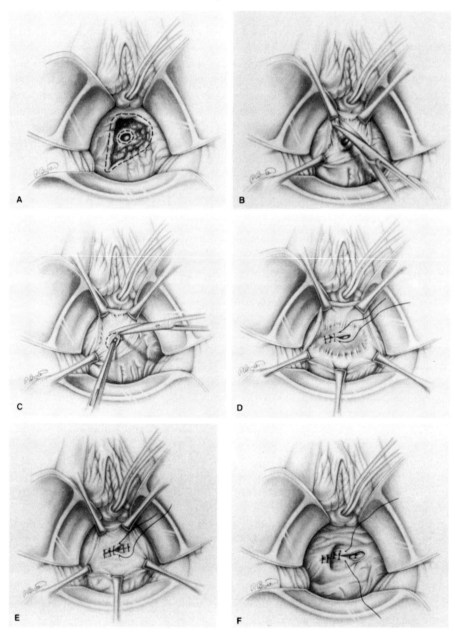

Figure 60.5.   Operation for a closure of a simple posthysterectomy vesicovaginal fistula by the Latzko technique. **A.** Ureters have been catheterized to prevent encirclement of a ureter by a suture. Incisions around the fistula opening and around the indurated vaginal mucosa margin are marked by the dotted lines. **B.** The vaginal mucosa is dissected back from the fistula opening for a sufficient distance to mobilize the bladder wall about the fistula. **C.** The fistula tract is sharply and completely excised. **D.** No. 3-0 delayed-absorbable interrupted mattress sutures taken parallel to the edge of the fistula tract are used as the initial suture line, inverting tissue into the bladder. The security of the closure should be tested by instillation of 100 to 200 ml dilute methylene blue or sterile milk into the bladder. **E.** Two or three additional suture layers should approximate the bladder muscularis broad surface without tension. No 3-0 delayed-absorbable interrupted mattress sutures should be used. **F.** The vaginal mucosa is closed transversely with interrupted no. 3-0 delayed-absorbable sutures.

for closure. Techniques of bringing in new tissue for support and neovascularization should be considered. These include mobilization of the bulbocavernosus muscle and labial fat pad, the gracilis muscle from the inner thigh, or an omental fat pad. A combined transvaginal-transvesical-transperitoneal approach may be needed.

Conclusion

In the United States and other developed countries in the world the first and essential step in limiting the morbidity of vesicovaginal fistulas is primary prevention by the correct performance of gynecologic operations. Secondary prevention depends on the recognition of bladder injury with correct repair of the injury at the operation of injury. If postoperative incontinence of urine develops, appropriate diagnostic studies must be done to determine the correct etiology.

There is no standard vesicovaginal fistula. There is considerable variation in etiology, size, location, and associated features. However, most vesicovaginal fistulas seen in the United States are relatively small, simple fistulas in the vaginal vault that result from unrecognized bladder injury during total hysterectomy, abdominal or vaginal, for benign gynecologic disease. These fistulas can usually be successfully repaired in the early postoperative period as soon as the diagnosis is made by using a simple transvaginal Latzko partial colpocleisis. When done correctly, the success rate should be between 90% and 95%.

SELECTED READINGS

Baker H.W: Selective indications for subtotal hysterectomy. *J Ky Med Assoc* 83:355, 1985.
Collins CG, Collins JH, Harrison BR, et al: Early repair of vesicovaginal fistula. *Am J Obstet Gynecol* 111:524, 1971.
Cruikshank SH: Early closure of posthysterectomy vesicovaginal fistulas. *So Med J* 81:1525, 1988.
Elkins TE, Drescher C, Martey JO, Fort D: Vesicovaginal fistula revisited. *Obstet Gynecol* 72:307, 1988.
Harrison KA: Obstetric fistula: One social calamity too many. *Br J Obstet Gynaecol* 90:385, 1983.
Kelly HA: The history of vesicovaginal fistula. *Trans Am Gynecol Soc* 37:3, 1912.
Latzko W: Postoperative vesicovaginal fistulas. *Am J Surg* 58:211, 1942.
Murphy M: Social consequences of vesicovaginal fistula in northern Nigeria. *J Biosoc Sci* 13:139, 1981.
Robertson JR: Vesicovaginal fistula: The gynecologist's responsibility. *Obstet Gynecol* 42:611, 1973.
Tahzib F: Epidemiological determinants of vesicovaginal fistulas. *Br J Obstet Gynaecol* 90:387, 1983.
Tancer ML: The post total hysterectomy (vault) vesicovaginal fistula. *J Urol* 123: 839, 1980.

61

Unrecognized Clamping of Ureter at Hysterectomy

Richard E. Symmonds

Case Abstract

A difficult abdominal hysterectomy, complicated by endometriosis and fibroids, had just been completed on a 37-year-old patient. After removal of the uterus and control of bleeding from deep within the pelvis, it was found that a Kelly hemostatic clamp had inadvertently been placed on a ureter and that the hemostat had been there for at least 30 minutes by the time the condition was discovered.

DISCUSSION

The continuing high incidence of ureteral injury with total abdominal hysterectomy (0.5% to 2%) is deplorable. Such injury can be almost completely avoided by the simple preliminary measure of demanding routine identification of the ureters above the level of disease as the initial step in every abdominal hysterectomy. The ureter then can be dissected down and displaced out of the diseased area, and injury can be either avoided or at least recognized. Regardless of experience or ability, any surgeon can injure the ureter during its dissection from the diseased area, but the injury should be recognized and immediately repaired to obviate a fistula. The insertion of ureteral catheters is not necessary for ureteral identification and may merely increase trauma to the ureter during its dissection, as noted by Talbert et al. Surgeons who do not have sufficient knowledge of the pelvic anatomy to practice routine and constant identification of the ureter should not operate in the pelvis. Once the injury has occurred, as with a clamp placed across the ureter for at least 30 minutes, the method of repair will be governed by (a) the location and severity of the injury (high or low on the ureter), (b) the nature of the disease process for which the hysterectomy was accomplished (infected, malignant), (c) the condition of the patient (critical, short-term prognosis), and (d) the training and experience of the operator. The surgeon who has little experience and knowledge regarding the proper management of ureteral injuries should obtain prompt consultation with someone knowledgeable in this area.

The clamp or ligature placed across (or around) the ureter should be promptly removed; generally, if removed within a few seconds of the time it was placed, tissue damage will be minimal and no repair is required. A ureteral catheter can be inserted to splint the area if desired. It can be inserted most easily by doing a simple anterior cystotomy, sliding the ureteral catheter up the ureter, and passing its lower end down through the urethra, where it can be tied to the urethral retention catheter; both catheters are left in place for approximately 10 days.

When the clamp has been placed across the ureter and allowed to remain in place for 30 minutes or longer, the damage to tissue if untreated will lead to necrosis and to either a ureteral stricture or fistula formation. Whereas simple trauma to the ureteral sheath or an incision in the ureter can be repaired with a few interrupted no. 4–0 chromic catgut sutures, this type of crush injury will require resection.

The location of the clamping injury is not stated in the present case; however, the ureter is frequently clamped or ligated at the pelvic brim level along with the infundibulopelvic ligament and ovarian vessels. At this high level, the repair is best accomplished by an end-to-end ureteroureterostomy. Both ends of a small ureter may need to be slightly spatulated to allow one to accomplish an accurate, somewhat oblique anastomosis. Excessive suture material should be avoided; perhaps no more than four to six interrupted sutures should be used. Each suture should include the ureteral sheath as well as the full thickness of the ureteral wall. Opinion is divided regarding the necessity of inserting a ureteral catheter for splinting; however, the author prefers to splint a ureteroureterostomy, inserting a ureteral catheter as noted above. There is no difference of opinion regarding the need to provide some form of extraperitoneal drainage down to the level of the anastomosis. A suction drain of the Hemovac type can be inserted through the abdominal wall retroperitoneally down to but not actually touching the anastomosis.

More frequently, the clamp will have been placed across the ureter at the level of the uterosacral ligament, uterine artery, or lateral vaginal angle. After resection of the damaged section of ureter, the continuity of the urinary tract can be best and most accurately restored by accomplishing a simple end-to-side ureteroneocystostomy, particularly when the injury has occurred in a deep, perhaps obese and sanguineous pelvis, where an end-to-end ureteroureterostomy may be difficult to accomplish. By doing an anterior cystotomy and inserting a finger in the bladder to "tent up" the most accessible portion of the bladder, the surgeon can quickly accomplish an end-to-side (mucosa-to-mucosa) anastomosis between the end of the ureter and the sidewall of the bladder. Any tension on the anastomosis must be avoided by mobilizing the bladder and displacing it upward toward the pelvic brim. Similarly, the upper segment of the ureter can be additionally mobilized or a "bladder hitch" can be accomplished to relieve tension on the anastomosis. A bladder hitch requires that the bladder be displaced upward and attached with interrupted absorbable sutures to the fascia of the iliopsoas muscle just lateral to the iliac artery bifurcation.

Generally, the urologist will advise (and accomplish) an antireflux type of ureteroneocystostomy (Politano-Leadbetter). The relatively inexperienced surgeon, when repairing a ureteral injury, probably should accomplish the more simple end-to-side anastomosis without an antireflux mechanism, because this will carry a lesser risk of producing subsequent obstructive problems.

Splinting a ureteroneocystostomy with a ureteral catheter is not necessary; however, the bladder should be drained with a transurethral catheter for 10 days. Again, some type of extraperitoneal suction drainage should be inserted down to but not touching the area of the ureteroneocystostomy.

When the ureteral injury has occurred in a patient whose condition is precarious or when the surgeon is not "comfortable" with ureteral surgery and immediate urologic consultation is not available, a temporizing method of managing the ureteral injury is advisable. A small Silastic catheter is brought out through an extraperitoneal stab wound in the abdominal wall—a "catheter ureterostomy." At least this will not do any additional harm, and it will protect the kidney until the patient's general condition has improved or until an experienced surgeon is available to accomplish a definitive repair. Similarly, with ureteral injury in a patient with a short-term prognosis (carcinomatosis, for instance), rather than doing a complex operation to repair or replace the ureter, one can merely ligate the proximal end of the ureter; this will produce prompt renal nonfunction and, in the absence of upper urinary tract infection, no significant clinical symptoms. If this is to be accomplished, it is absolutely essential to know that the patient has good renal function on the other side.

With the total abdominal hysterectomy technique, the admonition has always been to clamp parallel or close to the cervix and intrafascially to avoid ureteral injury. The passage of time has indicated that this has not been adequate either to prevent ureteral injuries or to promote their recognition. With endometriosis (as in the case presentation), with pelvic inflammatory disease, and with large uterine and broad ligament tumors, clamping close to the cervix or intrafascially may be impossible; similarly, with various types of uterine malignancy, intrafascial clamping is undesirable. Until it is taught and practiced that the routine identification of ureters, bladder base, and rectum represents an essential early step in the total abdominal hysterectomy technique, a high incidence of unrecognized injuries and fistula formation will continue with this operation.

SELECTED READINGS

Higgins CC: Ureteral injuries during surgery: A review of 87 cases. *JAMA* 199:82, 1967.

Lee RA, Symmonds RE: Ureterovaginal fistula. *Am J Obstet Gynecol* 109:1032, 1971.

Solomons E, Levin EJ, Bauman J, et al: A pyelographic study of ureteric injuries sustained during hysterectomy for benign conditions. *Surg Gynecol Obstet* 111:41, 1960.

Symmonds RE: Ureteral injuries associated with gynecologic surgery: Prevention and management. *Clin Obstet Gynecol* 19:623, 1976.

Talbert LM, Palumbo L, Shingleton H, et al: Urologic complications of radical hysterectomy for carcinoma of the cervix. *S Med J* 58:11, 1965.

62

Unilateral Postoperative Ureteral Obstruction

David H. Nichols

Case Abstract

A vaginal hysterectomy and repair were performed on a 43-year-old multipara to relieve a symptomatic genital prolapse. Each elongated uterosacral ligament was shortened about 1 inch and attached to the vaginal vault early in the operation. Following the hysterectomy, the ligaments were brought together in the midline by still another polyglycolic acid (Dexon) stitch placed beneath the vagina and posterior to the site of peritoneal closure. On the morning of the second postoperative day, the patient complained of pain in the right flank, and tenderness was demonstrated in the right costovertebral angle. The patient was afebrile. An infusion intravenous pyelogram was performed immediately, which demonstrated a normal collecting system on the left side, but appearance of the dye was delayed 10 minutes on the patient's right side, where a mild hydronephrosis and hydroureter with obstruction 3 to 4 cm from the ureterovesical junction were evident (Fig. 62.1). There were no positive findings on abdominal palpation.

DISCUSSION

Unilateral costovertebral tenderness in an afebrile postoperative patient is indicative of ureteral obstruction until proven otherwise. In the above instance, the obstruction was probably produced by ureteral kinking from the final but misdirected uterosacral ligament suture. Presence of the radiopaque dye in a dilated ureter suggests incomplete obstruction, since some urinary fluid flow is necessary to convey the dye into the ureter. Pain appearing on the second postoperative day instead of on the first suggests obstruction due to postsurgical edema and kinking of the ureter as from periureteral suture placement, rather than occlusion by a suture placed through or around the ureter. The absence of chills and fever speaks against a pyelonephritis.

Postoperative ureteral obstruction may be either "silent" or symptomatic and, if unrelieved, may result in ureterovaginal fistula, pyelonephritis, or destruction of the kidney. With ultimate absorption of the suture the obstruction may undergo spontaneous resolution. Renal atrophy or fistula formation is more common with complete obstruction, whereas in an incomplete obstruction ascending bacteria may result in acute pyelonephritis.

In the author's view, the costovertebral angles of every pelvic surgical patient should be palpated the evening of the day of surgery and any *unilateral* accentuation of

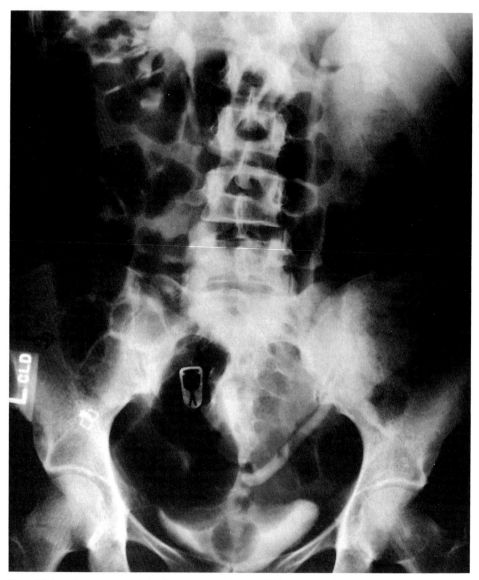

Figure 62.1.   Postoperative infusion intravenous pyelogram (IVP) showing dilation of right ureter with medial displacement and obstruction near the vault of the vagina.

pain promptly investigated. A diagnosis of possible postoperative ureteral obstruction should be confirmed or excluded by infusion pyelography as soon as it is suspected. If early in the postoperative period, the usual gastrointestinal preparation may be waived and a single intravenous injection of contrast material given, to be followed by 5-, 10-, and 20-minute radiographs, interpreted immediately. If the diagnosis of obstruction is confirmed, the obstruction should be promptly relieved with a splinting ureteral catheter or, failing this, deligation or ureteroneocystotomy, or percutaneous nephrostomy (4,5) 2 or

3 days later if a catheter still cannot be passed. If a catheter cannot be passed initially, the ureter is more likely occluded than kinked, with a more ominous prognosis. Delay only risks compounding the problem by increasing local edema and the possibility of upper urinary tract infection, further lessening the chance of successful subsequent passage of a splinting ureteral catheter.

The simplest treatment is prompt cystoscopic placement of a splinting ureteral catheter. The 25-cm 6F pigtail (1–3) stent is a good size and choice for the average adult female (Maynard JF: personal communication), although a range of sizes from which to choose should be available. It should be left in place until there has been adequate time for suture absorption. The length of time depends upon the type of suture material that was used in the primary procedure—in the range of 2 weeks for catgut and 1 to 2 months for polyglycolic acid suture. The pigtail catheter is a plastic catheter "with a memory," having a coil at each end. Using a stilette, one inserts one end into the renal pelvis and the other into the bladder. The catheter has multiple perforations through its wall to ensure adequate drainage. When the estimated time of suture absorption has been reached and excretory urography shows no evidence of obstructive uropathy, the catheter may be easily removed through an operating cystoscope by an endoscopic forceps in the hands of an experienced cystoscopist.

In the patient described in the abstract, a pigtail catheter was placed endoscopically the day the obstruction was diagnosed, relieving the obstruction. The patient was discharged on the eighth postoperative day, and the catheter was removed uneventfully through the cystoscope in an ambulatory facility several weeks later. The subsequent follow-up intravenous pyelogram was normal.

REFERENCES

1. Hepperlen TW, Mardis HK, Kammandel H: Self-contained internal ureteral stents: A new approach. *J Urol* 119:731, 1978.
2. Hepperlen TW, Mardis HK, Kammandel H: The pigtail ureteral stent in the cancer patient. *J Urol* 121:17, 1979.
3. Mardis HK, Hepperlen TW, Kammandel H: Double pigtail ureteral stent. *Urology* 14:23, 1979.
4. Mazer MJ: Permanent percutaneous antegrade ureteral stent placement without transureteral assistance. *Urology* 14:413, 1979.
5. Rutner AB, Fucilla I: Percutaneous pigtail nephrostomy. *Urology* 14:337, 1979.

63

Stitch Penetration of Bladder at Vaginal Hysterectomy and Repair

George W. Mitchell Jr.
Fred M. Massey

Case Abstract

A 70-year-old para II with symptomatic second-degree prolapse had a vaginal hysterectomy and repair. Although the urine was clear at the conclusion of the surgical procedure, it was bloody on the first postoperative day. There was no flank pain, examination of the costrovertebral angles was negative, and the patient was afebrile. Cytoscopy failed to demonstrate obvious laceration, showing only considerable edema of the base of the bladder. Although an intravenous pyelogram (IVP) was negative, the hematuria persisted.

DISCUSSION

Following a vaginal hysterectomy, with or without repair, it is customary to insert either a suprapubic or urethral catheter and to observe whether the urine that has accumulated during the procedure is clear. If the urine is examined microscopically, it will invariably show red blood cells, since this operation always causes some trauma to the bladder wall. When the urine is pink, it is probable that no serious injury has occurred, but, depending upon what has transpired during the operation, the surgeon may wish to be reassured by cystoscopy or by filling the bladder through the catheter to make sure that it is competent. Microscopic hematuria ordinarily persists for several days, but grossly bloody urinary drainage immediately following surgery, or occurring secondarily, is a sure sign that something is amiss, and investigation without delay is essential.

Hematuria occurring as a result of pyelonephritis is most unusual unless there has been partial occlusion of one of the ureters, and even then it is unlikely before the third or fourth postoperative day. In its full-blown form, pyelonephritis is associated with flank pain, chills, fever, anorexia, and general malaise, and a urine culture will be positive unless the ureter has been completely occluded. In the case under discussion, none of the classic signs and symptoms were present, and, because of the sequence of events, it is logical to conclude that the hematuria occurring on the first postoperative day was the result of direct injury to the bladder, with an outside possibility of some previously unsuspected occult intrinsic lesion in the bladder.

An IVP is the most appropriate test for ureteral patency and renal function in the postoperative phase, and this should be done prior to cystoscopy so that during the latter procedure the condition of the ureters is known and appropriate steps to determine the location and degree of injury to the ureters may be taken. The condition of the bladder should be checked with a cystoscopic instrument having a lens set at an angle of 30° to 45° so that the recesses of the organ may be easily seen. The urethra should be checked with a panendoscope, with the water or carbon dioxide running constantly to give the necessary distention. Rinsing the bladder several times may be necessary to evacuate clots and achieve adequate visualization. Clots tend to adhere to damaged areas or to stitches that have been placed through the bladder wall on the mucosal side, and they must be displaced with jets of water or a clot evacuator so that the extent of the damage can be accurately evaluated.

Few surgeons use nonabsorbable suture material for vaginal hysterectomy and repair, but some continue to place silk sutures at the urethrovesical neck, in accordance with the Kelly tradition. Nonabsorbable suture material is more commonly used for suprapubic suspension of the vesical neck, as in the Marshall-Marchetti-Krantz operation or the Burch modification. When a nonabsorbable suture penetrates the bladder or urethra, it can usually be visualized at cystoscopy. Such a suture can often be cut transvesically or transurethrally through the cystoscope, and it may retract out of the lumen, especially if a suprapubic suspension has been done. Failing that, an attempt should be made to pull the suture out after cutting it, and if this is unsuccessful, a retroperitoneal suprapubic cystostomy may be necessary to remove the offending ligature. Leaving such a foreign body in situ may cause intractable cystitis and eventual stone formation.

Absorbable synthetic sutures and catgut that have penetrated the bladder wall may also be easily identified by cystoscopy. Even though their life expectancy is relatively limited, these sutures cannot be left in situ, since they may give rise to symptoms of urgency bladder infection or even stone formation. Heavier synthetic sutures may last for a long time and are more likely to give long-term problems.

A laceration of the bladder should be repaired intraoperatively as soon as it is diagnosed, the only problem being that the surgeon must be certain that no portion of the ureter is included in the repair. Closure should be in two layers, each continuous to prevent leakage. Absorbable suture material should be used, and the inner layer, which includes the mucosa and immediately adjacent inner muscle, should be of the no. 3-0 or 4-0 size. Many gynecologists and urologists continue to prefer catgut for this layer because of its relative impermanence, but synthetic materials are also being used. The outer layer, which includes the outer muscle and whatever adventitial tissue is available, is also closed with absorbable material, synthetic or catgut. Injuries of this kind most commonly occur when the bladder is being mobilized from the anterior surface of the cervical isthmus. When this dissection is accomplished only with difficulty, the competency of the bladder should be tested at once by the transurethral introduction of some easily identified fluid like sterile milk, which does not stain the operative field, or methylene blue.

When a surgical laceration escapes detection and is discovered postoperatively by cystoscopy, there are two possible courses of action. The majority of minor lacerations will close spontaneously if the bladder is kept on constant drainage, and bleeding will usually stop. The indwelling catheter should be irrigated at least twice daily, or at any time when the flow of urine slows or stops, because of the possibility of its being plugged with blood clots. To avoid distention, no more than 30 to 50 cc of irrigating fluid should be injected. A hanging bottle of saline connected to a two-way catheter, forming a closed system, is best for this purpose. The indwelling catheter should remain for at least

2 weeks to allow good healing. A shorter period of time is considered sufficient by some surgeons, but the authors believe that more time is safer. If a small amount of bleeding continues but no fistula develops, the lacerated areas can be superficially fulgurated cystoscopically. This method is occasionally used by urologists for the closure of tiny vesicovaginal fistulas. Larger lacerations that sometimes occur during morcellation to remove a larger uterus vaginally are usually discovered during surgery, but, if not, should be repaired postoperatively by a suprapubic transvesical approach.

Whenever doubt exists about the possibility of bladder injury during surgery, continuous urinary drainage should be instituted and continued for longer than the usual 5 days. There is no harm in explaining to the patient that this is a safety precaution that is necessary because unexpected problems were encountered during surgery.

64

Bladder Management
at Postpartum Hysterectomy

R. Clay Burchell

Case Abstract

A para V at term was admitted in precipitate labor and gave birth 1 hour later. Moderate vaginal bleeding began postpartum and continued, despite massage of the uterus, oxytocics, and normal blood-clotting studies. In view of the diagnosis of uterine atony and the patient's parity, the decision was made after 2 hours to perform hysterectomy. At this time, the estimated postpartum blood loss was 600 to 800 cc.

When the bladder peritoneum was opened after the upper pedicles were ligated, it was considered virtually impossible to separate the bladder from the lower uterine segment because of large varices (1 cm in diameter) on the bladder and the uterus.

DISCUSSION

This case presents a dilemma for the operating surgeon. The patient obviously needs a hysterectomy and the operation is partially completed. A total hysterectomy, the most desirable procedure, appears to be difficult, dangerous, or impossible to perform. This is a recurrent problem with cesarean or postpartum hysterectomy. There is often a marked dilatation of veins on the lower uterine segment and on the bladder, particularly with multiparous patients. If these veins are torn, massive bleeding will result, yet it seems almost impossible to separate the tissues without tearing the veins.

Every obstetrician has noted the distention of veins on the anterior portion of the lower uterine segment at cesarean section. If these veins are observed carefully, it will be noted that there is less distention following birth of the baby. One study found that venous pressure varied between 30 and 3 cm of water (Burchell RC: unpublished data). High pressures between 18 and 30 cm of water were observed before birth, and pressures usually fell to approximately 3 cm of water after delivery.

Nevertheless, there is a good surgical solution if the operator possesses the required *knowledge* and *skill*. One must use sharp dissection and have a knowledge of bladder anatomy (3). This operative ability is not ordinarily required in obstetrics and gynecology, so it may not have been developed. Sharp dissection is best learned at an operation on a nonpregnant patient when there is no emergency. Detailed knowledge of the anatomy in this area is also necessary. The tissue layers between the cavity of the bladder and the cavity of the uterus are the bladder mucosa, the bladder muscularis, arteries and veins, the endopelvic fascia, the arteries and veins of the uterus, either the uterine myometrium or the cervical stroma (depending upon the specific area), and finally the endometrium or the endocervical glands (Fig. 64.1A).

The endopelvic fascia (vesicouterine or vesicocervical in this area) is always interspersed between veins of the bladder and uterus, providing a potential cleavage plane. This fascia appears as a loose areolar tissue condensed in some areas so as to essentially form ligaments (4, 5). This tissue is easily dissected by blunt dissection in the nonpregnant patient.

All tissues are more friable in pregnancy, so if large veins are present they will tear more easily than the fascia will separate. Hence, blunt dissection in the pregnant patient is likely to produce a cleavage plane through the venous plexus rather than in the natural fascial plane. Obviously this results in massive hemorrhage.

Dissection

For sharp dissection, traction is placed on the uterus in the direction of the patient's head. Traction is placed on the bladder at a 45° angle so that the vesicouterine peritoneum and fascia are placed on stretch and hence easily visualized (Fig. 64.1B). It is mandatory to grasp the bladder walls in order to complete this step. The main cause of injury and failure with sharp dissection is the operator's reluctance to grasp the bladder with an instrument that will not slip (toothed forceps, for example). With traction on both uterus and bladder, the endopelvic fascia will extend for a distance of approximately 2 cm between the organs (Fig. 64.1C). It is technically easy to sharply incise the fascial tissue with scissors by cutting *halfway* between the two organs. Even if there are large varices, the operator can incise *halfway* between bladder and uterine veins, completing virtually bloodless dissection.

As the dissection proceeds, the width of the fascial plane will diminish and the tissue will become more condensed. In the area of the internal os of the cervix, the distance between bladder and cervix is less than 1 cm and the fascial tissue is condensed into the so-called vesicocervical ligament. Nevertheless, there is always a space for bloodless sharp dissection if the operator has sufficient skill.

To remove the entire cervix (sometimes a problem with cesarean or postpartum hysterectomy) the dissection is carried to a point inferior to the cervix. Even a totally effaced cervix can be identified by either one of two methods. Both depend upon the fact that the cervix is always thicker than the vaginal wall (Fig. 64.2A). In one method the operator places a thumb in the vagina and a forefinger outside the vagina at a level below the cervix. If the fingers are approximated with some pressure and moved superiorly, an obstruction will be felt when the cervix is reached, no matter how well effaced it is (Fig. 64.2B). The other method is to place thumb and forefingers on the outside of the vagina anteriorly and posteriorly and repeat the same process (Fig. 64.2C).

Other Considerations

There are several other considerations with cesarean or postpartum hysterectomy. Sometimes there is marked vaginal bleeding from the vaginal cuff. This is seldom encountered in the nonpregnant patient. Bleeding can be controlled by placing ring clamps on the cuff. They are highly desirable in this situation because they compress a fairly large area, are gentle to tissues, and will not tear through. Clamps with teeth on them should not be used to control hemorrhage with friable tissues because they will only

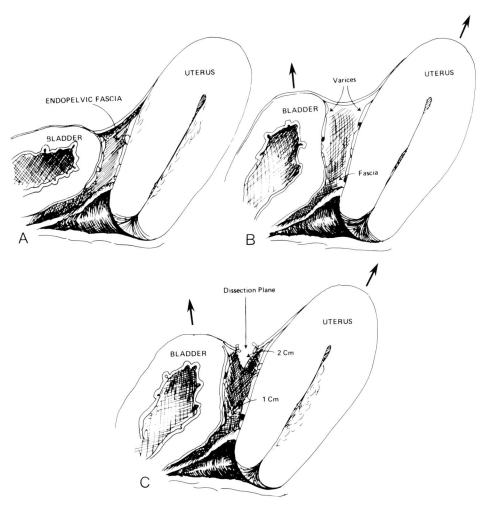

Figure 64.1. **A.** The endopelvic fascia is interspersed between the veins on the surface of the bladder and uterus. **B.** Traction on the bladder and uterus in tangential directions places the peritoneum on stretch so it can be sharply dissected. **C.** The fascial plane is wider (2 cm) and less dense near the fundus than close to the cervix (1 cm). There is always a bloodless cleavage plane for sharp dissection.

increase the hemorrhage by tearing the tissue. When the bleeding is particularly severe, the vaginal cuff can be immediately sutured as it is incised. These sutures can be fairly broad, extending 1 cm or more, but one should take great pains to ensure that there is no space between the individual figure-of-eight sutures.

Another consideration is whether a supracervical hysterectomy should ever be done. There is no doubt that the removal of the uterus, leaving the cervix intact, does avoid some of the difficulties with dissection of the bladder and may be necessary in rare instances. However, there are cogent reasons why the cervix should be removed. If the cervix remains there is danger of infection and subsequent pathology. If the operator has the surgical skill to remove the cervix, it can be done with very little difficulty.

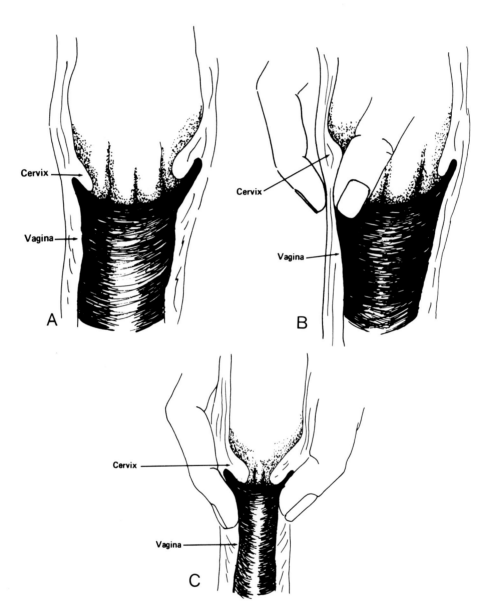

Figure 64.2.   **A.** The cervix is always thicker than the vaginal wall. **B.** The cervix can be palpated with one finger inside and one finger outside the vagina. **C.** The cervix can also be palpated with both fingers outside the vagina.

Another consideration is the desirability of intraoperative internal iliac artery ligation. Iliac ligation is possible, sometimes desirable, and sometimes but rarely necessary, with cesarean or postpartum hysterectomy (2). It should not be done prophylactically or *routinely* because it is unnecessary and will not necessarily prevent massive venous bleeding. The collateral circulation is so abundant in the human female that there can be considerable bleeding, even after iliac ligation (1). However, if bleeding cannot be controlled by conventional means, iliac ligation may be life-saving.

In summary, cesarean or postpartum hysterectomy is a formidable procedure because of the threat of hemorrhage and the apparent difficulty with bladder management. Bladder dissection is the most difficult aspect of the entire operation because it is the major source of hemorrhage. This difficulty is easily overcome if the operator possesses the prerequisite knowledge of bladder anatomy and the skill and courage to sharply dissect the bladder even with dilated veins. With this knowledge and skill (best learned previously when there is no emergency), the operating surgeon presented with the patient described in this abstract will never doubt his or her ability to proceed with the operation.

REFERENCES

1. Burchell RC: Arterial physiology of the human female patient. *Obstet Gynecol* 31:855, 1968.
2. Burchell RC: Internal iliac artery ligation: A series of 200 patients. *Int J Obstet Gynecol* 7:85, 1969.
3. Nichols DH, Milley PS: Clinical anatomy of the vulva, vagina, lower pelvis and perineum in gynecology and obstetrics. In: Sciarra (ed): *Gynecology and Obstetrics*, Vol. 1. Hagerstown, MD, Harper & Row, 1994, pp. 1–18.
4. Range RL, Woodburne RT: The gross and microscopic anatomy of the transverse cervical ligament. *Am J Obstet Gynecol* 90:460, 1964.
5. von Peham H, Amreich J: *Operative Gynecology*, Vol. 1. Philadelphia, JB Lippincott, 1934, pp. 166–197.

65

Large Uterine Leiomyomas and Stress Urinary Incontinence

Anne K. Wiskind
John D. Thompson

Case Abstract

Hysterectomy was recommended to a 45-year-old premenopausal patient with a large, symptomatic leiomyomatous uterus that extended halfway to the umbilicus. The patient was a heavy smoker with coexistent chronic bronchitis and severe, socially disabling stress urinary incontinence. The diagnosis was confirmed by pelvic examination, at which time a mild cystourethrocele was noted. The patient leaked copious amounts of urine while coughing in the standing position with a full bladder. Urodynamic studies confirmed the presence of genuine stress incontinence with no evidence of detrusor instability or voiding dysfunction.

DISCUSSION

Coexisting disease processes are commonly found in the female reproductive tract. Since uterine myomas occur in 20% to 25% of the adult female population, one might expect to encounter many women who have this condition. Urinary incontinence is estimated to affect at least 10 million American adults. The most common type of incontinence in women is genuine stress incontinence (GSI), defined as the involuntary loss of urine occurring when the intravesical pressure exceeds the maximum urethral pressure in the absence of a detrusor contraction. This often correlates with the patient complaint of the loss of urine during coughing, sneezing, laughing, and physical exercise and has the highest prevalence in women between the ages of 25 and 65 years. Thus one can expect to encounter patients with both of these conditions. Although the clinical manifestations of these two conditions may occur independently of the other, when both entities are progressively symptomatic the treatment requires individualized consideration and co-ordination of the surgical approach if indicated.

Anatomic Considerations

The base of the bladder rests on the lower uterine isthmus and cervix. The bladder trigone is below the level of the cervix and rests on the upper one-third of the anterior vaginal wall. In most cases of large uterine myomas, this anatomic relationship between the bladder and the uterus is unchanged. However, several conditions may alter this relationship. The anatomic distortion of the anterior uterine wall by myomas or the presence of a large cervical myoma can cause pressure against the bladder, resulting in the symptoms of frequency, urgency, or nocturia (Fig. 65.1). In extreme cases, urinary retention may result from the compression of the bladder and urethra against the symphysis pubis by a large, anterior myoma. The location of the bladder may also be altered to a more cephalad intra-abdominal position by the gradual, upward growth of uterine myomas out of the pelvis (Fig. 65.2). A similar condition may also be produced by a large myomatous uterus becoming impacted in the pelvis (Fig. 65.3).When an enlarging myoma causes obstruction at the vesical neck with chronic urinary retention, the detrusor muscle will hypertrophy and the bladder will enlarge, exactly mimicking the condition that exists in men with enlargement of the prostate. Under these circumstances, it is possible for the bladder to occupy the entire distance between the symphysis and the umbilicus. Although these anatomic alterations are uncommon, they must be kept in mind because they may increase the likelihood of bladder injury during surgery.

      The presence of GSI has no etiologic relationship to the uterine enlargement associated with leiomyomas. The anatomic changes in the levator ani muscles and the urogenital diaphragm contributing to GSI occur separately from the enlarging uterine corpus. In fact, lack of urethral support due to pelvic floor relaxation is only one factor responsible for urinary incontinence. An intact intrinsic urethral sphincter mechanism and intact autonomic nerve innervation to the pelvic floor muscles and the urethral sphincter also contribute to urinary continence.

      Extensive anatomic studies by DeLancey have shown that the urethra lies at an oblique axis to the horizontal, surrounded by the bladder above it, the space of Retzius and the pelvic bones anteriorly, and the levator ani muscles and the arcus tendineus

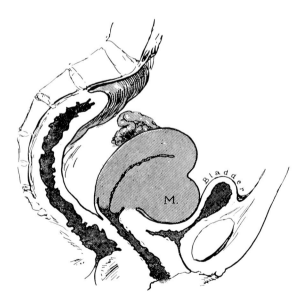

Figure 65.1. Occasionally, anterior myomas can cause pressure against the bladder, resulting in the symptoms of urinary urgency, frequency, or nocturia. In extreme cases, urinary retention may occur. (From HA Kelly, TS Allen: *Myomata of the Uterus.* Philadelphia, WB Saunders, 1909, with permission.)

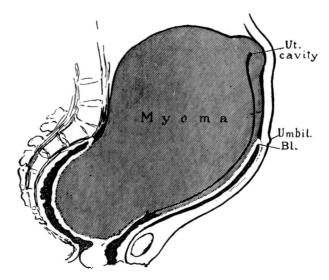

Figure 65.2. The bladder may become an abdominal rather than a pelvic organ as it accompanies the upward growth of a myoma out of the pelvis. This change in bladder location may increase the likelihood of bladder injury during surgery. (From HA Kelly, TS Allen: *Myomata of the Uterus.* Philadelphia, WB Saunders, 1909, with permission.)

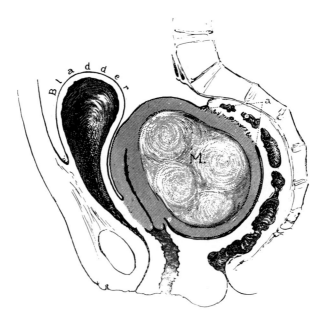

Figure 65.3. The impaction of a retroverted myomatous uterus in the pelvis may cause significant pressure against the bladder, displacing the bladder superiorly. (From HA Kelly, TS Allen: *Myomata of the Uterus.* Philadelphia, WB Saunders, 1909, with permission.)

fasciae pelvis laterally. Beneath the urethra is a single structural unit composed of the vaginal wall, the endopelvic fascia, the arcus tendineus fasciae pelvis, and the levator ani muscles, which provide the major support to the urethra. DeLancey and others theorize that stability of this layer allows the urethra to be compressed closed during increases in intra-abdominal pressure, and that laxity of this layer results in ineffective compression of the urethra and subsequent incontinence (Fig. 65.4).

The intrinsic integrity of the urethral sphincter mechanism depends on the function of the striated and smooth muscle of the urethral wall, as well as on the elasticity of the urethral wall connective tissue and submucosal blood flow. There may also be an element of extrinsic compression by the surrounding levator ani muscles. One-third of resting urethral pressure is due to vascular tone, one-third to smooth muscle, and one-third to striated muscle effects. The autonomic nervous system is responsible for maintaining the muscle tone of the urethral sphinter and the muscles of the pelvic floor. Nerve conduction studies of the pelvic floor show clear evidence of denervation injury in some patients with GSI and/or genitourinary prolapse.

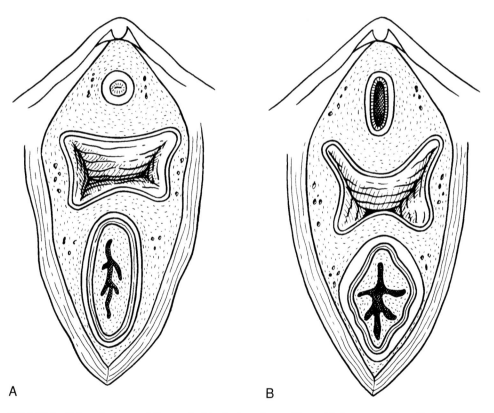

A   B

Figure 65.4.   Schematic representation emphasizing the importance of firm pelvic floor support to urethral function. **A.** The urethra, supported by a firm pelvic floor, compressed closed. **B.** Laxity of urethral support. Subsequently, this urethra remains open during increases in intra-abdominal pressure and incontinence occurs. (From AK Wiskind, SL Stanton: The Burch colposuspension for genuine stress urinary incontinence. Supplement to *Te Linde's Operative Gynecology.* Philadelphia, JB Lippincott, 1993, with permission.)

There is much debate over whether GSI is due to ineffective transmission of increases in intra-abdominal pressure to the urethra or to inadequate structural support of the urethra. It is likely that effective pressure transmission to the proximal urethra is dependent on effective urethral structural support. An exception to this may be in cases of a scarred, "drainpipe" urethra, where ineffective pressure transmission may be related to insufficient coaptation of the urethral mucosa rather than inadequate urethral structural support.

Therefore, the basic physiologic defects that occur in a patient with the combined problem of a large myomatous uterus and disabling stress urinary incontinence are usually unrelated to one another. However, objective urodynamic data on the effects of large uterine myomas on bladder function are limited. Only one study by Lancer and associates with 14 patients was found in the English-language literature addressing this topic. They found that uterine myomas may account for symptoms of urinary frequency, urgency, or nocturia. However, symptoms of stress or urge incontinence require more specific evaluation and treatment, since they are not related to uterine size.

Clinical Symptoms

The clinical features of uterine leiomyomas are variable. The symptoms are often dependent on the size, position, and number of myomas present. Although many are completely asymptomatic, an estimated 20% to 50% of myomas cause symptoms. The most commonly reported symptoms are menometrorrhagia and pelvic pain or pressure. Infrequently, uterine myomas are implicated in infertility or repeated pregnancy loss. Menstrual abnormalities affect approximately one-third of women with uterine myomas. The average menstrual blood loss of 35 to 55 cc per cycle may increase to 200 to 300 cc per cycle in the presence of a myomatous uterus. Several factors may account for this increase in menstrual flow. The increase in endometrial surface area of myomatous uteri has been correlated with the severity of bleeding. Others have suggested that anovulatory cycles associated with uterine leiomyomas are responsible for the menorrhagia. Using radiographic and histologic studies of uterine myomas, Farrer-Brown and associates have demonstrated that compression of venous plexi in the endomyometrium by the myomas causes congestion and dilatation of the subjacent endometrial venous plexi (endometrial venule ectasia), which probably plays a prominent role in abnormal uterine bleeding. Although uterine myomas are associated with menometrorrhagia, it is important to exclude other disease processes such as endometrial hyperplasia or carcinoma with an endometrial sampling as part of the evaluation in these patients.

Pelvic pain or pressure also affects about one-third of patients with uterine leiomyomas. However, such pain is usually attributable to coincident pelvic disease such as tubal inflammation, endometriosis, adenomyosis, ovarian neoplasms, or diverticulosis. A myoma in a retroverted uterus may cause dull back pain. Acute pain may be associated with carneous degeneration or torsion and necrosis of a pedunculated myoma. Severe abdominal pain may also develop in women with large myomas treated with gonadotropin-releasing hormone (GnRH) analogues. The pain is thought to be caused by acute necrosis of the myoma due to the GnRH analogue–induced hypoestrogenic state.

Pressure on the bladder by uterine myomas may cause sufficient symptoms of increasing urinary urgency, frequency, and nocturia to warrant hysterectomy. Certainly, the rare occurrence of acute urethral obstruction due to a myoma is an indication for intervention. Silent ureteral obstruction due to pressure by a large myoma at the pelvic brim is an uncommon finding, but can occur and is an indication for prompt surgical intervention. When hydronephrosis persists for an extended period of time, progressive blunting and irreversible deformity of the pyelocalyceal junction may lead to permanent renal damage. In most instances, however, brief periods of external ureteral pressure and partial obstruction at the pelvic brim do not produce lasting urinary tract abnormalities that persist after hysterectomy. The rectosigmoid colon rarely undergoes sufficient external pressure from an enlarged uterus to produce symptoms of constipation. Only in the occasional patient with an enlarged, incarcerated myoma in the cul-de-sac will the rectosigmoid undergo partial compression sufficient to produce bowel symptoms. Therefore, patients with uterine myomas should be counseled that treatment of the myomas is unlikely to improve bowel dysfunction.

There are differing opinions regarding the indications for hysterectomy for large asymptomatic uterine leiomyomas. There is general agreement that an asymptomatic myomatous uterus should be removed when there has been sufficient enlargement to obscure the clinical evaluation of the adnexal structures. Currently it is possible in some patients to assess the adnexa, as well as the uterine size, with pelvic ultrasound. This can be repeated at appropriate intervals (6 months) to confirm uterine size as well as ovarian status. However, since ovarian cancer is the most lethal gynecologic cancer, with a 30% overall 5-year survival rate, due principally to late stage at diagnosis, surgical exploration is indicated when adnexal pathology cannot be clearly differentiated from uterine myomas. In addition, rapid growth at any age or growth after menopause in the absence of estrogen therapy is an indication for surgical intervention because of the possibility of sarcomatous degeneration of a myoma. If a large, asymptomatic uterus is to be followed expectantly, it may be advisable to obtain an excretory urogram or a renal ultrasound to exclude silent ureteral obstruction and hydronephrosis.

There are few conditions more unacceptable to women than urinary incontinence. Stress incontinence is the sudden, precipitous loss of urine from increases in intra-abdominal pressure such as coughing, sneezing, laughing, and sudden changes in body position. Although the symptoms of stress incontinence may be infrequent and mild initially, the problem may become more troublesome with advancing age and increasing parity. The symptoms become disabling when the patient is required to wear a perineal pad for protection at all times and/or is unable to participate in normal activities. Stress incontinence may be associated with the symptoms of frequency, urgency, and nocturia, which are usually attributable to detrusor instability (DI). Such symptoms may also be related to uterovaginal prolapse, voiding dysfunction, and irritative bladder conditions. Certainly, the symptoms may also be due to an anterior myoma, when present. However, up to a third of patients will have mixed urinary incontinence with objective evidence of both GSI and DI. Such patients may benefit from anticholinergic therapy and timed voiding as part of their treatment plan. The poor correlation between urinary symptoms and urodynamic findings highlights the importance of obtaining urodynamic studies in all patients prior to surgery. A study by Sand et al. found that even patients with isolated complaints of stress incontinence had a 34.9% incidence of detrusor instability.

Preoperative Evaluation

A thorough preoperative evaluation is essential to determine the appropriate operation for an individual patient. The evaluation should begin with a detailed patient history, with particular emphasis on symptoms suggesting detrusor instability, neurologic disease, a fistula, voiding dysfunction, or recurrent cystitis. Previous gynecologic surgery must also be reviewed because significant vaginal scarring may result from previous colporrhaphy and incontinence procedures. Relevant gynecologic symptoms such as menometrorrhagia, dysmenorrhea, and prolapse should be evaluated, since they may influence the choice of operation. In addition, clinical review must include medical conditions that may complicate or contraindicate surgery. Patients with chronic pulmonary disease should have surgery at a time of optimal pulmonary function. Surgery may need to be deferred during winter months and allergy season, because severe repetitive coughing in the immediate postoperative period may compromise the repair.

Physical examination should include a careful screening neurologic examination, with particular emphasis on the S2–S4 spinal micturition center reflexes. These include the bulbocavernosus reflex, anal wink, cough reflex, and evaluation of anal sphincter tone. Careful bimanual examination should attempt to determine uterine size and the location of myomas encroaching on the bladder. The examination should evaluate adnexal pathology, as well as associated uterovaginal prolapse. Examination of the vaginal walls and uterine cervix with a Sims speculum at maximum Valsalva is a useful way to evaluate for genital prolapse, which occurs in up to half of patients with GSI. Accurate assessment of the degree of uterovaginal prolapse is an important clinical determination that must be made prior to selecting the appropriate operative procedure. Patients should be examined initially with a full bladder to demonstrate the physical sign of stress incontinence: that is, urine loss from the urethra simultaneous with physical exertion. The bladder should then be emptied to allow for a more accurate determination of pelvic pathology.

Assessment of vaginal capacity and mobility—in particular, easy elevation of the lateral vaginal fornices to a retropubic position—is an essential component of the preoperative evaluation in patients with stress incontinence, since this greatly influences the choice of operation (Fig. 65.5). Patients with a scarred, fixed anterior vaginal wall are unlikely to achieve any benefit from a vaginal, retropubic, or needle suspension procedure. The adequacy of estrogenization of the vaginal walls should also be determined, since this affects the suppleness and elasticity of the vaginal tissues and the sensitivity of the urethral sphincter alpha-adrenergic receptors.

Further investigations should be tailored to the individual patient. However, all patients should have a urine culture to exclude cystitis, uroflowmetry, and the measurement of residual urine volume. Subtracted multichannel cystometry with pressure/flow voiding studies should be performed in all patients preoperatively to confirm the objective, urodynamic diagnosis of GSI and to evaluate for coexistent detrusor instability and voiding dysfunction. Video cystourethrography, pelvic floor EMG, and cystoscopy may also be relevant studies in selected patients, particularly those with previous failed incontinence surgery and/or significant symptoms of frequency, urgency, or dysuria. Pelvic ultrasound, endometrial biopsy, and excretory urogram can be considered in patients with uterine leiomyomas as clinically indicated.

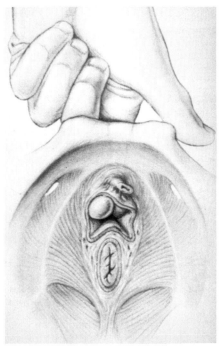

Figure 65.5. View of the pelvic floor showing the region of the urogenital diaphragm. The surgeon's finger elevates the paravaginal tissue to demonstrate the anatomic placement for each suture. Easy elevation of the lateral vaginal fornices to a retropubic position is an essential prerequisite for patients with GSI in whom an anterior colporrhaphy, retropubic bladder neck suspension, or needle suspension procedure is planned. (From Thompson JD, Rock JA (eds): *Te Linde's Operative Gynecology*, ed. 7. Philadelphia, JB Lippincott, 1992, with permission.)

The role of urethral pressure profilometry in the diagnosis and management of GSI is controversial. Although a low-pressure urethra (maximum urethral closure pressure [MUCP] < 20 cm H_2O) has been identified as a risk factor for failed retropubic surgery, there is significant overlap of MUCP parameters between continent and incontinent women, which limits its usefulness as a measure of urethral sphincter function. Furthermore, studies in patients with a MUCP < 20 cm H_2O and urethral hypermobility demonstrate surgical cure rates of 85% following a retropubic operation. This supports our supposition that it is the adequacy of vaginal capacity and mobility that should determine the choice of operation, not the urethral pressure profile.

Surgical Considerations

The choice of operation is determined by a variety of factors, including the uterine size and symptoms. associated adnexal or other pelvic pathology, the severity of the incontinence symptoms, the desire for future childbearing, and the degree of uterovaginal prolapse. The authors' usual choice of operation in the patient described in the case abstract would be a total abdominal hysterectomy, uterosacral ligament plication incorporating the posterior vaginal cuff (similar to the McCall's culdeplasty done vaginally), Moschcowitz culdoplasty, and Burch colpourethropexy through a low transverse Maylard or Cherney abdominal incision. Normal ovaries would be left in place unless there is a strong family history of ovarian cancer.

An abdominal hysterectomy is the preferred surgical treatment for a large myomatous uterus. Whereas vaginal hysterectomy is an ideal surgical approach for the removal of a smaller myomatous uterus (no more than 10 to 12 weeks in size), a larger uterus may prove to be a more hazardous surgical task by the vaginal route. The abdominal surgery may be tailored to the needs of the patient, including hysterectomy, myomectomy, and conservation of one or both ovaries. Support of the vaginal cuff and obliteration of a cul-de-sac defect should be performed in every hysterectomy. However, particular care is indicated when a retropubic operation for GSI is performed in conjunction with the hysterectomy. The incidence of enterocele and rectocele formation following the Burch operation ranges from 5% to 27%. It is unclear whether this prolapse is due to a disruption of the vaginal axis by the colpourethropexy, exposing the vaginal apex and the posterior vaginal wall to a greater degree of intra-abdominal pressure, or to an intrinsic weakness of the pelvic floor in these women. No risk factors for the development of the postcolpourethropexy prolapse have been identified, placing all patients at risk. Emphasis on the careful preoperative evaluation of genital prolapse and the correction of *any* existing prolapse at the time of colpourethropexy are paramount.

There have been over 100 operations described for the treatment of GSI. However, most of the operations fall into four general categories: (1) vaginal repair, including anterior colporrhaphy with Kelly plication and the vaginal paravaginal repair; (2) retropubic operations, including the Marshall-Marchetti-Krantz operation, the Burch colpourethropexy, and the paravaginal repair; (3) needle suspension procedures such as the Raz, Pereya, Gittes, and Stamey operations; and (4) suburethral sling procedures. More recently, laparoscopic bladder neck suspension and periurethral collagen injections have been added to the surgeon's techniques.

The Burch colpourethropexy is one of the most popular and successful operations used for the treatment of GSI. An adequate vaginal capacity and mobility of the anterior vaginal wall to a retropubic position are essential to success. Once the hysterectomy, vaginal cuff support, and culdoplasty have been completed, attention is directed to the retropubic space. Access to the space of Retzius may be facilitated by a low Maylard or Cherney incision (Fig. 65.6). The bladder is carefully dissected from the posterior aspect of the symphysis pubis. When there has been previous retropubic surgery, the bladder may be densely adherent to the symphysis, and sharp dissection with the scalpel or scissors is required.

Aided by the elevation of the lateral vaginal fornix by the surgeon's finger once the space of Retzius is exposed, one dissects the bladder medially off the paravaginal fascia (Fig. 65.7). Care should be taken to avoid dissection too near the urethra or vesicourethral junction to prevent surgical trauma to these delicate structures. Two to four pairs of no. 1 Ethibond (Ethicon, Inc., Somerville, NJ) are placed through the paravaginal fascia on either side of the bladder (Fig. 65.8). The most caudad suture is placed at the urethrovesical junction, and the remaining sutures are placed cephalad along the base of the bladder about 1 cm apart. The suture at the bladder neck serves to correct the GSI, and the remaining sutures support the bladder base and correct any cystocele. The sutures are then passed through the ipsilateral Cooper's ligament, with careful placement to allow the most natural elevation of the paravaginal fascia (Fig. 65.9). Once all the sutures have been placed through Cooper's ligament, they are tied. The most caudad sutures should be tied first, with the remaining sutures tied on alternating sides to ensure a balanced elevation.

It is common, and often desirable, to have a bridge of suture between the paravaginal fascia and Cooper's ligament. Excess elevation of the fascia may increase

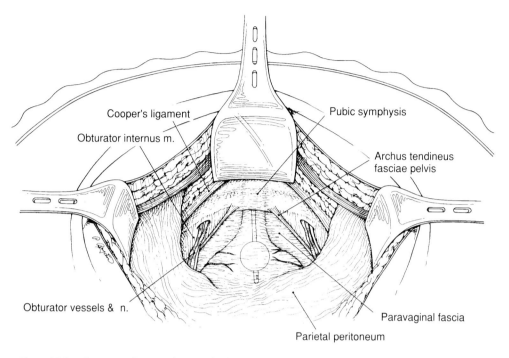

Figure 65.6. The space of Retzius. (From Wiskind AK, Stanton SL: The Burch colposuspension for genuine stress urinary incontinence. Supplement to *Te Linde's Operative Gynecology.* Philadelphia, JB Lippincott, 1993, with permission.)

the incidence of postoperative voiding dysfunction. In addition, ureteral obstruction due to kinking of the ureter from the acute elevation of the anterior vaginal wall has been reported, and there is a growing trend toward tying the sutures under less tension. The goal is simply to restore the urethra and the bladder to their normal position and to form a hammock of support under the bladder neck, while avoiding overcorrection of the defect.

Once the operation is completed and hemostasis achieved, cystoscopy can be performed after the patient is given 5 cc of indigo-carmine dye intravenously to evaluate for bladder injury and to confirm ureteral integrity. It is our preference to insert a suprapubic catheter through the dome of the bladder prior to closing the abdominal incision. Alternatively, postoperative urinary drainage may be provided satisfactorily with an indwelling Foley catheter. If residual venous bleeding is present, the space of Retzius should be drained by a suction drain. Once the abdominal incision is closed, any necessary repair of the posterior vaginal wall is then performed. It may be advisable to repair even mild, asymptomatic prolapse of the posterior vaginal wall, since even minimal weakness may be exacerbated by the colpourethropexy. It is rarely necessary to perform any vaginal repair of a cystocele following a retropubic colpourethropexy.

Postoperative complications following a Burch procedure include detrusor instability (17%), voiding dysfunction (2% to 25%), and the development of subsequent uterovaginal prolapse (26%). Ureteral obstruction, bladder and urethral injury, and fistula formation are rare. Some patients experience dyspareunia for 2 to 3 months following the operation, thought to be due to the change in the vaginal angle following surgery. On occasion, patients develop "hitch" pain in the groin at the site of the knots in Cooper's ligament.

Objective cure rates for the Burch operation range from 71% to 98% in a published series including at least 90 patients. When failures do occur, most are within the first year following the operation. Surgical outcome does not appear to be affected by a concomitant abdominal hysterectomy or by the degree of associated preoperative genital prolapse. Success following colpourethropexy does seem to be lower in patients with prior pelvic surgery, particularly previous failed incontinence operations.

Comparison of the colpourethropexy with other operations for GSI demonstrate better long-term results following the Burch operation than with the anterior colporrhaphy with Kelly plication. Although Beck has reported GSI cure rates greater than 90% utilizing the vaginal anterior repair, other have not achieved his success, reporting cure rates of only 36% to 69%. Because of these low long-term cure rates following anterior colporrhaphy with Kelly plication, many surgeons now favor a retropubic operation as a primary operation for GSI, and reserve the anterior colporrhaphy for the treatment of cystocele without GSI. An exception to this principle is an elderly patient with symptomatic genital prolapse and GSI in whom a vaginal repair is planned. In such

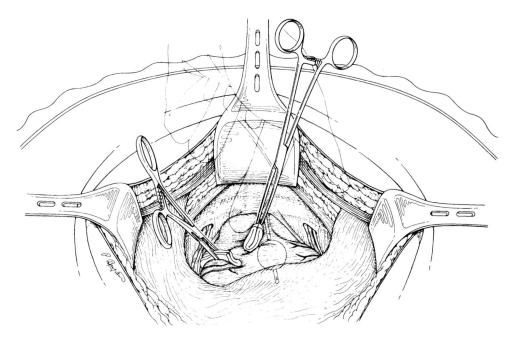

Figure 65.7.   With the forefinger of the surgeon's nondominant hand in the vagina elevating the lateral vaginal fornix, the bladder is dissected medially off the paravaginal fascia. The sponge stick on the right is holding the bladder medially. The sponge stick on the left is held by the assistant to hold peritoneal contents cephalad. (From AK Wiskind, SL Stanton: The Burch colposuspension for genuine stress urinary incontinence. Supplement to *Te Linde's Operative Gynecology.* Philadelphia, JB Lippincott, 1993, with permission.)

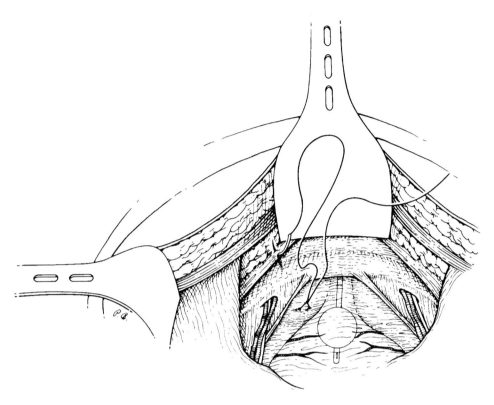

Figure 65.8. The most caudad suture is placed at the level of the bladder neck, perpendicular to the vaginal axis, full thickness through the paravaginal fascia, and tied. The suture is then placed through the ipsilateral Cooper's ligament to allow the most natural elevation of the paravaginal fascia. (From AK Wiskind, SL Stanton: The Burch colposuspension for genuine stress urinary incontinence. Supplement to *Te Linde's Operative Gynecology*. Philadelphia, JB Lippincott, 1993, with permission.)

circumstances, an extensive anterior colporrhaphy with Kelly plication, if done correctly, often cures the urinary stress incontinence. However, if a patient requires an abdominal operation for pelvic pathology, a retropubic operation would be the procedure of choice for the treatment of concurrent GSI.

Recent attention has focused on the paravaginal defect repair for the treatment of GSI. Although this operation is not designed to treat GSI but to correct the specific anatomic defect of the separation of the endopelvic fascia between the lateral edge of the vagina and the arcus tendineus fasciae pelvis ("the white line"), subjective incontinence cure rates of 95% to 97% following this repair have been reported. The key to the success of the operation is to identify preoperatively which patients have a lateral paravaginal defect. Few studies reporting the objective efficacy of this procedure have been reported, and no comparative studies have evaluated the Burch colpourethropexy with the paravaginal defect repair.

Advocates of endoscopic needle suspension procedures claim that they are quicker, easier, and associated with less perioperative complications than retropubic operations. They also have equivalent short-term continence rates (about 90%) compated with the Burch procedure. However, the continence rates of the needle suspension procedures do not seem to hold up as well over time, with 5-year cure rates averaging 70%. In contrast, continence rates following the Burch procedure remain essentially unchanged at 5 years compared with 1 year postoperatively.

Suburethral sling operations are indicated for patients with severe GSI who have significant vaginal scarring and/or intrinsic urethral weakness due to trauma, pelvic irradiation, or congenital problems that preclude the performance of any type of vaginal suspension operation. Postoperative complications include voiding dysfunction, detrusor instability, and sling erosion. In particular, postoperative voiding dysfunction is a significant complication, and patients should be prepared for prolonged catheter drainage or self-intermittent catheterization following surgery. The use of a bulbocavernosus flap may help prevent sling erosion in patients with compromised periurethral vascularization due to excessive scarring or prior pelvic irradiation. A suburethral sling may be performed in conjunction with an abdominal hysterectomy for uterine leiomyomas in the unusual circumstance of inadequate vaginal capacity or mobility for a retropubic suspension operation. A combined abdominal and vaginal approach is usually required.

Periurethral collagen injections are also effective treatment for patients with GSI who have intrinsic urethral weakness and little urethral mobility. This approach is indicated in

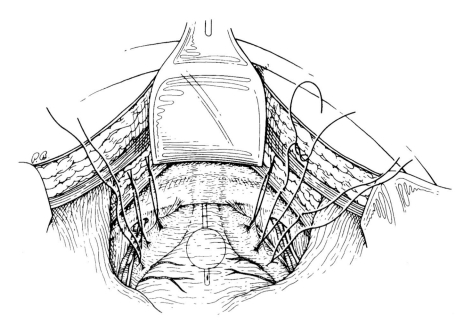

Figure 65.9. Once all the sutures are in place bilaterally, they are tied. The most caudad sutures are tied first; then the remaining sutures are tied on alternating sides to ensure a balanced elevation. A suture bridge may be present between the paravaginal fascia and Cooper's ligament. (From AK Wiskind, SL Stanton: The Burch colposuspension for genuine stress urinary incontinence. Supplement to *Te Linde's Operative Gynecology*. Philadelphia, JB Lippincott, 1993, with permission.)

patients who are unfit for major surgery, who decline it, or who have failed previous incontinence surgery. However, patients often require retreatment after 2 years. If a patient with significant GSI requires major abdominal surgery to treat a large uterine leiomyoma, more definitive treatment of the stress urinary incontinence may be achieved surgically.

Although the authors feel that the patient described in the abstract is best treated with an abdominal hysterectomy and Burch colpourethropexy as described, a number of other options may be considered. Should the patient have significant menometrorrhagia associated with the uterine leiomyomas, resulting in severe iron deficiency anemia, she may benefit from preoperative GnRH analogue therapy to induce ammenorrhea and allow the restoration of an appropriate preoperative hematocrit, facilitated by oral iron therapy. An added benefit may be a reduction in size of the leiomyomatous uterus, which may allow a vaginal approach to be considered. The role of laparoscopy-assisted vaginal hysterectomy (LAVH) with culdoplasty, followed by laparoscopic colpourethropexy, is unknown at present. Maintenance of a adequate pneumoperitoneum to allow a laparoscopic colpourethropexy to be performed after completion of the LAVH is but one of the problems to be considered.

To perform a laparoscopic urethropexy, four trocar sites are usually required. The anterior peritoneum is incised medial to the umbilical ligament and the space of Retzius is entered. Sutures of no. 2-0 Ethibond (Ethicon, Inc., Somerville, NJ) are placed through the paravaginal fascia, stapled to Cooper's ligament, and tied. An alternative method is to utilize an endoscopic stapling device and staple a Gore-Tex® (W.L. Gore Co., Flagstaff, AZ) strap to the paravaginal fascia and Cooper's ligament. Preliminary studies indicate that this procedure can be done safely by the skilled pelviscopic surgeon; however, no long-term studies are available yet to evaluate the efficacy, morbidity, and expense of this procedure compared with a standard transabdominal approach.

SELECTED READINGS

Abrams P, Blaivas JG, Stanton SL, et al: Standardization of terminology of lower urinary tract function. *Neurourol Urodynam* 7:403, 1988.

Beck RP, McCormick S: Treatment of urinary stress incontinence with anterior colporrhaphy. *Obstet Gynecol* 59:269, 1982.

Bergman A, Ballard CA, Koonings PP: Comparison of three different surgical procedures for genuine stress incontinence: Prospective randomized study. *Am J Obstet Gynecol* 160:1102, 1989.

Bergman A, Koonings PP, Ballard CA: Negative Q-tip test as a risk factor for failed incontinence surgery in women. *J Reprod Med* 34:193, 1989.

Bergman A, Koonings PP, Ballard CA: Primary stress urinary incontinence and pelvic relaxation: Prospective randomized comparison of three different operations. *Am J Obstet Gynecol* 161:97, 1989.

Bowen LW, Sand PK, Ostergard DR, et al: Unsuccessful Burch retropubic urethropexy: A case-controlled urodynamic study. *Am J Obstet Gynecol* 160:452, 1989.

Burch JC: Cooper's ligament urethrovesical suspension for stress incontinence. *Am J Obstet Gynecol* 100:764, 1968.

Burch JC: Urethrovaginal fixation to Cooper's ligament for correction of stress incontinence, cystocele, and prolapse. *Am J Obstet Gynecol* 81:281, 1961.

Buttram VC Jr, Reiter RC: Uterine leiomyomata: Etiology, symptomatology, and management. *Fertil Steril* 36:433, 1981.

Carey MP, Dwyer PL: Position and mobility of the urethrovesical junction in continent and in stress incontinent women before and after successful surgery. *Aust N Z J Obstet Gynaecol* 31:279, 1991.

Delancey JOL: Structural support of the urethra as it relates to stress urinary incontinence: The "hammock hypothesis." *Am J Obstet Gynecol* 1994; 170:1713–1720.

Drutz HP, Baker KR, Lemieux MC: Retropubic colpourethropexy with transabdominal anterior and/or posterior repair for the treatment of genuine stress urinary incontinence and genital prolapse. *Int Urogynecol J* 2:201, 1991.

Eriksen BC, Hagen B, Eik-Nes SH, et al: Long-term effectiveness of the Burch colposuspension in female urinary stress incontinence. *Acta Obstet Gynecol Scand* 69:45, 1990.

Farrer-Brown G, Beilby JOW, Tarbit MH: The vascular patterns in myomatous uteri. *J Obstet Gynecol* 77:967, 1970.

Farrer-Brown G, Beilby JOW, Tarbit MH: Venous changes in the endometrium of myomatous uteri. *Obstet Gynecol* 38:743, 1971.

Fowler JE Jr: Experience with suprapubic vesicourethral suspension and endoscopic suspension of the vesical neck for stress urinary incontinence in females. *Surg Gynecol Obstet* 162:437, 1986.

Haylen B, Sutherst J: *The Incidence and Treatment of Uterovaginal Prolapse Associated with Genuine Stress Incontinence.* Proceedings of the 17th Annual Meeting of the International Continence Society, Bristol, 1987.

Hertogs K, Stanton SL: Mechanism of urinary continence after colposuspension: Barrier studies. *Br J Obstet Gynaecol* 92:1184, 1985.

Hilton P, Stanton SL: A clinical and urodynamic assessment of the Burch colposuspension for genuine stress incontinence. *Br J Obstet Gynaecol* 90:934, 1983.

Hilton P, Stanton SL: Urethral pressure measurement by microtransducer: The results in symptom-free women and in those with genuine stress incontinence. *Br J Obstet Gynaecol* 90:919, 1983.

Iosif CS: Retropubic colpourethrocystopexy. *Urol Int* 37:125, 1982.

Karram MM, Bhatia NN: Management of coexistent stress and urge urinary incontinence. *Obstet Gynecol* 73:4, 1989.

Kelly HA: Incontinence of urine in women. *Urol Cutan Rev* 17:291, 1915.

Kelly HA, Cullen TS: *Myomata of the Uterus.* Philadelphia, WB Saunders, 1909, p. 365.

Kennedy WT: Incontinence of urine in the female, the urethral sphincter mechanism, damage of function, and restoration of control. *Am J Obstet Gynecol* 34:576, 1937.

Kil PJM, Hoekstra JW, van der Meijden APM, et al: Transvaginal ultrasonography and urodynamic evaluation after suspension operations: Comparison among the Gittes, Stamey and Burch suspension. *J Urol* 146:132, 1991.

Kohorn EI: The surgery of stress urinary incontinence. *Obstet Clin North Am* 16:841, 1989.

Koonings PP, Bergman A, Ballard CA: Low urethral pressure and stress urinary incontinence in women: Risk factor for failed retropubic surgical procedure. *Urology* 36:245, 1990.

Lam TC, Hadley HR: Surgical procedures for uncomplicated ("routine") female stress incontinence. *Urol Clin North Am* 18:327, 1991.

Langer R, Golan A, Neuman M, et al: The effect of large uterine fibroids on urinary bladder function and symptoms. *Am J Obstet Gynecol* 163:1139, 1990.

Langer R, Ron-EL R, Neuman M, et al: The value of simultaneous hysterectomy during Burch colposuspension for urinary stress incontinence. *Obstet Gynecol* 72:866, 1988.

Marshall VF, Marchetti AA, Krantz KE: The correction of stress incontinence by simple vesicourethral suspension. *Surg Gynecol Obstet* 88:509, 1949.

NIH Consensus Conference: Urinary incontinence in adults. *JAMA* 261:2685, 1989.

Penttinen J, Lindholm EL, Kaar K, et al: Successful colposuspension in stress urinary incontinence reduces bladderneck mobility and increases pressure transmission to the urethra. *Arch Gynecol Obstet* 244:233, 1989.

Richard AC, Edmonds PB, Williams NL: Treatment of stress urinary incontinence due to paravaginal fascial defect. *Obstet Gynecol* 57:357, 1981.

Richardson DA, Ramahi A, Chalas E: Surgical management of stress incontinence in patients with low urethral pressure. *Gynecol Obstet Invest* 31:106, 1991.

Sand PK, Bowen LW, Panganiban R, et al: The low pressure urethra as a factor in failed retropubic urethropexy. *Obstet Gynecol* 69:399, 1987.

Sand PK, Hill RC, Ostergard DR: Incontinence history as a predictor of detrusor stability. *Obstet Gynecol* 71:257, 1988.

Shull BL, Baden WF: A six-year experience with paravaginal defect repair for stress urinary incontinence. *Am J Obstet Gynecol* 160:1432, 1989.

Smith ARB, Hosker GL, Warrell DW: The role of partial denervation of the pelvic floor in the aetiology of genitourinary prolapse and stress incontinence of urine: A neurophysiological study. *Br J Obstet Gynaecol* 96:24, 1989.

Smith ARB, Hosker GL, Warrell DW: The role of pundendal nerve damage in the aetiology of genuine stress incontinence in women. *Br J Obstet Gynaecol* 96:29, 1989.

Stanton SL: Colposuspension. In: Stanton SL (ed): *Surgery of Female Incontinence.* New York, Springer-Verlag, 1986, p. 95.

Stanton SL: Stress incontinence: Why and how operations work. *Urol Clin North Am* 12:279, 1985.

Stanton SL, Cardozo LD: A comparison of vaginal and suprapubic surgery in the correction of incontinence due to urethral sphincter incompetence. *Br J Urol* 51:497, 1979.

Stanton SL, Cardozo LD: Results of the colposuspension operation for incontinence and prolapse. *Br J Obstet Gynaecol* 86:693, 1979.

Stanton SL, Williams JE, Ritchie D: The colposuspension operation for urinary incontinence. *Br J Obstet Gynaecol* 83:890, 1976.

Tanagho EA: Colpocystourethropexy: The way we do it. *J Urol* 116:751, 1976.

Timmons MC, Addison WA: Choice of operation for genuine stress incontinence. *Curr Opin Obstet Gynecol* 3:528, 1991.

Vancaillie TG, Schuessler W: Laparoscopic bladderneck suspension. *J Laparoendoscopic Surg* 1:169, 1991.

Varner RE, Sparks JM: Surgery for stress urinary incontinence. *Surg Clin North Am* 71:1111, 1991.

Vollenhoven BJ, Lawrence AS, Healy DL: Uterine fibroids: A clinical review. *Br J Obstet Gynaecol* 97:285, 1990.

Wall LL: Clinical evaluation of the incontinent patient. In: Thompson JD, Rock JA (eds): *TeLinde's Operative Gynecology,* ed. 7. Philadelphia, JB Lippincott, 1992, p. 887.

Wiskind AK, Creighton SM, Stanton SL: The incidence of genital prolapse after the Burch colposuspension. *Am J Obstet Gynecol* 167:399, 1992.

Wiskind AK, Stanton SL: The Burch colposuspension for genuine stress urinary incontinence. In: Thompson JD, Rock JA (eds): Supplement to *TeLinde's Operative Gynecology,* ed. 7. Philadelphia, JB Lippincott, 1993. 1(11).

66

Urinary Stress Incontinence in a Young Patient Who Wants More Children

W. Glenn Hurt

Case Abstract

Progressively socially disabling urinary stress incontinence was present in a 27-year-old para V who had expressed a firm desire to have more children. Positive findings on pelvic examination included marked hypermobility of the urethra, a moderate-sized cystocele and rectocele, and a retroverted uterus in first-degree prolapse.

DISCUSSION

The basic evaluation of all patients seen in consultation because of urinary incontinence begins with a general history and physical examination supplemented by an incisive urologic history (1), a urologically oriented neurologic examination, and a detailed pelvic examination with special attention to the integrity of the pelvic support systems. Demonstration of incontinence is an essential part of the evaluation. A postvoid residual urine measurement is made to determine bladder efficiency, and the specimen is sent for urinalysis and/or culture to ensure that there is no infection. The Q-tip test (2) is helpful in demonstrating proximal urethral mobility. Cystometry should be performed to estimate bladder volume and to determine neurologic control of the micturition reflex. This basic evaluation may enable the clinician to make the diagnosis of urinary stress incontinence with added confidence. Findings during the basic evaluation may indicate the need for endoscopy, additional urodynamic testing, radiologic studies, and further consultation.

It is particularly helpful if the patient will come to the initial evaluation with a representative urinary diary and a listing of food intolerances, drug allergies, and current medications. Some physicians furnish the patient with a gynecologic-urologic questionnaire to be completed at home and made a part of the patient's history.

If the evaluation of this patient results in a final diagnosis of socially disabling pure urinary stress incontinence and if she has a firm desire to have more children, she should be counseled regarding what is known of the etiology and pathophysiology of this disorder. The patient should also be informed of the advantage of a concerted effort to develop compensatory continence mechanisms through nonsurgical therapy until she completes childbearing, with full realization that surgery ultimately may offer the only real cure. Since vaginal delivery is thought to contribute to the development of urinary stress incontinence and since it is recognized that the first surgical attempt at correction of the disorder is the one most likely to succeed, the physician should outline a plan for the nonsurgical management of urinary stress incontinence and encourage the patient to complete childbearing as soon as is reasonable.

All patients with urinary incontinence need counseling regarding dietary indiscretions, especially if there is obesity and excessive fluid intake. Since some acid foods (tomatoes, strawberries, etc.) and those containing caffeine (coffee, tea, chocolates, etc.) may irritate the bladder, they should be ingested in moderation or eliminated from the diet. Bacteriuria, whether symptomatic or asymptomatic, cervicitis, and vaginitis must be treated. Medications which the patient takes and which may contribute to urinary incontinence (diuretics, phenothiazines, etc.) should be scrutinized. Special attention should be given to the treatment of chronic respiratory and metabolic diseases. These problems often necessitate consultation with other physicians. Bladder retraining may be necessary to adjust the patient's voiding schedule. The patient also may have to limit some activities associated with daily lifestyle (jogging, tennis, etc.), and should embark upon an honest attempt at Kegel's exercises (3,4).

Kegel's perineal resistive exercises should be taught to postpartum patients as prophylaxis against the development of urinary stress incontinence. They will help many patients with urinary stress incontinence compensate to such a degree that surgery may be postponed. The first step in teaching a patient Kegel's exercises is to teach her awareness of the function of the pubococcygeus muscle. Once this is learned, with the examining finger on the medial margin of the pubococcygeus at the level of the urethra, the patient should be told to "1) squeeze the vaginal muscles upon the palpating finger, 2) draw up or draw in the perineum, 3) contract or draw up the rectum as though checking a bowel movement, and 4) contract the perineal muscles as though interrupting the flow of urine while voiding." Once this is learned, the pubococcygeus should be contracted for 3 to 4 seconds, 15 times in a row, at least 6 times a day for at least 3 months. In addition, the patient should learn to contract the pubococcygeus *prior* to physical efforts which may cause sudden increases in intra-abdominal pressure (coughing, laughing, sneezing, lifting, awkward movements, etc.).

The alpha-adrenergic stimulating drugs phenylpropanolamine, imipramine, and phenylephrine and the general adrenergic stimulator ephedrine can increase the smooth muscle tone of the urethra and be useful in treating urinary stress incontinence. The beta-adrenergic blocker propranodol has theoretic usefulness but is rarely used for this problem.

Tampons, Smith-Hodge and ring pessaries, and other devices have been recommended for the relief of urinary stress incontinence (6). Their success in providing socially acceptable continence is variable and unpredictable. To buy time, they may be tried if care is taken to prevent excessive drying of the vagina, pressure necrosis, and the inflammation and ulceration which may be associated with their use.

In cases of socially disabling urinary stress incontinence, the author prefers a modification of the Burch colpourethropexy (1) as the primary surgical procedure, and is even more convinced that this is the procedure of choice for the patient who insists upon preserving childbearing potential. The operation was designed to correct mild and moderate cystocele; its durability can be improved by using permanent suture materials.

In this particular case, the surgeon would have to use his or her best judgment about entering the peritoneal cavity to obliterate the cul-de-sac and/or suspend the uterus prophylactically. Although these procedures may realign the uterus and prevent the development of an enterocele, which is a recognized complication of a Burch procedure, they may cause adhesions and infertility. Likewise, the surgeon would have to use his or her judgment about the need for correction of the "moderate rectocele." If a rectocele repair is to be done, the author would not do it until all other procedures had been completed.

The author is not aware of any articles in medical literature that deal specifically with the route of delivery of an infant in a patient who becomes pregnant and must be delivered after successful surgical correction of urinary stress incontinence. Krantz (5) has stated that after the Marshall-Marchetti-Krantz procedure "pregnancy may be anticipated without difficulty and vaginal delivery, while not preferred, is not contraindicated." Given what we know about the etiology and pathophysiology of urinary stress incontinence and the importance attached to cure by the first operation, the author would not hesitate to recommend an elective cesarean section, preferably prior to the onset of labor, for all patients needing delivery who have had a successful operation and cure of their urinary stress incontinence.

REFERENCES

1. Burch JC: Urethrovaginal fixation to Cooper's ligament for correction of stress incontinence, cystocele and prolapse. *Am J Obstet Gynecol* 81:281–290, 1961.
2. Crystle CD, Charme LS, Copeland WE: Q-tip test in stress urinary incontinence after repair operations. *Obstet Gynecol* 38:313–315, 1971.
3. Kegel AH: Progressive resistance exercises in the functional restoration of the perineal muscles. *Am J Obstet Gynecol* 56:238–248, 1948.
4. Kegel AH: Stress incontinence and genital relaxation. In: Walton JH (ed): *Ciba Clinical Symposia*. Summit, NJ, Ciba Pharmaceutical Products, 4:35–51, 1952.
5. Krantz KE: The Marshall-Marchetti-Krantz procedure. In: Stanton SL, Tanagho EA (eds): *Surgery of Female Incontinence*. New York, Springer Verlag, 1980, pp. 47–54.
6. Norton C: Pads and mechanical methods. In: Stanton SL (ed): *Clinical Gynecologic Urology*. St. Louis, CV Mosby, 1984, pp. 499–510.

67

Inability to Void Following Vesicourethral Sling Procedure

David H. Nichols

Case Abstract

Severe and socially disabling recurrent urinary stress incontinence was found in an obese patient with chronic bronchitis and emphysema.

A vesicourethral sling procedure was advised and was accomplished using a modified Goebell-Frangenheim-Stoeckel technique employing a strip of fascia lata.

The transurethral catheter was removed on the fourth postoperative day, and although otherwise comfortable, the patient was unable to void. She was catheterized repeatedly during the next 24 hours, after which the transurethral catheter was replaced. It was removed again on the morning of the eighth postoperative day, and despite a strong desire and conviction that the bladder would function, the patient was still unable to void. Although straining hard as by a Valsalva maneuver, she could express only a few drops of urine.

DISCUSSION

One presumes that a normal detrusor pressure had been determined preoperatively. A "hypotonic" bladder, so diagnosed, would predispose to an overflow incontinence masquerading as urinary stress incontinence, for which the treatment might be detrusor stimulation as by bethanecol (Urecholine) in a therapeutic dose (10 to 25 mg, three times daily). This condition might be encountered in a patient with multiple sclerosis, central nervous system lues, or diabetic neuropathy. If it has been determined that the postvoid residual urine volume is greater than 100 cc, self-catheterization at least three times daily would help to restore the baseline of a periodically empty bladder. This should be continued often for a very long time until the residual urine volume obtained is consistently less than 60 cc. The Mentor female plastic disposable catheter is an excellent instrument the patient can learn to use for this purpose.

The surgeon must review the list of daily medications that a patient is taking to determine whether any alpha-adrenergic blockers are being consumed, as in the treatment of coexistent hypertension. Should this be found, alternate antihypertensive therapy should be employed and the patient's urodynamics appropriately restudied.

Inability to void following a retropubic suburethral sling procedure generally occurs when the tension under which the sling has been fixed is too great, and an actual mechanical obstruction of the urethra has been produced. In most instances the sling has been initially fixed too tightly; either the operator misjudged the proper tension, or more likely the sling itself was too short and excess tension was produced consequent to fixing the ends of the sling to the rectus aponeurosis.

This problem might be avoided by more thoughtful consideration of the initial tension at which the sling should be placed—observing Moir's suggestion that it be placed only tightly enough to "take out the wrinkles and ruckles that are present" within the sling (1) (Fig. 67.1).

If the sling has been fashioned from a strip of Mersilene mesh (never tape) it may be precut to any desired length up to 12 cm. If, however, the operator has chosen fascia lata, and the strip is too short and can be fixed in place only by applying an excess degree of tension, it is possible to lengthen the sling before it has been fixed in place, as shown in Figure 67.2.

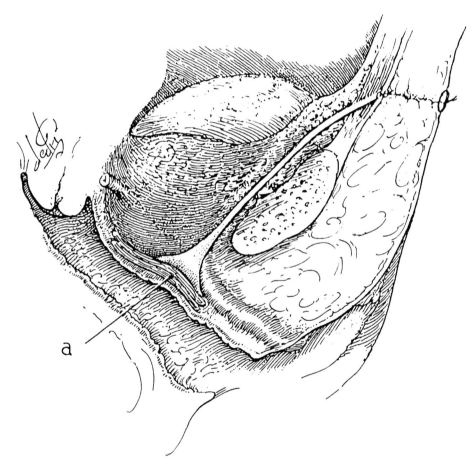

Figure 67.1.   The gauze hammock is shown fixed in place beneath the vesicourethral junction and the bladder. The ends have been attached to the rectus aponeurosis, and the incision in each groin closed. The vaginal portion of the hammock has been insulated from the vagina by a two-layer vaginal lapping procedure (A).

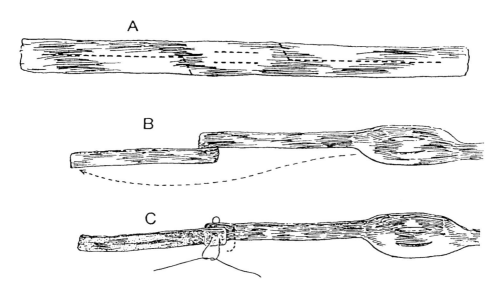

Figure 67.2. **A.** A means of increasing the length of the fascia strip is shown. Incisions are made along the path of the *dotted lines.* **B.** This is folded back without loss of continuity. **C.** A single stitch is placed to fix the folded fascia in place. The same procedure is accomplished on the opposite end of the fascial strip. If an increase in the thickness of the central belly of the strip is desired, it may be incised, as shown by the *two dotted lines* in the center of the strip **(A).** This widened belly may be anchored in place by a few sutures beneath the vesicourethral junction at the time the vaginal portion of the sling is placed.

Although there is considerable postoperative edema immediately following a surgical sling procedure, this generally subsides by the fourth or fifth postoperative day and by itself is not a common cause of postoperative inability to void. Replacing the catheter (preferably using one which is silicon coated to reduce mucosal edema) for a day or two will allow residual edema to subside further. However, if the patient is still unable to void and the bladder is neurologically normal, one must presume a mechanical obstruction from the sling. Because there are a few persons who habitually void by contracting their rectus abdominis muscles instead of relaxing them, one should ascertain from the patient's history that this is not the case. If it is, the voiding habits of such a person must be changed and the patient taught to relax when voiding.

The treatment of a significant mechanical obstruction requires that it should be relieved promptly by freeing *one* end of the sling from its attachment to the rectus aponeurosis within a few days of the initial surgery; if this was the cause of the inability to void, the patient will invariably be relieved. Interestingly, the patient will generally remain continent, because by the fifth or sixth postoperative day there is enough healing around the sling to hold its central belly more or less in place. The opposite end of the sling still elevates the vesicourethral junction, but the pathologic obstruction has been relieved.

After 2 months from the original surgery, the fibrosis and healing around the sling will probably be so great that the tension may not be relieved by cutting or freeing the sling at the site of its attachment to the rectus aponeurosis. If this is the case, the sling may be transected through a transvaginal incision lateral to the midline, thus avoiding the site of the previous incision into the vagina. If necessary, this may be followed by stretching the urethra with an appropriately sized dilator, which will also permit the urethra to "rock" beneath the pubis. Transvaginal cutting of the sling does increase the potential risk of infection by exposing the wound to the considerably mixed bacterial flora of the vagina.

This complication should not exist if the sling has not been initially placed under too much tension. The degree of tension requires precise judgment: if too loose the incontinence will not be relieved, and if too tight the patient will be unable to void comfortably.

The vesicourethral junction may be replaced to a proper retropubic pelvic position by inserting a firm intravaginal packing at the conclusion of the vaginal portion of the operation and prior to fixing the abdominal ends of the sling to the rectus aponeurosis. When the vaginal portion of the operation has been completed, the abdominal ends of the sling may be fixed to the rectus aponeurosis with minimal tension.

A mild or partial degree of obstruction appears to be generally transient, since over a period of time the patient tends to develop increased detrusor tone sufficient to permit intravesical pressure to exceed intraurethral pressure at the time of voiding. Patients so inclined may be taught self-catherization using the flexible plastic Mentor catheter for the female urethra. The technique is "clean," but not sterile, and the patient may boil and reuse the catheter as necessary. This is particularly helpful for the patient in whom inability to void adequate amounts is thought to be the result of transient postoperative edema, which will subside with healing. Some operators prefer to use a suprapubic catheter regularly instead of a transurethral one. This is certainly an acceptable approach to postoperative bladder drainage but would of itself not relieve urethral obstruction. If the latter is present and the patient is persistently unable to void following clamping of the suprapubic catheter, the treatment of the problem would be outlined as above.

REFERENCE

1. Moir JC: The Gauze Hammock Operation. *J Obstet Gynaecol Br Commonw* 75:1, 1968.

SELECTED READINGS

Nichols DH: The Mersilene mesh gauze-hammock in repair of severe or recurrent urinary stress incontinence. In: Taymor ML, Green TH (eds): *Progress in Gynecology*, Vol. 5: New York, Grune & Stratton, 1970.
Nichols DH: The sling operations. In: Cantor EB (ed): *Female Urinary Stress Incontinence*. Springfield, IL, Charles C. Thomas, 1979.
Ridley JH: *Gynecologic Surgery—Errors, Safeguards, Salvage*, ed. 2. Baltimore, Williams & Wilkins, 1981.

68

Suburethral Sling Rejection

Stephen B. Young

Case Abstract

A polytetrafluoroethylene suburethral sling (Gore-Tex® soft tissue patch) was inserted in a 62-year-old multiparous female weighing 240 pounds and measuring 5 feet tall. The indication was recurrent genuine stress incontinence (GSI) with a low-pressure urethra (maximum urethral closure pressure of 14 cm H_2O) in the presence of chronically increased intra-abdominal pressure secondary to marked obesity, as well as a 46-pack-a-year cigarette history with concomitant chronic cough and asthma. The patient had undergone two prior anterior colporrhaphies for stress incontinence and was markedly disabled secondary to her recurrent GSI. The surgery and early postoperative course were completely uncomplicated, with normal voiding, complete continence, and no local vaginal symptoms.

Beginning 2 months after the operation, the patient experienced persistent vaginal bleeding and discharge. Large quantities of polypoid granulation tissue were removed from the anterior vaginal wall incision site where it had been closed in two layers of interrupted no. 2–0 polyglycolic acid suture (Dexon). During the next 4 months, recurrent granulation tissue was removed or cauterized on multiple occasions without success. Finally, at 8 months after the operation, the central belly of the Gore-Tex® patch became palpable through an open anterior vaginal wall.

DISCUSSION

Sling procedures using autologous and more recently synthetic materials have developed over the past 85 years as a very effective treatment for both recurrent GSI and as a primary procedure in those patients at high risk for failure of a standard urethropexy. Since 1951, the search for a perfectly strong and inert synthetic material has progressed through Nylon and Mersilene tape, to gauze hammocks of Mersilene or Marlex, to Dacron and Vicryl mesh, and most recently to Silastic bands and Gore-Tex® patches (3). The tape was quickly abandoned because the narrow 0.5-cm slings obstructed and sometimes transected urethras. Professor J. Chasser Moir and more recently Professor David Nichols have successfully utilized a wider piece of Mersilene mesh rather than tape, cutting it into the shape of a hammock 2.5 to 3 cm wide at the central belly (4). This Mersilene gauze hammock more widely and evenly distributes the tension over the entire proximal urethra and distal bladder, thus rendering the sling nonobstructive. It obstructs the urethrovesical junction only at the moment of physical stress when its lateral arms sutured to the anterior rectus fascia are pulled cephalad.

Concerns regarding severe scar formation secondary to fibroblastic infiltration through the large interstices of the Mersilene mesh have limited its wide acceptance. The prospect of the difficult task of excising a densely scarred, infected Mersilene mesh sling has prompted urogynecologic investigators to seek a material with less tendency toward fibroblastic infiltration. Silastic and Gore-Tex® remain freer from surrounding tissues. Thus, in instances of inappropriate sling tension, infection, or rejection, the Silastic and Gore-Tex® materials are more easily approached for adjusting tension or removing the sling.

The Gore-Tex® suburethral sling has an 85% cure rate, and the complications are delayed voiding and poor healing of the anterior vaginal wall over the graft (1). The sling reaction and removal rate with the Gore-Tex® patch has recently been reported as high as 23% (2). In 24 of 115 patients (21%) the Gore-Tex® sling was removed because of tissue reaction, the site being vaginal in 18, abdominal in 8, and in both sites in 2 patients. The reactions occurred before 1 month in 5 patients, between 1 and 3 months in 12 patients, between 3 and 6 months in 3 patients, and beyond 6 months in 4 patients. The incontinence cure rates following sling removal were 74% subjectively and 65% objectively. In another study of 45 patients, six slings (13%) required removal secondary to graft infection and/or vaginal mucosa erosion (5). Though most patients following Gore-Tex® sling removal have reportedly remained continent, the postsling symptoms of significant vaginal bleeding and discharge in addition to the need for a second surgical procedure make this complication distressing.

Over the past 3 years, the author's clinic has inserted 83 Mersilene mesh suburethral slings and has not as yet had to remove a single one. One patient has had four episodes of unilateral suprafascial *Staph aureus* groin infection; the one inguinal sling arm

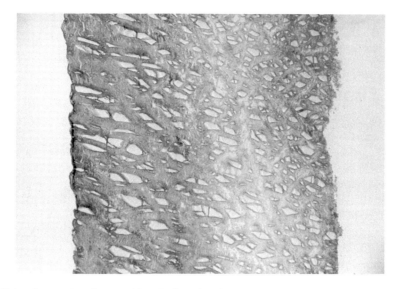

Figure 68.1. Cross section of removed Gore-Tex® patch, H & E stain; 25 × magnification. The W.L. Gore company reported as follows: "Histological analysis of the soft tissue patch sling confirmed your findings of infection. Gram-positive cocci were evident within the soft tissue patch interstices directly beneath the surfaces. A degenerated cell-neutrophilic granulocyte-protein matrix was associated with the bacteria. Both Gore-Tex soft tissue patch surfaces were essentially devoid of biological material."

and its sinus tract was excised 6 months ago and the patient has remained completely continent and symptom-free. Three patients have had one episode of superficial wound infection which resolved completely and did not recur. Overall cure rates have been 92% by 1 year postoperative urodynamics. Forty-two patients responded to a postsling questionnaire 10 to 36 months postoperatively; 34 (81%) were totally stress continent, 6 (14%) reported total stress continence except for an occasional minimal leak, 1 patient (2%) described rare morning stress incontinence with a full bladder only, and 1 patient (2%) with a preoperative drainpipe urethra reported no improvement. Further experience may confirm that Mersilene mesh has a far lower risk of sling rejection than Gore-Tex®.

Case Resolution

The patient presented in the abstract was returned to the operating room 8 months after the sling was installed and the central belly of the sling was excised vaginally (Fig. 68.1). However, the symptoms persisted and the patient developed a draining sinus from the right groin incision. Four months later the inguinal arms of the Gore-Tex® were removed along with the sinus tract via groin incisions. Following this second procedure, the patient healed completely and had no further vaginal symptoms. After an initial period of recurrent urinary incontinence, she became completely dry.

REFERENCES

1. Bent AE: Management of recurrent genuine stress incontinence. *Clin Obstet Gynecol* 33:358-366, 1990.
2. Bent AE, Ostergard DR, Zwick-Zaffuto M: Tissue reaction to expanded polytetrafluoroethylene suburethral sling for urinary incontinence: Clinical and histologic study. *Am J Obstet Gynecol* 169:1198-1204, 1993.
3. Horbach NS: Suburethral sling procedures. In: Ostergard DR, Bent AE (eds.): *Urogynecology and Urodynamics*, ed. 3. Baltimore, Williams & Wilkins, 1991, Chapter 41.
4. Nichols DH: *Vaginal Surgery*, ed. 3. Baltimore, Williams & Wilkins, 1989, Chapter 5.
5. Summit RL, Bent AE, Ostergard DR, Harris TA: Suburethral sling procedure for genuine stress incontinence and low urethral closure pressure: A continued experience. *Int Urogynecol J* 3:18-21, 1992.

SUGGESTED READINGS

Hohenfellner R, Eckhard P: Sling procedures. In: Stanton SL, Tanagho EA (eds): *Surgery of Female Incontinence,* ed. 2. Berlin & Heidelberg, Springer-Verlag, 1986, Chapter 7.
McGuire EJ, Wan J: Pubovaginal slings. In: Hurt WG (ed.): *Urogynecologic Surgery.* Gaithersberg, MD, Aspen Publishers, 1992, Chapter 5–5.

69

Persistent Stress Urinary Incontinence After Retropubic Sling Procedure: Pharmacologic Management

Michael P. Aronson

Case Abstract

A 63-year-old obese, hypertensive para IV on multiple medications, including conjugated estrogen and prazosin, was seen for a 2-year history of severe recurrent urinary incontinence. She had had a vaginal hysterectomy with anterior and posterior colporrhaphies in the distant past. The patient's physical examination revealed a grade 2 rotational descent of the bladder neck. Multichannel urethrocystometry with urethral pressure profilometry revealed marked stress urinary incontinence, no evidence of detrusor instability, and a low maximal urethral closure pressure with poor stress pressure transmission. The patient underwent a retropubic sling procedure. On postoperative day 5, she voided well with small residuals and was discharged. Subsequently, the patient reported stress-related incontinence with mild symptoms of detrusor instability. A repeat urodynamic study revealed improved, but still low normal, urethral pressures with improved stress pressure transmission. The patient was changed from prazosin to a different antihypertensive medication with some improvement. The patient was then started on imipramine, after which she became completely continent.

DISCUSSION

All urinary continence is ultimately a problem in fluid dynamics. The outlet, or urethral, pressure must be maintained above that in the bladder or the patient will be incontinent. Continence therefore depends on the ability of intra-abdominal forces to transmit to the proximal urethra and on the inherent intraurethral pressure itself. Multiple anatomic and physiologic factors contribute to the development of urethral pressures. There are many surgical, pharmacologic, and hormonal options available to enhance those pressures. The above case illustrates several of them well.

Anatomic and Physiologic Factors

The anatomic location of the urethrovesical junction in relation to the pelvic floor is widely recognized as crucial to the maintainence of continence. Loss of the normal supports to the anterior vaginal wall, bladder, and urethra can lead to loss of equal and simultaneous transmission of increases in intra-abdominal pressures to the bladder and

318

the proximal urethra. This loss of pressure advantage at the outlet leads to spillage of vesicular contents. Most surgical procedures for correction of genuine stress urinary incontinence, including this patient's prior anterior colporrhaphy, are designed to elevate the urethrovesical junction into a position to receive intra-abdominal forces.

In addition to the anatomic relations of the bladder neck, the inherent pressure within the urethra plays an important role in maintaining continence. The anatomy and physiology of the female urethra are quite complex (3,12,2). A full discussion is beyond the scope of this chapter, but a simplified functional model can be examined. Resting intraurethral pressure develops from three distinct sources: striated muscle, smooth muscle, and a vascular, mucosal effect.

A three-portion, striated, urogenital sphincter muscle surrounds the urethra for approximately 80% of its length. This striated muscle acts as a unit and is composed of predominantly slow-twitch fibers largely under voluntary control. Its contribution to urethral pressures can be lost secondary to mechanical damage or denervation injury. Sometimes its contribution can be enhanced by pelvic floor exercises.

Deep to this striated muscle is a thin circular and a well-developed longitudinal smooth muscle layer. This smooth muscle is under autonomic control, primarily by alpha-adrenergic innervation. Because of its concentration of alpha-adrenergic receptors, the smooth muscle contribution to urethral pressures can be decreased with alpha-adrenergic blockers or enhanced with alpha sympathomimetics. Estrogen may increase the number of these receptors.

The smooth muscle of the urethra surrounds an arteriovenous complex which underlies the urethral mucosa itself. This plexus can fill and empty. Interruption of its arterial supply has been shown to decrease urethral pressures. The contribution to urethral pressures of this component can be lost to estrogen deprivation atrophy in the menopausal patient (5). Conversely, urethral pressures can be enhanced with exogenous estrogens.

Retropubic Sling Procedures and the Low-Pressure Urethra

In this case, the patient had recurrent stress incontinence with low urethral pressures demonstrated with multichannel urodynamics and urethral pressure profilometry. Not all patients with recurrent incontinence require a retropubic sling procedure, but those with low urethral pressures respond well to this approach. A retrospective study of patients undergoing a Burch retropubic urethropexy found that those with low-pressure urethras failed their surgery three times more often than those with normal preoperative urethral pressure profiles (13). One investigator found that 75% of patients who failed incontinence surgery had urodynamic evidence of low urethral pressures (8). The same investigator demonstrated a greater than 90% subjective cure rate in this same population after a retropubic sling procedure (9). Overall subjective cure rates in collected series of retropubic sling procedures range from 60% to 100%. Objective cure rates range from 70% to 95%.

Previous incontinence surgery is a major predisposing factor for a low-pressure urethra. This is particularly true of anterior colporrhaphy, which can disrupt the laterally entering blood and nerve supply to the urethra if it is skeletonized during the procedure. This leaves a devitalized and scarred urethra which cannot function normally even when properly positioned. Low urethral pressures are not limited to previously operated patients and should be ruled out in older patients with new-onset incontinence. Continent patients with massive prolapse should have low urethral pressures ruled out to prevent unmasking potential "hidden incontinence" during repair of their prolapse. Retropubic sling procedures should also be considered for patients with severe chronic obstructive pulmonary disease, obesity, congenital tissue weakness, or a strenuous or athletic lifestyle.

Retropubic sling procedures have been performed for over three-quarters of a century. Over the years there have been many modifications of this operation in terms of sling materials (both organic and synthetic), attachment points, and surgical technique. This patient had a Mersilene mesh sling performed in the manner described by Nichols (10). No matter what material or technique is used, the most crucial part of the procedure is judging the tension on the sling itself. Numerous methods have been described to facilitate this decision, including the use of intraoperative cystoscopy, intraoperative urethral pressure measurements, pull through of inflated balloon devices, and assessment with progressive dilators. A vaginal packing technique as described in the above reference was used in this case. It is important to acknowledge that all these methods share the limitation of being performed on an anesthetized patient in the lithotomy position and cannot accurately reflect the anatomy and physiology of the nonparalyzed patient during her activities of daily living.

Evaluation

While postoperative urodynamic studies in general consistently show improvement in the stress pressure transmission ratios, the maximum urethral closure pressure and functional urethral length may be increased, decreased, or left unchanged by a retropubic sling procedure (7,11,6). The success or failure of the procedure does not appear to correlate with the latter two parameters. A correlation has been shown between improved pressure transmission ratios in the proximal urethra and surgical success (11,6).

This patient voided easily after her surgery but demonstrated stress incontinence within weeks. Her repeat urodynamic study showed improvement of her cough transmission ratio and minimal improvement of her urethral pressures. This patient, however, had another factor contributing to her low urethral pressures and perhaps her incontinence. She was taking prazosin.

Pharmacologic Management

Prazosin (Minipress) is a popular antihypertensive agent which selectively blocks postsynaptic alpha-1 adrenergic receptors on arteriolar smooth muscle, thereby lowering the peripheral vascular resistance. Like any alpha-adrenergic blocker (such as phenoxybenzamine), it decreases urethral smooth muscle contractility and also relaxes the vascular bed underlying the urethral mucosa, with a subsequent decrease in urethral pressures.

In 1990, Wall and Addison published a case report documenting resolution of stress incontinence as well as a substantial increase in urethral pressures and functional urethral length in a hypertensive patient after discontinuance of prazosin (14). In 1992, Dwyer and Teele reported on 1335 women evaluated in their urodynamics unit (4).

Fifty-eight (4.3%) were taking prazosin. Twenty-five of 45 patients had their incontinence improved or cured by stopping prazosin. Seven of those cured had follow-up urodynamics with results consistent with those reported by Wall and Addison.

This patient was taken off prazosin and showed some improvement, but she continued to have mild stress incontinence as well as some symptoms of detrusor instability. She was started on an alpha-adrenergic stimulating agent in an effort to further enhance her inherent urethral pressures. Studies of three commonly used alpha-sympathomimetic drugs—imipramine, phenylpropanolamine, and ephedrine—have shown improvement or cure in more than half of patients treated with mild to moderate stress incontinence (1). Because of this patient's mild detrusor instability, imipramine was chosen since it also demonstrates an anticholinergic effect, which would address these symptoms. Throughout this interval, this patient continued to take exogenous estrogen as she had preoperatively. The patient became, and remains, completely continent.

Summary

This patient had residual stress urinary incontinence after a retropubic sling procedure. Her urethral pressures and stress pressure transmission were close enough to the continent state to allow medical manipulation of her inherent urethral pressures to make her continent. Had this not been the case, surgical options such as tightening of one arm of her sling, replacement of her sling, periurethral collagen bulk injections, or artificial sphincter placement could have been considered.

REFERENCES

1. Castleden CM, George CF, Renwick AG, Asher MJ: Imipramine: A possible alternative to current therapy for urinary incontinence in the elderly. *J Urol* 125:318, 1981.
2. DeLancey JOL: Correlative study of paraurethral anatomy. *Obstet Gynecol* 68:91, 1986.
3. DeLancey JOL: Structural aspects of the extrinsic continence mechanism. *Obstet Gynecol* 72:296, 1988.
4. Dwyer PL, Teele JS: Prazosin: A neglected cause of genuine stress incontinence. *Obstet Gynecol* 79(1):117, 1992.
5. Fantl JA, Wyman JF, Anderson RL, Matt DW, Bump RC: Postmenopausal urinary incontinence: Comparison between non-estrogen supplement and estrogen supplement women. *Obstet Gynecol* 71:823, 1988.
6. Hilton P: A clinical and urodynamic study comparing the Stamey bladder neck suspension and suburethral sling procedures in the treatment of genuine stress incontinence. *Br J Obstet Gynaecol* 96:213, 1989.
7. Horbach NS, Blanco JS, Ostergard DR, et al: A suburethral sling procedure with polytetrafluoroethylene for the treatment of genuine stress incontinence in patients with low urethral closure pressure. *Obstet Gynecol* 71:648, 1988.
8. McGuire EJ: Urodynamic findings in patients after failure of stress incontinence operations. *Prog Clin Biol Res* 78:351, 1981.
9. McGuire EJ, Lytton B: Pubovaginal sling procedure for stress incontinence. *J Urol* 119:82, 1978.
10. Nichols DH: Recurrent urinary stress incontinence. In: Nichols DH, Randall CL: *Vaginal Surgery*, ed. 3. Baltimore: Williams and Wilkins, 1989, 109–124.
11. Rottenberg RD, Weil A, Brioschi PA, Bischof P, Frauer F: Urodynamic and clinical assessment of the Iyodura sling operation for urinary stress incontinence. *Br J Obstet Gynaecol* 92:829, 1985.
12. Rud T, Anderson KE, Asmussen M, Hunting A, Ulmsten U: Factors maintaining the intraurethral pressure in women. *Invest Urol* 17:343, 1980.
13. Sand PK, Bowen LW, Panganiban R, Ostergard DR: The low pressure urethra as a factor in failed retropubic urethropexy. *Obstet Gynecol* 69:399, 1987.
14. Wall LL, Addison WA: Prazosin-induced stress incontinence. *Obstet Gynecol* 75:558, 1990.

70

Inability to Void Four Months After Needle Suspension Surgery

Edward J. McGuire

Case Abstract

An 81-year-old woman complained of intermittent urge incontinence and inability to void volitionally 4 months following a needle suspension procedure for urinary stress incontinence. Examination demonstrated a "well-supported" urethra.

DISCUSSION

Inability to urinate following needle suspension, retropubic suspension, or sling procedures is not unusual; some 15% to 30% of patients are in varying stages of urinary retention 10 days to 2 weeks after such procedures. Although a general perception exists that hypersuspension or elevation of the urethra can lead to problems with emptying, there are no prospective data on particular surgical techniques which would prevent urinary retention from occurring. Retention is more likely to occur in the elderly because detrusor muscular strength and functional capacity decrease with age. It is possible that difficulty with voiding occurs when a given suspension induces more urethral resistance than a particular bladder can handle or overcome.

The ability of the detrusor to overcome urethral resistance is unknown, since we have no accepted method to measure urethral resistance during voiding, except as that process is related to an elevation in detrusor pressure during micturition. If no detrusor contraction can be elicited during a urodynamic evaluation, it is impossible to establish a diagnosis of obstructive uropathy objectively, even though that may exist.

On the other hand, women unable to urinate 6 to 8 weeks following a needle suspension operation are unlikely to spontaneously resolve that problem, and thus surgical relief of the condition should be considered. Patients with severe urethral incontinence often urinate by abdominal pressure alone, and of course that is impossible after an adequate suspension operation has been performed. If one can urinate effectively using abdominal pressure alone, then some degree of stress incontinence will also be present. A normal (or surgically achieved normal) stress-competent urethra will not leak at any abdominal pressure, and thus voiding by straining is not possible following an operation that repairs urethral hypermobility or poor function. Therefore, the careful evaluation of a patient "unable to void" has one overriding goal: to determine as nearly as possible whether this is a patient without detrusor function. In that case the patient will be better off using intermittent catheterization for life in lieu of recurrent stress incontinence, since stress incontinence, surgically induced, will be required for her to resume "voiding" by abdominal pressure. Patients with detrusor activity are not a problem, since release or takedown of the hypersuspension is all that is required even if that is not always easily achieved.

Historical Hints Regarding Reflex Contractility

Symptoms are an unreliable index of the presence of obstruction or of true reflex bladder contractility. For example, the symptom scores used for males in an effort to partially quantitate the degree of obstructive uropathy associated with benign prostatic hypertrophy have been higher for women with stress incontinence than for men with a presumptive diagnosis of prostatism. Nevertheless, the presence of urge incontinence after a suspension often indicates reflex detrusor contractility, particularly if this occurs in women who are unable to void volitionally. In other words, women who are surprised by sudden wetting in certain circumstances postoperatively, and who are still required to use intermittent catheterization to empty the bladder or who are relying on suprapubic tube drainage, are usually obstructed at the bladder outlet. Urgency and frequency alone, without incontinence and pain, are not indicative of detrusor contractility. These symptoms may result from malposition or eroded sutures, which may need removal, but they are not specific for obstruction of an otherwise capable detrusor.

Age definitely has a bearing on detrusor function. Younger women can usually, but not always, be assumed to have reasonable detrusor contractile function.

Physical Findings

The urethra is typically hypersuspended with the vesical neck in an unusually high position. The vagina will be found to be pulled toward the top of the symphysis on either side of the urethra and vesical neck. Endoscopy is usually difficult, with the axis of the urethra being angled sharply anteriorly toward a point midway between the umbilicus and pubic symphysis, rather than in the normal nearly horizontal course of the urethra. In long-term obstruction the bladder may look trabeculated, but that change also occurs in the aging bladder and is, by itself, an unreliable sign of obstruction. Tenderness at palpation of the suture or bolster sites on either side of the urethra may lead to an early decision to remove sutures and bolsters, but that finding does not indicate that the patient will resume normal voiding after urethrolysis. It does suggest that relief of pain may be obtained by removing the sutures and bolsters.

Urodynamic Evaluation

For an unequivocal diagnosis of obstructive uropathy, bladder pressure at the time of volitional micturition, with the external sphincter relaxed, must be greater than 30 cm H_2O, and the bladder outlet should open poorly or not at all at that time. The rise in bladder pressure must clearly be the result of a detrusor contraction, and not a Valsalva maneuver. To positively identify all of these changes, a video urodynamic study, with at least two pressure channels, is usually required. Pressure flow studies help if the bladder pressure is elevated at the time when the flow rate is highest, but normative data for females are not very extensive, and the test is plagued by artifacts. Flow rates alone are not helpful, since they do not allow the differentiation of poor voiding related to obstruction from that related to detrusor hypofunction or nonfunction.

Clinical Decision Making

On purely clinical grounds, a patient voiding normally prior to the operation, who cannot void at all after 4 months, who has either urge incontinence or so-called bladder spasms (painful bladder contractions associated with extreme urgency), *and* who also demonstrates a hypersuspended urethra on the basis of physical examination and endoscopy, can be presumed to suffer from obstructive uropathy. Although this diagnosis is not 100% accurate, it is reasonably close.

Urethrolysis

The transvaginal approach to loosening the urethral suspension is quick, avoids the operative trauma and difficulty of a suprapubic approach, and yet allows the operator to freely mobilize the urethra within its fibrous fascial envelope. The author uses a vertical incision over the urethra or two lateral incisions similar to the incisions and dissection used for needle bladder neck suspension operations. The dissection should be deliberately kept superficial to the periurethral fascia as the vaginal mucosa is lifted off that underlying structure, even if the offending sutures and bolster material are deep to that plane. The dissection is carried laterally until, the maneuver described by Raz, the retropubic space is entered on both sides. This frees the urethra and its envelope of fascia and allows for excellent mobility. The degree of mobility can be assessed by placing traction on the Foley catheter and noting the degree to which the urethra moves posteriorly into the vagina. If the urethra is still relatively fixed, continued sharp dissection of the adherent bands lateral to and, if necessary, anterior to, the urethra can be done to effect free mobilization. If sutures or bolsters have been a source of pain or inflammation, an effort to remove them should be made at this point. Often the sutures can be palpated in the retropubic space and grasped with a right-angle clamp, cut, and removed. Occasionally one needs to open the individual or collective suprapubic wound(s) and remove the suture material and bolsters there as well. Sutures anchored with bolster material placed in the periurethral tissue will not pull out from above, and the bolsters must generally be removed by sharply dissecting them from the surrounding tissue.

Recently surgeons have begun using synthetic material to bolster needle suspension suture fixation or as "slings" placed behind the urethra. When Gore-Tex® is used beneath or adjacent to the urethra or to bolster the purchase of the sutures in the rectus fascia, a dense inflammatory process makes removal extremely difficult. Nevertheless, if obstructive uropathy is present, any foreign body in the paraurethral area must usually be removed to relieve the obstruction.

Operative Outcome

In the author's experience normal and reasonably normal voiding usually occurs within 1 to 2 days after urethrolysis. Residual urine volumes are checked by instituting intermittent catheterization. Very occasionally, after urethrolysis, normal voiding resumes over a 1- to 2-week period following discharge from the hospital. The author does not have any reasonable explanation for why, in some patients, it takes some time to resume voiding. Also, infrequently but occasionally, patients who have an initial good result from a total urethrolysis return with obstructive uropathy. On examination the urethra is again found to be hypersuspended. The author knows of no perfect solution to this problem, except to redo the urethrolysis. Some surgeons have advocated wrapping the urethra in omentum or a labial fat graft, but no prospective study to demonstrate the efficacy of these techniques presently exists.

If intermittent catheterization is chosen as a long-term method of management, bladder pressure to those volumes obtained by catheterization must be less than 20 cm H_2O. This indicates a "safe" bladder as far as the upper urinary tract is concerned.

SELECTED READINGS

Chancellor MB, Kaplan SA, Axelrod D, Blaivas JG: Bladder outflow obstruction versus impaired contractility: Role of uroflow. *J Urol* 145:810, 1991.

Foster HE, McGuire EJ: Management of urethral obstruction with transvaginal urethrolysis. *J Urol* (in press).

Kelly MJ, Zimmern PE, Leach GE: Complications of bladder neck suspension procedures. *Urol Clin North Am* 18:342, 1991.

Labasky RF, Leach GE: Failure of operations for stress urinary incontinence: Evaluation and treatment. *Advances in Urology* 3:107, 1990.

Lose G, Jorgensen L, Mortensen SO, Molstead-Pedersen L, Kristensen JK: Voiding difficulties after culpo suspension. *Obstet Gynecol* 69:33, 1987.

Raz S: *Atlas of Transvaginal Surgery.* Philadelphia, WB Saunders, 1992.

Richardson DA, Bent AE, Ostergard DR, Cannon P: Delayed reaction to the Dacron buttress in urethropexy. *J Reprod Med* 29:689, 1993.

SECTION VII

INTESTINAL PROBLEMS AND INJURIES

71

Right Lower Quadrant Pelvic Abscess

Leslie W. Ottinger

Case Abstract

A 57-year-old nullipara gave a history of recurrent episodes of progressively more severe right lower quadrant abdominal pain and fever of six almost monthly intervals. These were accompanied by loss of appetite and nausea without vomiting, and a progressive chronic constipation. During the episodes of pain the abdomen became somewhat distended, but the condition had generally responded to several days of bedrest and broad-spectrum antibiotics. However, the patient had recently been experiencing spiking temperature elevations to 102°F, and some leukocytosis at 28,000, mostly polymorphonuclear leukocytes.

Convinced that this persistent and very tender, fixed, right adnexal ill-defined mass, slowly enlarging to its present 8-cm diameter, represented a chronic recurrent pyosalpinx, the surgeon determined that the patient was a candidate for surgery. At laparotomy, performed through a Pfannenstiel incision, a watery, purulent exudate was encountered in the peritoneal cavity, along with dense fibrinous adhesions between the large and small bowel, making exposure of the pelvis exceedingly difficult. Digital exploration of the deep right lower quadrant pelvic thickening was undertaken, and the examining finger broke through the wall of an abscess cavity from which a large quantity of copious, thick, creamy green exudate emerged. Digital exploration of the abscess cavity appeared to demonstrate thickened, shaggy walls composed, for the most part, of the edematous walls of both large and small intestine. The pelvic organs were not visualized, and the surgeon wondered about the source of the abscess and what to do next.

DISCUSSION

Based on a history of monthly recurrent episodes of sepsis and the presence of a tender right pelvic mass, this surgeon favored a clinical diagnosis of a chronic recurrent pyosalpinx. Then acute signs of worsening infection led to an urgent operation. In fact, if the gastrointestinal symptoms are attributed to secondary bowel inflammation, the picture would seem generally consistent with the diagnosis. It was not necessarily incorrect to proceed to a laparotomy, although the surgeon no doubt would come to wish that other diagnoses had been ruled out by preoperative tests and studies. In fact, to go ahead with drainage is the first step, whatever the underlying cause, and it is usually possible to establish the etiology at the time of operation.

The surgeon, by a safe, blunt dissecting technique, entered and drained a large abscess cavity. The wall was made up of loops of intestine. Fibrous adhesions made further exploration difficult. Seeking the underlying cause of the abscess under the described circumstances would be unwise and would risk injuring a normal segment of intestine, perhaps with a resultant fistula. The surgeon should place a large passive drain, bringing it out through a separate small incision in the right lower quadrant. This would keep a tract open for liquification and drainage of the exudate in the walls of the cavity and of a fistula should one form. Next, attention to preventing a wound infection is important. Useful measures include intraoperative parenteral antibiotics, careful hemostasis, thorough irrigation of the wound, and closure, as far as possible, of all open spaces. With respect to this last point, the Pfannenstiel incision is perhaps not the best choice when the surgeon expects to encounter sepsis. Other measures to be considered are antibiotic solution irrigations of the wound and delayed closure of the skin and subcutaneous layer.

Since the cause of the abscess was not established at the time of surgery, several diagnoses will need to be ruled out during the postoperative period. Should a fistula ensue, this task will be simplified. Without this, a CT scan would be a good place to start. Contrast studies and endoscopy will help to rule out a lesion in the sigmoid colon, cecum, and terminal ileum.

The following are the diagnoses other than pelvic inflammatory disease that need to be ruled out and that might have been given more attention in the preoperative evaluation:

1. Appendicitis with a chronic abscess
2. Diverticular abscess of the sigmoid colon
3. Perforated carcinoma of the sigmoid colon
4. Chronic inflammatory bowel disease, colon or ileum
5. Perforated cecal carcinoma or diverticulum
6. Idiopathic pelvic abscess, perhaps from an occult foreign body

All except the idiopathic abscess will require a further operation, appendectomy being a possible exception. Although recurrence of appendicitis will occur in approximately 20% of cases where only drainage was performed, some patients may prefer to accept this risk rather than undergo an elective appendectomy.

72

Injury to Bowel During Pelvic Surgery

George W. Mitchell, Jr.
Fred M. Massey

Case Abstract 1: Transabdominal Injury

A total abdominal hysterectomy with bilateral salpingo-oophorectomy was being performed on a 36-year-old patient with severely symptomatic disability from advanced pelvic endometriosis.

Because of the long-standing severity of the condition, the hysterectomy was difficult, especially since surgical dissection proceeded in the tissues around the cervix. The cul-de-sac had been obliterated by the disease, and cleavage planes were difficult to establish. As soon as the uterus had been removed, it was evident that a 2-cm longitudinal rent had been made through the full thickness of the anterior rectal wall near the vaginal apex.

DISCUSSION

When a difficult pelvic operation is in prospect, it is essential for the surgeon to determine, to the extent possible, whether or not the bowel is likely to be involved. This is particularly true when endometriosis is palpable in the posterior pelvis adjacent to the rectal wall, when the secondary manifestations of pelvic inflammatory disease are known to be present and adherent masses palpable, when the presence of ovarian carcinoma is suspected, and in all instances when the patient has had multiple previous pelvic surgical procedures. Pelvic operations may also be necessary on patients who are known to have intrinsic bowel problems such as Crohn's disease, ulcerative colitis, and diverticulitis. In all of these circumstances, some type of preoperative bowel workup is indicated, and this should include at minimum proctosigmoidoscopy or barium enema. Selected patients should also have an upper intestinal endoscopy and barium studies.

If direct bowel involvement is diagnosed preoperatively or there is a strong possibility of bowel injury during surgery, preoperative preparation of the bowel is indicated. Even if no bowel problems are anticipated, decompression of both the large and small intestine greatly facilitates pelvic surgery and is routinely accomplished by a mild cathartic the evening before and an enema the morning immediately prior to surgery. Nurses should be instructed to be certain that all of the fluid injected into the rectum is recovered before discontinuing the enema. More rigorous bowel preparation consists of cleansing enemas until clear and the oral administration of a drug, such as neomycin and erythromycin base, to lower the intraluminal bacterial content of the intestine. Various different solutions have been proposed for the enemas, including some containing anti-bacterial drugs, but plain water is probably just as effective. A good rule is to prepare the bowel when there is the slightest doubt about the need to do so. After a rigorous bowel preparation, electrolytes should be checked, and an intravenous solution with potassium should be started if there is evidence of dehydration.

At the operating table, the pelvic surgeon should always protect the intestine from injury. Even relatively minor nicks and abrasions have been shown to increase the risk of postoperative intestinal obstruction. In packing the bowel out of the operating field, care should be taken not to exert undue pressure, not to handle the bowel directly with forceps, and not to release intestinal adhesions by blunt dissection. If the rectosig-moid is prolapsed and adherent to the lower pelvis, its attachments to the pelvic organs should be severed by careful sharp dissection and the lateral peritoneal reflection cut as high as is necessary to allow adequate upward mobilization. Attempts to free the intestine by avulsing it from its attachment often cause injury either to the bowel wall or to the mesentery. Packing should be accomplished when the patient has had enough relaxing drug to permit it to be done easily. Nitrous oxide distends the bowel and should not be used in these circumstances. The anesthesiologist should be kept informed of problems. To attempt to pack the bowel against persistent downward pressure will increase the chances of postoperative ileus, if it does not cause immediate bowel injury. As in the case of the rectosigmoid, adherent ileum in the pelvis should be mobilized by sharp dissection and bleeding points carefully ligated or fulgurated following relocation upward.

Direct injury to the bowel may be quite accidental, making the need for constant inspection of the viscera adjacent to the operative site imperative, or it may be the result of a calculated risk when tissue planes are absolutely unreadable and progressive dissection is essential for the successful completion of the operation. An intrafascial enucleation of the cervix is helpful in preventing rectal injury. This is particularly true when there are dense adhesions caused by endometriosis between the anterior surface of the rectum and the posterior surfaces of the cervix and vagina, as in the case described. Early recognition of such injury is important to avoid spillage of bowel contents, and closure should be undertaken immediately unless the primary surgical procedure is at a critical stage or there is an additional emergency, such as excessive blood loss, which takes priority.

In the case under discussion, the 2-cm vertical rent in the anterior surface of the rectum should have been carefully debrided and closed in the same plane with interrupted sutures about 3 mm apart, set in such a way that the mucosa and the immediately adjacent seromuscular layer would be inverted. Profuse leakage from the opening should be controlled by a proximal rubber-shod intestinal clamp. A two-layer closure of an opening this small would be technically difficult and would add little to the competence of the closure. The caliber of the rectum is so large that a vertical closure seldom constricts the lumen significantly. Most surgeons would use nonabsorbable suture material for the closure, some preferring nylon or other synthetic material and some preferring silk. The preference here is for the latter. The other difficult question in this type of situation is whether the rectal tissues being closed are so disrupted or fibrous, as a result of endometriosis, that they will not heal. The odds are that a small opening will heal well, but, if the opening is large, creating a tissue deficiency, or if serious disease such as carcinoma is present, making successful closure unlikely, an attempt might be made to approximate the edges and cover the closure with a portion of the greater omentum. However, a temporary diverting colostomy at the level of the descending colon should also be done. Diverting sigmoid colostomies have the advantage of better patient acceptance because of the passage of formed stools, but the disadvantage that their location might eventually complicate the process of secondary rectal repair requiring mobilization of the sigmoid colon. Had the ovaries not been removed prior to the injury to the bowel, oophorectomy should have been seriously considered before closure to prevent future bowel problems due to endometriosis, provided that the necessary consent had been obtained.

Following closure of an unplanned opening through the full thickness of the rectal wall or elsewhere in the colon, most surgeons would institute some type of drainage, especially if there had been overt spillage of feces into the peritoneal cavity. Suction drainage is preferred over the old Penrose drain, and the tube should be brought out, retroperitoneally if possible, through a stab wound in either lower quadrant, where it should be fixed to the skin with sutures.

Drains should never be brought out through the original incision and should be left in for no longer than 24 to 48 hours, since they serve only to provide an immediate portal for infected material which might otherwise collect to form an abscess. If left in longer, they act as foreign bodies and channels for the reentry of bacteria.

Injuries to the small intestine in the course of pelvic surgery should also be closed as soon as possible. Horizontal tears are best closed in the same plane, but vertical or diagonal tears, if they are long and through the full thickness of the bowel wall, should be closed in the horizontal plane to avoid constriction of the lumen. In most instances, a single-layer closure will suffice, using interrupted nonabsorbable suture material and carefully inverting the edges of the mucosa and the adjacent seromuscular layer. Necrotic tissue should be trimmed before the closure. The patency of the lumen should be tested by squeezing the thumb and forefinger together from either side of the suture line. Occasionally, injuries occur as a result of the necessity to separate small bowel loops damaged by irradiation. The blood supply to damaged loops should be evaluated to determine whether the bowel is viable and whether a closure will remain competent. If this is questionable, or if the injuries are multiple but confined to a specific segment, resection of that segment and stapled functional end-to-end anastomosis or hand-sewn end-to-end anastomosis constitutes the procedure of choice.

Attempts have been made to determine the viability of injured bowel by sending biopsies to the pathology laboratory, but this is usually not helpful. Ten cc of 10% fluorescein may be given intravenously and a Wood's light used to evaluate the vascularity of the affected area. When the patient's condition is poor, resection of the small bowel difficult, and injuries multiple—a combination most often associated with irradiation damage—sidetracking the involved area by side-to-side anastomosis of the proximal and distal loops while leaving the damaged intestine in situ may be expedient. Obviously, this is not possible if the affected area is necrotic. While the abdomen is still open for verification of placement, the anesthesiologist can insert a nasogastric tube.

Prior to closure, the peritoneal contents should be irrigated, especially if there has been gross spillage of fecal material. Although some surgeons prefer to use antibiotics in the irrigating solution, there are no data to suggest that this is superior to normal saline. It is appropriate, however, to start such patients intraoperatively on antibiotic therapy on the assumption that peritonitis is certain to occur otherwise. Although the predominant organism is *Escherichia coli*, good broad-spectrum coverage can be obtained with a combination of a cephalosporin and an aminoglycoside. Intravenous fluids should be continued for at least 3 days, and the patient should be permitted nothing by mouth until normal bowel sounds have returned and she is passing flatus per rectum. Vital signs should be monitored for the early possibility of septic shock, should some virulent organism such as beta-hemolytic streptococcus be the invader. Peritoneal signs should also be carefully followed and the wound inspected daily. After a contaminated case, some surgeons prefer to leave the skin and subcutaneous tissues open, with sutures placed for secondary closure. Others drain the subcutaneous space superficially at either end of the closed incision. The preference here is for primary closure unless the contamination at the time of injury has been great, in which case secondary closure should be done. The risk of postoperative wound infection is significantly increased and should be promptly treated when it occurs. Local redness, heat, pain and swelling, and an elevation of temperature suggest the need for drainage. The incidence of dehiscence of the wound is also increased.

When normal bowel sounds return and the patient begins to pass gas per rectum, a liquid diet may be started. If this is well tolerated, the diet may be graduated rapidly to soft and then to regular fare. If ileus persists or there is evidence of partial mechanical obstruction, the patient should be permitted nothing by mouth, and a nasogastric tube should be inserted for continuous decompression. Failure to use a nasogastric tube for abdominal distention or persistent ileus can result in perforation of the intestinal closure. On some services, postoperative enemas are used routinely to expedite evacuation of gas and the return of normal peristalsis. These and cholinergic drugs are strictly contraindicated when there has been an injury to the large or small bowel or when the appendix has been removed. When symptoms of obstruction persist or when there is evidence of spreading peritonitis, long-tube drainage should be instituted if nasogastric suction fails, and surgical reexploration of the abdomen should be considered. Total parenteral nutrition should be instituted when it seems likely that oral feeding will have to be long deferred. Gastrostomy or feeding jejunostomy may also be necessary to improve the nutritional status.

Case Abstract 2: Accidental Proctotomy at Vaginal Tubal Ligation

Colpotomy was performed to perform a transvaginal tubal ligation. The initial incision in the vault of the vagina was made directly into an unprepared rectum, covering the operative field with fecal material. As the operator attempted to close the defect with some side-to-side interrupted stitches in the rectum, it was evident that a small opening had been made in the peritoneum of the cul-de-sac.

DISCUSSION

To enter the posterior cul-de-sac with precision, using needle, scalpel, or scissors, it is logical first to identify the approximate inferior margin of the cul-de-sac of Douglas. This can be done in several ways, the most efficient being to circumcise the cervix at the junction of the posterior portio with the vaginal mucosa and, with strong upward traction on the incised cervical margin, to sweep the vagina and rectum away from the isthmus, using a forefinger covered by a layer of gauze. With this method it is difficult to miss the right plane, and the peritoneum will eventually protrude between the rectal muscle and the posterior surface of the uterus. To provide the necessary mobility when the cul-de-sac is shallow, it may be necessary to sever the lateral vaginal mucosa from its cervical attachment as well. This technique should be used for posterior colpotomy for tubal ligation, but, since it takes time and colpotomy can usually be accomplished without it, many experienced surgeons prefer to estimate the most likely spot for the incision.

While the posterior lip of the cervix is drawn toward the pubis with heavy traction, a midline vertical fold of vagina, about 2 inches from the portio, is pulled downward toward the introitus with forceps. The grasping point should be distal to any obvious high rectocele. A triangle of vaginal mucosa, outlined by the tenaculum, the forceps, and the posterior wall of the cervix, is thus exposed. The incision is made with curved scissors, points turned upward, into the vertical fold about midway between the tenaculum and the forceps and directed toward the posterior cervix. Some surgeons prefer to enter the peritoneum with one cut of the scissors, but safety dictates a more cautious approach, first cutting through both layers of the vagina, noting whether rectal fibers are present, and then proceeding upward, exploring with the scissors and using blunt dissection to mobilize rectal muscle downward until the peritoneum is opened. Bleeding points on the rectal muscle are fulgurated or ligated. A retractor can then be inserted into the peritoneum and any type of exploration feasible for that area carried out.

The third method, suitable for beginners or when disease or anatomic defect seems to obliterate the posterior cul-de-sac, is to proceed as above but to explore the rectum directly through the anus, with a forefinger covered with a second glove. This will assure the surgeon that the planned culdotomy is well above the rectal mucosa or that he or she should modify his or her approach to suit the anatomic situation.

In the event the rectal wall is entered but not the rectal mucosa, a few interrupted absorbable sutures, placed to invert torn edges, should serve to close the defect. Straight Lambert-type sutures are best because they invert the edges, and, to prevent their pulling through, they should not be tied at maximum tightness. A smooth approximation is all that is needed. When the injury penetrates the rectal mucosa, a similar closure is done through all layers. One layer of sutures is sufficient unless the margins of the rent are badly mangled, in which case the rectum should be widely mobilized from the undersurface of the vagina and closed with as many sutures as necessary to ensure competence. The vagina mucosa, when closed, acts as a back-up layer. Synthetic sutures of no. 2-0 size are best for this type of repair, but the catgut used by many senior surgeons is still acceptable. The minimum number of sutures to effect the closure successfully should be used.

Since inadvertent proctotomy in the course of posterior culdotomy is uncommon, major preoperative bowel preparation is not ordered routinely for such cases, but enemas should be given, not only to clear the bowel of feces, but also to avoid rectal distention. In the case under discussion, the immediate contamination of the field by feces suggests that enemas were not given or that they were not properly evacuated. When gross contamination occurs, it should be sucked out of the field as rapidly as possible and an attempt made to seal the defect temporarily, either with a finger or a loosely placed figure-of-eight suture, while the extent of the damage is considered and a decision made regarding what should be done next. Most accidental rectal openings are below the peritoneal reflection; in fact, it is difficult to make a surgical opening in the intraperitoneal portion of the rectum. Opening the peritoneum at the same time that the rectum was opened strongly suggests a careless initial incision by the surgeon, and this action introduces the possibility of postoperative peritonitis.

An immediate decision should have been made not to do the tubal ligation, in order to avoid further contamination higher in the pelvis. The rectal opening should have been closed as outlined above, removing any temporary suture that might have been placed unless it was presumed to be adequate. A difference of opinion exists as to whether the peritoneum should be drained or closed primarily. The decision should be based on the degree of contamination. If a drain is to be used, it should be of the suction type. To prevent its slipping out, the drain can be kept in place by a single, fine, plain catgut suture through the drain and the edge of the peritoneum, not more than 2 mm from the edge, from which it can be easily pulled out. After the rectal closure, the vagina should be closed around the drain with interrupted sutures and a loose vaginal pack left in the posterior vagina to obliterate dead space. Temporary diverting colostomy is seldom indicated when inadvertent proctotomy occurs below the peritoneal reflection, since the closure will usually heal without fistula formation. Only if a significant opening is made above the peritoneal reflection, the local damage around the proctotomy site is extensive, or the tissues have been irradiated should colostomy be considered.

Postoperatively, the patient who has suffered such a surgical accident will soon be wide awake and inquiring about the operation. An immediate full disclosure of exactly what happened is indicated. The patient should be told that, even though another hospitalization will be required and another anesthesia, the tubal interruption must be postponed until after any possible complications. The patient should not be fed solid food until wound healing is ensured. For the first week, an elemental diet that is largely absorbed in the jejunum should be given, and for 2 weeks thereafter, a low-residue diet. The drain and vaginal pack should not be left in longer than 24 hours. In the authors' opinion, antibiotics should be given but should not be continued for more than 24 to 48 hours. The authors' preference is to administer therapeutic antibiotics if the temperature remains elevated for 2 successive days or if signs of pelvic peritonitis develop.

73

Unexpected Clamping of Small Bowel During Hysterectomy

John H. Isaacs

Case Abstract

A 70-year-old patient with procidentia was undergoing a vaginal hysterectomy. A partial colectomy because of diverticulitis of the sigmoid colon had been performed 5 years previously. There were adhesions of small bowel to the left cornual angle prior to the removal of the uterus. The operative procedure, being photographed, was momentarily halted while the photographer changed tape and refocused the camera. When surgery was resumed 10 minutes later, it was evident that the Heaney forceps on the right cornual angle of the uterus had included 2 inches of small bowel that previously had not been noticed at this site. The bowel had not been opened.

DISCUSSION

The literature on intestinal injury during gynecologic surgery is scant. A search of the literature of the past 10 years has revealed only two articles published on the subject (1). Krebs's article reported that 128 incidents of intestinal injury occurred in his institution from 1973 to 1982. Vaginal operations led to bowel injury in 11 of 965 cases (1.1%). The principal reason, as in this case, was adhesions from previous surgery. In the discussion of Krebs's paper, Droegemueller points out that it is not lack of knowledge that leads to intestinal injury but rather incompetence during the surgical procedure. This may well have been what happened with this patient.

This mishap might have been avoided if the surgeon had had good visualization. Before the first Heaney clamp was placed across the cornual angle of the uterus, care should have been taken to dissect any adhesions that were attached to the uterine fundus or to the proximal portion of the round ligament, ovarian ligament, or fallopian tube. Since these adhesions can be either on the anterior or posterior surface of any of these structures, careful scrutiny of the area is mandatory before the Heaney clamp is applied. One safeguard is to ligate the first pedicle, leaving the suture long and tagged with a hemostat. In this way, there is no clamp in the way that might add further difficulty in clamping the opposite cornual angle. In spite of these precautions, accidents do happen and must be rectified.

The situation in this case is an area of bowel that has been crushed and consequently devitalized (Fig. 73.1). If this tissue is left as is it will undoubtedly necrose and the bowel will perforate in 24 to 48 hours, with a resulting enterovaginal fistula at best

Figure 73.1. Heaney clamp across the round ligament, ovarian ligament, fallopian tube, and including a segment of small bowel.

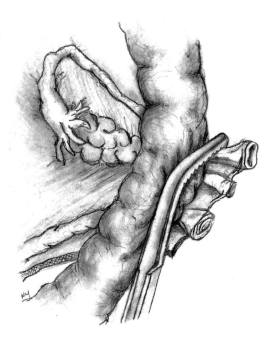

or an operative death at worst. Major small bowel fistulae are associated with a mortality rate of approximately 20% to 30%.

Since we must assume that the surgeon is aware of the gravity of the situation, methods of correction must be considered. In various textbooks and the literature through 1993, no specific guidelines are offered for managing this situation. The two articles mentioned earlier (by Krebs and by Parys) may be helpful. Three possibilities exist. First, one can open the abdomen and resect the damaged portion of the bowel and possibly do an end-to-end anastomosis. This, in the author's view, would represent far too much surgery for the problem at hand and should be done only if it is technically impossible to repair the damage via the vaginal route. The second option is to resect the crushed section of bowel, as it is exposed through the vagina, and close the bowel in two layers. This would contaminate the operative field and increase the chances of postoperative morbidity. There would also be the risk that the repaired enterostomy site might not heal, causing leaking and subsequent complications. The ideal (third) choice would be to remove the Heaney clamp and dissect the remaining adhesions between the small bowel and the adnexa. The Heaney clamp could be reapplied to the adnexal pedicle and ligated. The portion of bowel which has been damaged could be steadied with two Babcock clamps and the damaged area inspected closely (Fig. 73.2). Since the bowel has been crushed but not opened, the damaged portion could be inverted using several interrupted no. 00 black silk sutures or polyglycolic acid sutures through the seromuscular layers of the normal bowel on each side of the devitalized portion (Fig. 73.3) of ileum. This should promote secure healing, since the healing process depends on approximation of the serosal surfaces. This technique may reduce the lumen of the small bowel (Fig. 73.4) but should not really interfere with normal bowel function. Over time the bowel lumen will enlarge to equal that of the adjacent bowel.

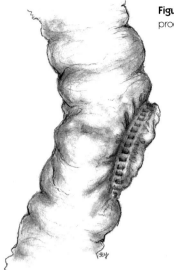

Figure 73.2.   The damaged section of small bowel showing the crush mark produced by the Heaney clamp.

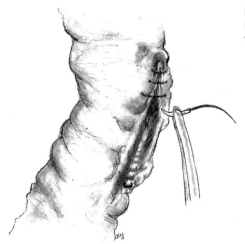

Figure 73.3.   The devitalized bowel has been invaginated and healthy serosal surfaces are approximated with interrupted no. 00 black silk sutures.

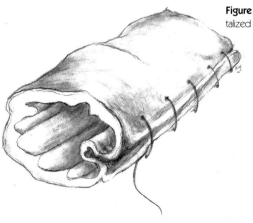

Figure 73.4.   Cross section of the small bowel after the devitalized area has been invaginated.

REFERENCES

1. Krebs HB: Intestinal injury in gynecologic surgery: A ten-year experience. *Am J Obstet Gynecol* 155:509–514, 1986.
2. Parys BT: Effect of hysterectomy on bowel function (letter). *Br Med J* 299:979, 1989.

SELECTED READINGS

Barber HR, Graber EA: The intestinal tract in relation to obstetrics and gynecology. *Clin Obstet Gynecol* 15:650, 1972.

Hardy JD: Surgical complications. In: Sabiston D (ed): *Textbook of Surgery.* Philadelphia, WB Saunders, 1981.

Howkins J, Stallworthy J: *Bonney's Gynaecological Surgery,* ed. 8. Baltimore, Williams & Wilkins, 1974.

Irvin TT: Techniques of anastomosis in gastro-intestinal surgery. In: Rod G, Smith R (eds): *Atlas of General Surgery,* ed. 3. London & Boston, Butterworths, 1981.

Käser I, Iklé FA, Hirsch HA: *Atlas of Gynecological Surgery.* New York, Thieme Stratton, 1985.

Simmons SC, Luck RJ: *General Surgery in Gynaecological Practice.* Oxford & Edinburgh, Blackwell Scientific Publications, 1971.

74

Rectovaginal Fistula

John J. Mikuta

Case Abstract

Spontaneous delivery and right mediolateral episiotomy and repair were followed by considerable rectal pain throughout the patient's hospitalization. A fecal impaction was broken up the day before discharge, and considerable edema and tenderness of the anterior rectal wall were noted. At a dimple at the base of the anterior rectal wall, a small loop of suture was palpable. The patient was discharged.

At 6-week postpartum checkup the patient complained that she had difficulty controlling rectal gas, and a copious purulent and almost constant vaginal discharge required sanitary protection. Although the episiotomy had healed, a 0.5-cm defect surrounded by granulation tissue was noted between the vagina and the top of an anal crypt.

DISCUSSION

The sequence of events in this particular case suggests very strongly that the causative factor in this patient's case was probably a combination of a rectal suture and the trauma associated with a fecal impaction as well as removal. Rectal sutures following episiotomy repair are not at all uncommon. If they are discovered at the time the repair is completed, it can be relatively simple to cut the suture and leave it be. On the other hand, there are probably many times when unidentified sutures in the rectum at the time of episiotomy repair are never discovered and appear to cause no significant problems. If catgut suture had been used in the repair the possibility of subsequent development of fistula would be much less than if a synthetic suture material was used. This is because catgut is absorbed much more quickly than is synthetic suture material.

A fistula that is discovered 6 weeks after delivery and episiotomy should not be repaired immediately, but the repair should be delayed anywhere from 4 to 6 months. This will allow reduction of the inflammatory reaction, an increase in the blood supply to the area, and time for maximal scar tissue delineation to occur prior to making the attempt at repair. In the meantime, again depending on the size of the fistula, the patient may be made more comfortable by being placed on a low-residue diet. The patient should reduce the intake of foods that have a tendency to produce intestinal irritability and that may increase the amount of gas or create a more liquid type of stool. Another problem is resumption of sexual activity if the patient is concerned about the esthetic effect of the fistula or about the escape of gas during intercourse. Such factors may be controlled by either the use of condoms by the male or by the use of enemas or douches prior to intercourse.

For a very small fistula as described here, it is very important to know whether the fistulous opening leads into the bowel at an angle or whether it is straight, and also whether it involves the anal sphincter. In the former case, the repair is relatively straightforward. The latter would require incision through the muscle of the anal sphincter to remove all of the scar of the fistula prior to performing the repair.

Assuming that the anal sphincter is intact, one can prepare the patient for the standard layer-by-layer repair. After the appropriate waiting period and a careful examination with probing of the fistula to determine its direction and length, it is very helpful to proctoscope the patient to be sure that there is no intrinsic bowel disease. A fistula associated with Crohn's disease may be very difficult to repair successfully and may be associated later with other fistulas in the perianal area.

Preoperative preparation should include mechanical cleansing of the bowel with laxatives and enemas to remove as much fecal material as possible. Bowel preparation using neomycin orally may be given over a period of 3 days, although some individuals recommend instillation of neomycin just prior to surgery after a thorough mechanical cleansing of the bowel has been done for several days. A liquid diet 24 hours prior to surgery will help to reduce bowel contents.

The surgical principles involved in a repair of a rectovaginal fistula include having a wide enough ellipse of normal vaginal mucosa removed to guarantee that the underlying tissues that remain will be free of scar and freely mobile. The rectal mucosa then is closed by no. 3-0 chromic catgut, avoiding entry into the lumen of the bowel and inverting the rectal mucosa into the rectal lumen. A second layer approximates the rectal muscularis and fascia, and the final layer approximates the vaginal mucosa. The second layer is generally of a longer-lasting standing material such as Vicryl or Dexon.

Postoperatively the patient is kept on a low-residue diet for several days until spontaneous evacuation of the bowel occurs. Laxatives and enemas are avoided, as is digital examination of the rectum.

There may be variations in the technique depending on the location of the fistula. At times a fistula that involves the anal sphincter is best handled by producing a fresh fourth-degree tear, excising the fistula completely, and then doing a fresh repair, approximating the rectal mucosa and the anal sphincter and reconstituting the perineal body. In patients who have an old third- or fourth-degree laceration where the anal sphincter has retracted laterally on either side, the Warren flap operation has for years been a standby. A flap is created that essentially constitutes the posterior vaginal wall, with part of the base of the triangle being the areas at which the anal sphincter edges create a puckering of the perianal tissues. A flap is created from this mucosa above which the sphincter edges are approximated. The sphincter edges must be free of scar and fully mobilized. The rectal fascia and the levator ani muscles are approximated over this midline, and then the perineal body is reconstituted to complete the repair.

Today many surgeons, in carrying out this complete perineal repair, use a simple layer method. Instead of creating the flap, they simply remove the tissue, identify the sphincter ends, and then approximate the denuded tissue to reconstitute the anterior rectal wall down to the level where the sphincter has been placed.

There are times when the sphincter has been retracted for such a long period of time that approximation of the sphincter ends creates a significant narrowing of the anal canal. An excellent way to avoid this problem is to make a counter-sphincterotomy away from the site of the repaired sphincter edges and remove the tension from the repair site, as described by Miller in the 1930s (1).

The final question is when to do a colostomy. Fecal diversion may be necessary in patients who have a fistula of significant size and constant soilage is occurring, and if a waiting period must be observed before a repair is attempted. This would be especially true of large fistulas or a fistula located high up in the vagina. This type is usually produced by entry into the rectum at the time of abdominal or vaginal hysterectomy. These colostomies are generally undertaken for patient comfort and can be replaced after the fistula is repaired.

There are also times when the repair fails and when, in order to have optimal bowel preparation and the healthiest possible environment for the repair, a colostomy should be carried out. Although this may be disagreeable to the patient, the fact that it may improve the potential for successful repair may provide a sufficient incentive for the patient to agree to the procedure.

REFERENCE

1. Miller NF, Brown W: The surgical treatment of complete perineal tears in the female. *Am J Obstet Gynecol* 34:196, 1937.

SELECTED READINGS

Mengert WF, Fish SW: Anterior rectal wall advancement. *Obstet Gynecol* 5:262, 1955.
Nichols DH, Milley PS: Surgical significance of the rectovaginal septum. *Am J Obstet Gynecol* 108:215, 1970.
Nichols DH, Randall CL: *Vaginal Surgery*, ed. 3. Baltimore, Williams & Wilkins, 1989.
Warren JC: A new method of operation for the relief of rupture of the perineum through the sphincter and rectum. *Trans Am Gynecol Soc* 72:322, 1882.

SECTION VIII

PELVIC CANCER SURGERY

75

Carcinoma of the Vulva with Coexistent Genital Prolapse

George W. Morley

Case Abstract

A 39-year-old married homemaker with multiparous relaxation of the vagina, mild urinary stress incontinence, and a retroverted, slightly enlarged uterus had a 1.5-cm invasive squamous cell carcinoma of the right labium majus. A single, hard, immovable lymph node was palpable in the right groin.

DISCUSSION

It is interesting to note that this patient is only 39 years of age, since invasive carcinoma of the vulva is seen more commonly as a clinical entity in the older age population. This lesion is, however, seen occasionally in younger patients; therefore, one should be prepared to carry out appropriate diagnostic tests when a lesion of this type is seen in this age group. The treatment of choice for this patient is radical vulvectomy and bilateral groin lymph node dissection and pelvic lymph node exploration. Certainly a frozen section should be carried out on the suspicious groin lymph node; should this be positive, then some gynecologic oncologists would carry out a retroperitoneal pelvic lymph node exploration at this time. The issue of whether this patient should be treated with postoperative pelvic irradiation is not within the scope of this discussion.

The question raised in this abstract is an interesting one in that it becomes a question of clinical judgment as to whether surgery for two different and unrelated problems should be performed at "one sitting." With more sophisticated anesthetic methods and with improved surgical techniques, certainly this question enters the realm of possibility. Much experience has been reported in the surgical literature throughout the last decade, and many authors feel that "double" surgery for unrelated pathologic conditions carries with it very little risk. This seems to be especially true when one considers intra-abdominal procedures such as hysterectomy and cholecystectomy.

In regard to this case, the answer seems quite simple, since the patient has only "mild" urinary stress incontinence and the uterus is only "slightly" enlarged. In this patient, the author would be much more concerned with possibly altering surgical techniques as they relate to the primary problem in an attempt to preserve the clitoral tissue without jeopardizing the patient's chance for survival. This, of course, would increase the operating time. It is possible that too much tissue was removed in performing the radical vulvectomy part of the procedure. This question can only be resolved by gynecologic oncologists, who see a significant number of these patients each year, and in clinics where close follow-up is a major part of their effort. It must be remembered, however, that the conventional therapy as indicated above is the treatment of choice until the results from these principal investigators are in.

If one is considering more surgery for this patient, then certainly "cosmetic" vulvoplasty should be given attention. Certain rotational or transpositional flap techniques could be included in the primary procedure in an attempt to gain an improved cosmetic result. To date, most gynecologic oncologists have deferred this part of the procedure because of (a) lack of experience, (b) limited technical possibilities, and (c) poor results. Furthermore, a number of these patients develop functional abnormalities—such as misdirected micturition, introital stenosis, or marked pelvic relaxation—which requires surgical correction in the future. It is at this time that some type of vulvoplasty can be considered.

This abstract might have read: "moderate stress urinary incontinence and grade 2 uterine prolapse with a symptomatic rectocele, and the patient wants something done." This makes the discussion more controversial. If the patient were 75 years of age, the answer would be easier and the author would probably deny her request.

Even in the 39-year-old patient, given the risk of additional surgery and another anesthetic and realizing that abdominal and pelvic surgeons are less hesitant today to do unrelated surgeries at one time, there is one overwhelming point that supports the decision not to perform combined surgery in this patient. It has often been reported that wound infection and wound disruption are the most common complications following radical pelvic surgery for an existing invasive carcinoma of the vulva. This militates against doing any additional elective surgery on these patients. The rectal area is difficult to sterilize, and, in its close proximity to the operative site, this may, in itself, be a reason for the high incidence of groin wound breakdown. One could, however, do a perineorrhaphy at the time of closure of the posterior vulvar wound to correct this patient's symptomatic rectocele. In addition, one might consider an anterior colporrhaphy in an attempt to correct the stress urinary incontinence symptoms. The author would draw the line at this point, being strongly opposed to entering the peritoneal cavity via the vaginal hysterectomy and to entering the space of Retzius with all its vascularity in performing a retropubic urethropexy.

In the future, should the incidence of wound disruption in radical vulvectomy and groin lymph node dissection decrease significantly, then the treatment of the symptomatic pelvic relaxation could be seriously considered—especially in a 39-year-old patient. This patient may want something done, but her desires could suddenly change if she experiences a significant postoperative complication. This combined surgical approach would be difficult to defend in other arenas.

A number of less conservative gynecologic surgeons would not hesitate to do a radical vulvectomy and groin lymph node dissection followed by a vaginal hysterectomy, and anterior colporrhaphy or possibly a retropubic urethropexy, a posterior colpoperineorrhaphy, and even a sacrospinous ligament suspension of the vaginal apex if indicated—especially in a 39-year-old patient. More than likely, the patient would do well; however, if she became morbid, it could be very significant. The author would probably not be influenced much by the patient's age. Many physicians say that they took a chance in a young patient and did thus and so. We must remember it is the patient who takes the chance. It seems wiser to avoid the "blue-plate special" or the "package deal" as a convenience to the patient when one might place the patient in significant jeopardy.

Carcinoma of the Vulva with Coexistent Genital Prolapse—A Contrasting View

Augusto G. Ferrari
Luigi Frigerio

Case Abstract 1

A 66-year-old woman (gravida II, para II) presented with a painful, ulcerated lump 4 cm in diameter on the right labium majus. She also demonstrated a large cystocele (third degree, according to Halfway System (HWS) classification) (1) with moderate uterine descensus (first degree). Vulvar biopsy was positive for invasive squamous cell carcinoma.

The patient underwent a radical "en bloc" vulvectomy with bilateral and retroperitoneal pelvic lymphadenectomy. Vaginal hysterectomy and McCall culdeplasty (6) were performed, followed by an anterior colporrhaphy combined with pubourethral ligament plication (Nichols procedure) (7). A bilateral skin flap transposition from the internal thigh was employed to correct the perineal defect.

Pathology revealed squamous cell carcinoma of the right vulva that extended to the clitoris (maximal thickness 14 mm, invading subcutaneous fat). Lichen sclerosus was found on marginal areas. Staging T2 N1 M0 (stage III, Federation of International Gynecologists and Obstetricians) was related to metastatic involvement of one right inguinal node. Uterine and cervical specimens were negative for metastatic disease.

The patient's postoperative course was complicated by superficial wound breakdown on the right inguinal margin. She received 5000 cGy of pelvic and groin irradiation. Sixty months after diagnosis the patient remained without evidence of recurrent disease. She was still continent with good vaginal vault suspension in spite of moderate cystocele (first degree).

DISCUSSION

Radical vulvectomy combined with en bloc dissection of the groin lymphatics may be performed by removing the area of the femoral nodes without the skin of the inner thigh (Fig. 76.1). This procedure reduces the risk of postoperative wound breakdown. When frozen section is positive for metastatic involvement of Cloquet's nodes, extraperitoneal gland dissection of the iliac, obturator, and hypogastric nodes could be necessary.

Closed Jackson-Pratt suction systems ensure appropriate drainage of retroperitoneal fluid, thus decreasing the risk of lymphocyst and infection.

Figure 76.1.   Modified removal of femoral nodes without the thigh skin. The *vertically striped area* represents the surgical incisions and specimen. The *pointed triangles* indicate the area of groin dissection without sacrifice of overlying skin. The *dotted line* marks the inguinal ligaments: the fascial incision for extraperitoneal lymphadenectomy extends just above the line from the external inguinal ring to the anterior superior spine. *(P.* Pubic symphysis. *ASIS.* Anteriorsuperior iliac spine.)

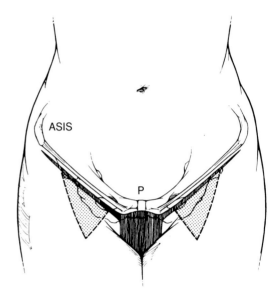

Total vaginal hysterectomy was employed to restore normal anatomy and to correct vaginal prolapse. After a V-shaped resection was done of the high posterior vaginal wall, a McCall culdeplasty suspended the posterior vaginal fornix to the uterosacral ligaments, closing the cul-de-sac. Two no. 2–0 polyglycolic acid sutures are generally used for the McCall procedure, and a no. 2–0 polydiaxinone suture is used for peritoneal closure, involving the vault as high as possible.

The anterior vaginal wall is correctly mobilized after anterior median colpotomy. Pubourethral ligament plication using polydioxanone (PDS) suture (no. 2–0) in the authors' experience prevents the appearance of "de novo" stress incontinence after prolapse correction (4).

A marking pen outlines the flap area, which should be approximately 20% longer than the defect to decrease tension. Skin flaps are not isolated from their own blood supply, and the tip of the flap is moved to the tip of the defect (2). In one study, the 5-year survival rate fell from 90% in patients with no node involvement to 57% for cases with a single regional node involvement (9). Patients showing an intracapsular positivity or a size of metastasis less than 5 mm have a 5-year cancer-related survival of almost 90%, whereas patients showing a metastasis larger than 15 mm or an extracapsular site have a 20% survival rate (8).

Estrogen cream therapy may be given to reduce local effects of radiotherapy.

Case Abstract 2

A 74-year-old diabetic woman (103 kg and 158 cm) presented with symptoms of vulvar itching and severe genuine stress incontinence (third degree) (3). Severe anterior vaginal wall prolapse extended to the introitus at rest (1). The patient noticed the appearance of a lump in the left labium majus. Vulvar biopsy and fine needle aspiration cytology were both conclusive for invasive squamous cell carcinoma with high keratoblastic activity. Modified radical vulvectomy with bilateral inguinal lymphadenectomy was performed by different inguinal incisions (5).

Genuine stress incontinence was corrected using a modified Raz procedure (Fig. 76.1) with four-corner bladder and urethral suspension (10). No. 0 Prolene sutures were tied to the abdominal fascia after surgical preparation of the space of Retzius (Fig. 76.3). Pathology revealed poorly differentiated squamous cell carcinoma grade IV. Tumor invasion (6.5 mm) was evident in periclitoral skin and lichen sclerosus transformation was focally present in the surgical margins. All node specimens were negative for metastatic disease (T2 N0 M0). Urinary retention was treated by Foley catheterization until spontaneous micturition (26 days after operation).

One year later the patient had a moderate lymphoedema of the inferior left limb. She was still continent but complained of slight urge incontinence in the morning.

The patient was still alive 36 months after surgery with no evidence of recurrent disease.

DISCUSSION

Severe genuine stress incontinence may be accompanied by large cystocele in patients with paravaginal (lateral) defect. Successful gynecologic surgery in presence of grade III or IV cystocele will depend much upon the adequacy of bladder neck suspension and upon the ability to restore the anterior vaginal wall anatomy.

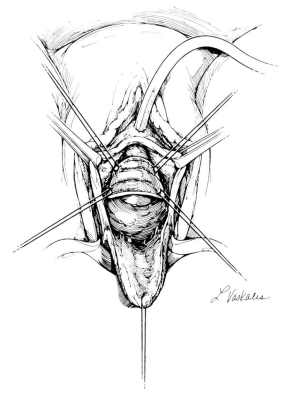

Figure 76.2. An inverted V-shaped incision in the anterior vaginal wall was previously performed and the four corners of the preserved vaginal island are anchored with individual sutures of no. 0 Prolene.

Radical vulvectomy and groin dissection may be done through separate incisions placed 2 cm below and parallel to the inguinal ligament (extending from the anterior superior iliac spine to the pubic tubercle). The outcome following triple-incision technique surgery is essentially equal to that of en bloc dissection in early-stage disease (5). This modified procedure reduces the morbidity and permits a 2-cm incision in the midline just above the superior margin of the pubic bone (4). Under finger control in the Retzius space a ligature carrier is guided to the vaginal area. The suspending sutures are pulled upward to the suprapubic incision (Fig. 76.3).

When the suspending sutures are tied upward, the bladder neck should close properly. The colporrhaphy is then completed, excess tissue of the vaginal wall is excised, and the vagina is closed from side to side to insulate the rectangular island of the Prolene-anchored vaginal wall. Cystoscopy may be performed to confirm the correct closure of the bladder neck, ruling out bladder damage and ureter injury.

In clinical practice vulvar carcinoma may be combined with severe genital prolapse because of the prevalence of those pathologies in elderly women. Sometimes this condition is complicated by the presence of severe stress incontinence. Surgical

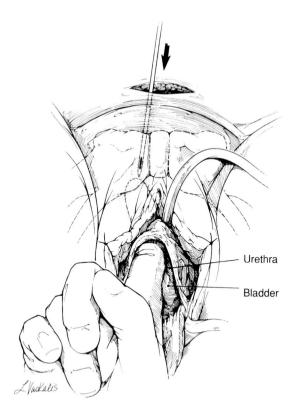

Urethra

Bladder

Figure 76.3.   The operator's index finger, sweeping the bladder and urethra medially, exposes the space of Retzius. The ligature carrier is guided by finger control from the suprapubic to the vaginal area.

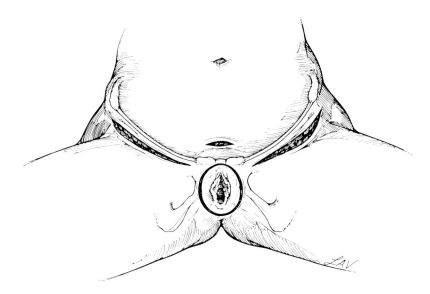

Figure 76.4.   Modified radical vulvectomy and groin dissection through separate incisions. A 2-cm incision is made in the midline above the superior margin of the pubic bone. The suspending sutures will pass at the midline over the abdominal fascia.

resection of the vulvar cancer induces vaginal correction of severe genital prolapse with or without urinary incontinence. Pubourethral ligament plication in accord with the Nichols procedure may prevent or correct slight urinary incontinence during surgical correction for prolapse.

A four-corner vaginal sling for urethrovesical suspension (Raz procedure) in the authors' experience is the easier and more practical method (compared to autologous or heterologous slings) for surgical correction of severe urinary incontinence. In fact, this approach is simplified by a previous suprapubic incision combined with a modified radical vulvectomy with inguinal separate incisions.

REFERENCES

1. Baden WF, Walker T: Grading support loss: The halfway system. In: Baden WF, Walker T (eds): *Surgical Repair of Vaginal Defects,* Vol. 2. Philadelphia, JB Lippincott, 1992, pp. 2, 13.
2. Crukshank SH: Reconstructive procedures for the gynecologic surgeon. *Am J Obstet Gynecol* 168(2):469–475, 1993.
3. Ferrari A, Baresi L, Frigerio L: A grading model for stress urinary incontinence. *Urology* 1:76, 1986.
4. Frigerio L, Ferrari A, Celli A, et al: Kelly–Kennedy suspension and pubourethral ligament plication for the prolapse correction. In: Montorsi M, Granelli P (eds): *Lecture Book II.* Twenty-sixth World Congress of the International College of Surgeons. Milano, Monduzzi Editore, 1988.
5. Helm CW, Hatch K, Austin M, et al: A matched comparison of single and triple incision techniques for the surgical treatment of carcinoma of the vulva. *Gynecol Oncol* 46:150, 1992.
6. McCall ML: Posterior culdeplasty: Surgical correction of enterocele during vaginal hysterectomy: A preliminary report. *Obstet Gynecol* 10:595, 1957.
7. Nichols DH: Techniques of colporrhaphy. In: Nichols DH, Randall CL: *Vaginal Surgery,* ed. 3. Baltimore, Williams & Wilkins, 1989.

  8. Origoni M, Sideri M, Garsia S, Carinelli S, Ferrari A: Prognostic value of pathological patterns of lymph node positivity in squamous cell carcinoma of the value stage III and IVA FIGO. *Gynecol Oncol* 45:313–316, 1992.
  9. Podratz KC, Symmonds RE, Taylor WF, et al: Carcinoma of the vulva: Analysis of treatment and survival. *Obstet Gynecol* 61:63, 1983.
 10. Raz S: Surgical therapy for urinary incontinence. In: Raz S (ed): *Atlas of Transvaginal Surgery.* Philadelphia, WB Saunders, 1992.

77

Radical Vulvectomy — One Node Positive

Philip J. DiSaia

Case Abstract

A 70-year-old patient, in otherwise good health, had a radical vulvectomy with bilateral superficial node excision because of a grade II invasive squamous cell carcinoma about 1.5 cm in diameter involving the inner surface of the right labia majora. Although no nodes were palpable, a bilateral inguino-femoral lymph node dissection was accomplished and one node of 20, from the patient's right, but not the node of Cloquet, was positive for metastatic disease.

DISCUSSION

The patient described has a small invasive squamous cell cancer of the vulva and is discovered to have only one positive lymph node in the ipsilateral groin dissection (Fig. 77.1). Several questions arise: (a) Should the contralateral groin have been dissected? (b) Should the deep pelvic nodes be excised, and if so, should the dissection be done on one or both sides? (c) Are further diagnostic studies appropriate? (d) What additional therapy should be advised?

Over the last decade, clinicians have been tailoring therapy in vulvar cancer to the diseased state, often avoiding extended surgical procedures. This statement is especially true for small lesions such as this case presents. In this case the groin dissection could be restricted to the right side (ipsilateral) because the patient's lesion was less than 2 cm and lateralized. With lateralized lesions less than 2 cm in diameter, the contralateral groin nodes are rarely involved, unless extensive lymph node involvement is found with a small central lesion. It is invariably an anaplastic primary tumor which is the source. If the contralateral side had not been dissected, a program of close observation for at least 2 years would be practiced at the author's institution because experience has shown that good salvage can be attained with delayed inguino-femoral node dissections in patients who subsequently develop palpable groin nodes.

In the author's experience, the prognosis for patients with clinically negative groins who are found to have one positive inguinal node is very similar to that of patients with negative nodes. A similar outcome was reported by Boyce et al. in a review of all patients with one positive groin node: a 78% 2-year survival rate was compared to an 82% recurrence-free interval in all patients with negative nodes. On the basis of these observations, one could omit the pelvic lymphadenectomy on the uninvolved side, since several studies have shown that pelvic node involvement does not occur in the absence of ipsilateral inguinal nodal metastasis.

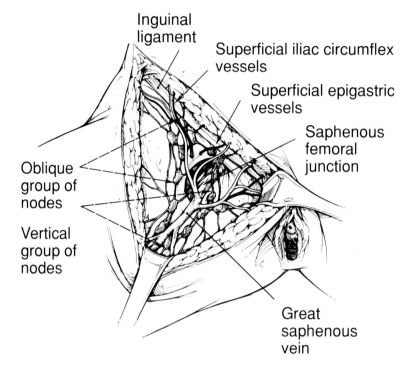

Figure 77.1.   Anatomy of the superficial groin.

Further diagnostic studies should be considered. Since this patient is asymptomatic and undoubtedly had a preoperative chest x-ray, the only recommendation would be a computerized tomography (CT) scan of the abdomen and pelvis with intravenous contrast to outline rare distant metastases, especially in the retroperitoneal lymph nodes of the pelvic and para-aortic chains. The cost effectiveness of even this recommendation could be questioned. Lymphangiography should not be considered because an inguino-femoral lymphadenectomy results in ligation of the main lymphatic channels from the leg to the pelvis and periaortic nodes, resulting in a very poor study.

Adjuvant therapy in the form of chemotherapy or radiation therapy is not necessary in this case. Chemotherapy for vulvar squamous cancer is not very effective and hardly appropriate in a patient with such a good prognosis. The issue of adjuvant radiation therapy to the groins and pelvis is not nearly as well defined. The analysis of a Gynecologic Oncology Group study suggested that survival with postoperative radiation therapy for patients with positive groin nodes in whom the deep pelvic nodes were not dissected was as good as that for patients who underwent pelvic lymphadenectomy. The real issue is the probability that the patient has a positive pelvic node balanced against the morbidity and expense of radiation therapy. The probability of a positive pelvic node in all patients with positive inguinal nodes is 20%. With only one positive inguinal node and a small central lesion, this probably falls to less than 5%. In addition, experience has shown that only 20% of patients with positive pelvic nodes survive 5 years following therapy. Therefore, the author's preference in this case would be to omit all adjuvant therapy unless the CT scan was positive.

SELECTED READINGS

Boyce J et al: Prognostic factors in carcinoma of the vulva. *Gynecol Oncol* 20:364–377, 1985.

Figge D, Tamimi H, Greer B: Lymphatic spread in carcinoma of the vulva. *Am J Obstet Gynecol* 152:387–392, 1985.

Franklin EW, Rutledge FN: Prognostic factors in epidermoid carcinoma of the vulva. *Obstet Gynecol* 37:892–901, 1971.

Homesley HD et al: Radiation therapy versus pelvic node resection for carcinoma of the vulva with positive groin nodes. *Obstet Gynecol* 68:733, 1986.

Morris JM: A formula for selective lymphadenectomy: Its application to cancer of the vulva. *Obstet Gynecol* 50:152–158, 1977.

78

Carcinoma of the Vulva with Postoperative Inguinal Wound Breakdown

George W. Morley

Case Abstract

A radical vulvectomy with en bloc bilateral superficial inguinal lymphadenectomy had been performed on a 62-year-old, 276-lb, diabetic through a large "butterfly"-type incision, with primary closure of all exposed surfaces. Preoperative biopsy had shown an invasive, well-differentiated squamous cell carcinoma, 1 × 2.5 cm, on the medial aspect of the left labium majus.

On the third postoperative day, the inguinal skin flaps were swollen and inflamed and the incisional edges were dusky colored. The patient was, and remained, afebrile.

When the skin sutures were removed on the fifth postoperative day, the wounds were grossly purulent, and the skin flaps in the inguinal areas pale white, becoming necrotic, and well demarcated from the adjacent viable skin. After debridement, the underlying soft tissues, covered with thick, creamy, purulent exudate, were widely exposed. A foul-smelling odor was present.

DISCUSSION

Wound breakdown in a patient who has undergone a radical vulvectomy and bilateral groin lymph node dissections is the most common complication encountered in the treatment of invasive carcinoma of the vulva (4). This complication is frightening to the patient and worrisome to the more junior physicians caring for the patient, but patients respond satisfactorily to appropriate conservative measures once the wound is adequately exposed and treated accordingly. This patient had a significant lesion of the vulva, classified as stage II because the lesion was greater than 2 cm (Fig. 78.1) in diameter and it was necessary to do an extensive procedure to control the malignant process.

A review of the literature and personal communications indicates that the inguinal wounds following this procedure break down to some degree in approximately 50% to 75% of the cases. It has even been stated that if the wound does *not* break down to some degree then an adequate enough procedure probably has not been performed.

In the series at the University of Michigan, approximately 50% of the wounds break down to some extent. Often these wounds become infected locally without any associated febrile episodes. However, it is important to open the wound more adequately once this complication is recognized so that appropriate treatment can be carried out. All

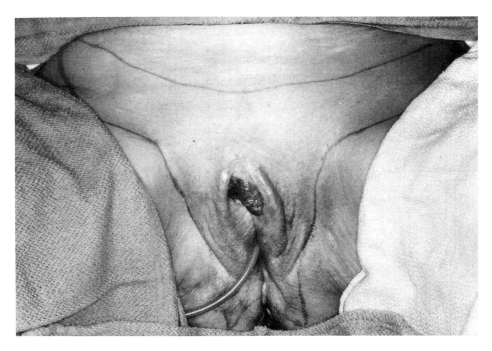

Figure 78.1.   Invasive carcinoma of the vulva, stage II (lesion greater than 2 cm in diameter, involving the clitoris and paraclitoral tissue). "Butterfly" incision is also outlined.

patients undergoing this procedure are treated with prophylactic broad-spectrum anti-biotics. Infrequently, a significant cellulitis will occur, and these patients must be treated more aggressively utilizing appropriate therapeutic doses of chemotherapeutic agents.

In discussing this complication of radical vulvectomy and groin lymph node dissection, one must first consider the question, "Could it be prevented?" The literature describes many techniques for the type of incision to be used in performing the groin lymph node dissection on these patients. Whether one selects a "butterfly" type of incision or uses a separate inguinal incision for the lymph node dissection does not seem to matter significantly. The author has used a "butterfly" incision (Fig. 78.1) previously and now reserves it for clitoral and paraclitoral lesions as well as for the advanced lesions seen at the University of Michigan.

In the future, with patients seeking medical attention earlier, physicians will see early stage I disease more frequently. In these cases, it is perfectly appropriate to use the "3-in-1" incision with the vulvar tissue and the right and left groin lymph node tissue being removed through three separate incisions, especially when the clitoral tissue is not involved.

The author has used separate groin incisions with undermining of the skin flaps in the past, but for several years has employed for most cases the full thickness type dissection in the groins with significantly less wound breakdown. For an adequate full thickness dissection of the groins, the width of the skin incision must approximate 7 cm at its greatest point to ensure an adequate dissection of the lymph node-bearing tissue. On the other hand, if the undermining technique is utilized, then one must be certain to remove all of the tissue lying deep to Camper's fascia, again to ensure removal of all the superficial groin lymph nodes. As stated above, this technique does increase the incidence of skin flap loss through infection and necrosis.

Several steps help reduce significant wound breakdown. First of all, while in the operating room, it is useful to "freshen up" the skin scars and the underlying subcutaneous tissue after completion of this rather lengthy dissection. The incisions are then closed in layers using one of a variety of absorbable sutures. The skin edges are approximated at wide intervals between the sutures to encourage adequate drainage of the wound. A pressure dressing is then applied in an attempt to reduce fluid accumulation and to immobilize the wound flaps as effectively as possible to encourage wound healing. A number of surgeons dress the wounds open to allow closure by secondary intention.

The patients are placed in a semi-Fowler's position for 48 hours to reduce the tension on the suture line. They are strictly confined to bed for approximately 72 hours. All of these patients have previously been placed on prophylactic anticoagulant therapy, and they are urged to move around in bed at frequent intervals.

One of the most controversial issues is whether to drain the wounds once the procedure is completed. The author does not use drains in these wounds and has had no reason to regret this decision. This approach is supported by a number of gynecologic oncologists, but a number of surgeons also believe to the contrary.

A word of caution must be made in regard to the dissection of the mons veneris tissue overlying the symphysis pubis. It seems advisable to leave a small amount of fatty tissue on the periosteum in this area so that the periosteum is not traumatized. There have been a few isolated reports of osteitis pubis secondary to an overly aggressive dissection of this area, and this complication is extremely difficult to treat satisfactorily. Frequently, the area overlying the symphysis cannot be closed primarily. This should cause no concern, and this part of the wound is dressed with appropriate packing.

The use of skin grafts in this area is not recommended since all of these wounds ultimately heal, primarily with linear scarring overlying the symphysis, as is seen in the groin wounds (Fig. 78.2). The use of skin grafts further prolongs the operative procedure in these elderly patients, and the result is somewhat disfiguring because there is no underlying fatty tissue in the region of the skin grafts.

If the wound has not healed satisfactorily and the common complication of wound breakdown is encountered, then an aggressive approach to its treatment is to be outlined. As stated before, these wounds should be opened up completely to the extent of the infection so that adequate therapy can be applied. Debridement is carried out periodically to "freshen up" the wound edges to rid the exposed area of the necrotic membrane. These wounds are packed three times daily, and the patients are placed in a whirlpool bath for 30 minutes twice daily to stimulate wound healing. Silver nitrate, potassium permanganate, Elase, and various antibiotic ointments have been used in the past, but their efficacy has been challenged. Applications of honey to these open wounds is recommended periodically by the more junior staff caring for these patients, and it does

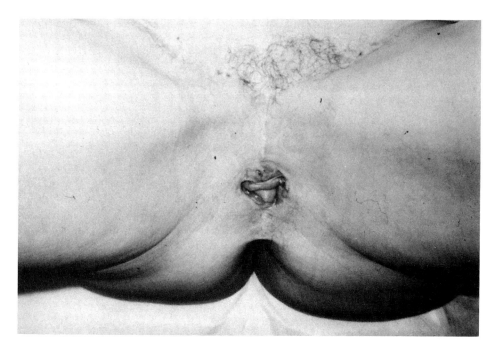

Figure 78.2. Invasive carcinoma of the vulva treated 3 months previously by radical vulvectomy and groin and pelvic lymphadenectomy. Note linear scarring, which represents complete healing.

have some merit. In the undiluted form, honey is considered to be bactericidal, and it is thought not to support pathogenic organisms (1). Skin grafts should not be used in these areas, at least until the infection is cleared and the wound is granulating in well. The indications for the use of skin graft at this time seem to be very limited.

One must exercise great caution, however, in the debridement of the diabetic patient since their potential for wound healing is compromised. Although debridement is good 90% of the time, there is a 10% untoward response, since debridement itself also causes some tissue destruction. In the diabetic patient, one must be sure that the necrotic area is well demarcated before carrying out aggressive debridement.

At the University of Michigan, once the wounds have started to heal and the infection is cleared, the patient becomes increasingly active in self-care. The nurse in charge instructs the patient on the dressing changes and packing of the wounds. Once the patient is comfortable with this self-care program, she is ready for discharge from the hospital. The median hospital stay for these patients is about 21 days; however, if the wounds do not break down, the patient can usually be discharged approximately 2 weeks after surgery.

Other complications should be mentioned in the postoperative care of these patients. Rarely do any of them encounter a thromboembolic complication to the surgery. This is somewhat surprising, since not only are these patients elderly and strictly confined to bed postoperatively for a short period of time, but the surgery directly involves the femoral and often the pelvic venous system. One should always be alerted to the possibility of pulmonary embolization and act accordingly. As stated above, all of these patients are treated with prophylactic anticoagulant therapy, which is continued until they are actively ambulated in the postoperative period.

The risk of hemorrhage, particularly from the groin region, is ever present in these patients, but this again is an unusual complication. The major blood supply to the leg is exposed when performing the deep groin lymph node dissection and certainly must be protected following the initial dissection. This is accomplished with closure of the cribriform fascia over the vessels. Alternatively, if the dissection is extensive, the sartorius muscle can be transplanted from its lateral insertion into the anterior iliac spine and lateral third of the inguinal ligament with an attachment to the medial portion of Poupart's ligament, thus being placed to overlie these vessels.

On infrequent occasions, a groin lymphocyst will be encountered in the postoperative period. These "cysts" usually can be prevented by being certain that all of the vessels are clamped and tied throughout the dissection. If this complication does occur, it can be treated rather conservatively with intermittent aspiration of the lymph fluid followed by pressure dressings. The surgical approach to the control of this complication is rarely, if ever, necessary.

In regard to delayed complications, chronic lymphedema of the lower extremities seems to be the only one that appears with any significant frequency. Although most of these patients do not complain of any particular discomfort from this complication, they are terribly self-conscious about the resultant deformity and appearance of the "fat" leg. In an attempt to avoid this, elastic stockings (at least up to the knee) should be worn postoperatively every day for at least 6 months, and other conservative precautions should be outlined. Recently, the author's institution has been preserving the saphenous vein during the groin lymph node dissection; whether this will aid in reducing the incidence of chronic lymphedema remains to be seen.

In closing, it must be remembered that the breakdown of the wounds in patients undergoing radical vulvectomy and groin lymph node dissection is the most common complication encountered in patients going through this procedure; yet, it must be realized that the 5-year survival rate of women treated in this way is most satisfactory. From a collaborative review, one estimates that the 5-year survival rate for patients having no positive inguinal lymph nodes is approximately 90%. If one groin lymph node is involved with metastatic disease, the 5-year survival rate is reduced to approximately 85%. If more than one node is involved, the overall survival rate is reduced to around 50%. In the future, surgeons must not only improve the survival rates, but must focus attention on various surgical techniques and care of wounds that reduce the incidence of this fairly common complication.

Probably the most significant recent modification of technique has been in the area of incisions. In the past 10 to 15 years, fortunately, the lesions seen are much more often classified as either stage I or early stage II. In this group of patients, as mentioned earlier, the separate "3-in-1" incision is preferred to the "butterfly" incision. With this preservation of normal tissue, the postoperative morbidity and complications are lessened significantly.

REFERENCES

1. Cavanagh D, Beazley J, Ostapowicz F: Radical operation for carcinoma of the vulva: A new approach to wound healing. *J Obstet Gynaecol Br Commonw* 77:1037, 1970.
2. Morley GW: Infiltrative carcinoma of the vulva: Results of surgical management. *Am J Obstet Gynecol* 124:874, 1976.
3. Morley G: Surgery for vulvar cancer. In: Nichols D (ed): *Gynecologic and Obstetric Surgery,* St. Louis, Mosby–Yearbook, 1993, pp. 286–296.
4. Way S: Carcinoma of the vulva. *Am J Obstet Gynecol* 79:692, 1960.

79

Vulvar Paget's Disease Involving Anal Skin

John H. Isaacs

Case Abstract

The vulvar biopsy of a 42-year-old married woman with a long history of vulvar pruritis was diagnosed as typical extramammary Paget's disease. A skinning vulvectomy was planned. The area to be excised extended over the perineum and perianal skin.

DISCUSSION

The treatment of Paget's disease of the vulva is to remove all of the involved area plus a margin of at least 2 cm of normal skin surrounding the entire lesion. Since the Paget cells may well extend horizontally along the hair follicles, the apocrine and eccrine sweat glands, and the sebaceous glands, the skinning vulvectomy should extend deep enough into the superficial layer of the subcutaneous fat to remove all of the adnexal structures.

For the sake of discussion, it must be assumed that in this patient there is no underlying separate adenocarcinoma of the vulva, coexisting squamous cell carcinoma of the anus, or a visceral adenocarcinoma of the rectum, since these would require a more radical procedure. Such cases have been reported (3). We must further assume that this is a typical Paget's disease, which is usually a slowly progressive indolent localized process.

After the involved area has been completely excised, a large raw surface, which includes the area around the perineum and anal skin, must be covered. Such an area can be covered with a split-thickness skin graft taken from the buttock, lower abdomen, or upper thigh. The skin from the donor site should be placed on a Derma carrier II with a 1.5 to 1 expansion ratio and then meshed by running the skin through the Meshgraft Skin Expander (Fig. 79.1).

After the skin has been meshed, it is placed over the raw surface, including the raw area of the perineum and surrounding the anal canal. Since the blood supply is plentiful in this area, the chances of success are almost 80% to 90%. The graft is fixed laterally to the external skin margins, medially to the introitus, and posteriorly to the skin at the anal verge. The author uses no. 00 Dexon for this purpose. The graft is further stabilized by interrupting stitches, fixing the graft to the underlying raw surface (Fig. 79.2). The skin graft is covered with multiple saline-soaked gauze balls; gauze dressings are then placed over the gauze balls. This stent is held in place by heavy black sutures anchored to

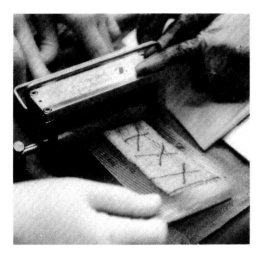

Figure 79.1. The donor skin has passed through the Meshgraft Skin Expander. Note the meshing pattern on the donor skin.

the skin (Fig. 79.3). The patient must remain at bedrest for at least 5 to 7 days with a Foley or suprapubic catheter in place. The bowel should have been thoroughly cleansed prior to surgery. An elemental diet and an antispasmodic should prevent a bowel movement for the first few days, thus reducing the chance of infection (Fig. 79.4).

The author has used this technique on numerous occasions and has not had any severe complications or any vaginal or anal strictures. If there is a lack of "take" around the perineal area, a full-thickness pedicle graft can be utilized (Figs. 79.5 and 79.6).

Wide local excision as described may not always be possible. Thirlby et al. (5) described a case involving the anal verge in all four quadrants. They concluded that wide local excision would require circumferential excision, including rectal mucosa. In their opinion, a skin graft would have healed poorly and resulted in anal stenosis. The question of chemoradiotherapy versus abdominoperineal resection was considered. It was decided to use radiotherapy to a total dose of 5000 cGy. Five-fluorouracil 1000 mg/m^2 × 4 days, mitomycin-C 7.5 mg/m^2 was also given. There has been no evidence of recurrence.

Since recurrences are not unusual, close follow-up is mandatory. Any recurrent sites may be treated with further excision and skin grafting with primary closure of pedicle grafts depending on the site of the recurrence. Small areas of recurrence may also be treated by CO_2 laser, but whether this will cause complications later is as yet unknown.

Addendum

Since 1988, follow-up of patients treated for vulvar Paget's disease has shown that the recurrence rate is much higher than anticipated, and the problem presented at the beginning of this chapter should receive more consideration. Surgical excision of the area must be complete, but the simple vulvectomy must be carried down to a depth of at least 0.5 cm of subcutaneous tissue to be certain there is no invasive lesion (2). Also, the extent of the disease must be completely defined by frozen-section margins. In such instances, additional intraoperative resections may be necessary. Stacy et al. reported no recurrences in 3 to 8 years of follow-up (4). They also noted that patients with anal mucosal involvement had associated mucinous adenocarcinoma of the rectum.

Figure 79.2. Meshed skin graft fixed in place over the raw surface of the vulvar and perianal area.

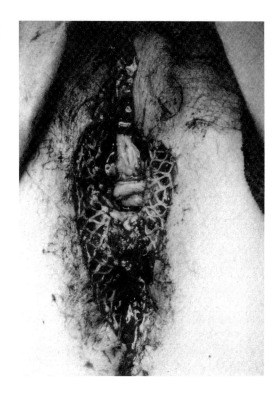

Figure 79.3. Gauze stent covering the skin graft and held in place with black silk sutures.

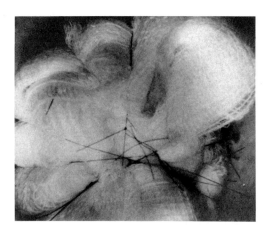

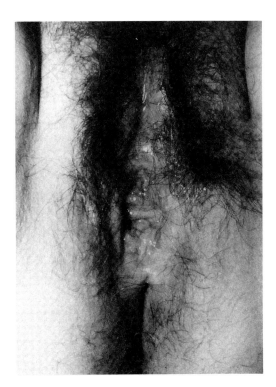

Figure 79.4.   Vulvar and anal area approximately 3 months after the skin graft has been applied.

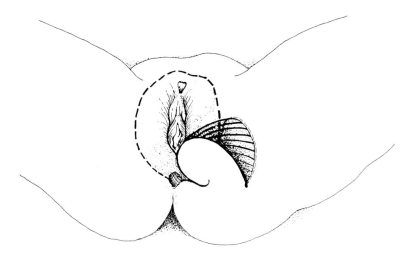

Figure 79.5.   A pedicle graft has been shifted to cover the perineum and perianal area.

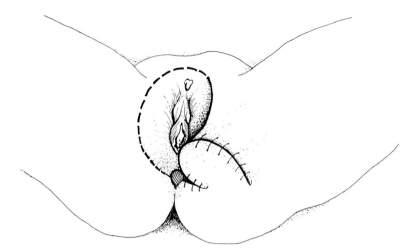

Figure 79.6.   Pedicle graft sutured in place. A similar pedicle graft can be raised for the contralateral side.

Patients with extramammary Paget's disease have a high recurrence rate and morbidity. As suggested by Besa et al., radiotherapy may be considered as an alternate to further surgery or for anyone wishing to avoid surgery (1).

References

1. Besa P, Tyvin AR, Delclos L, Edwards CL, Ota DM, Wharton JT: Extramammary Paget's disease of the perineal skin: Role of radiotherapy. *Int J Radiation Oncol Biol Phys* 34:73–76, 1993.
2. Feuer GA, Shevchuk M, Calanog A: Vulvar Paget's disease: The need to exclude an invasive lesion. *Gynecol Oncol* 38(1):81–89, 1990.
3. Jensen SL, Sjolin KE, Shokouh-Amiri MH, Hagen K, Harling H: Paget's disease of the anal margin. *Br J Surg* 75:1089–1092, 1988.
4. Stacy D, Burrell MO, Franklin EW: Extramammary Paget's disease of the vulva and anus: Use of intraoperative frozen-section margins. *Am J Obstet Gynecol* 155(3):519–523, 1986.
5. Thirlby RC, Hammer CJ, Galagan KA, Travaglini JJ, Picozzi VJ: Perianal Paget's disease: Successful treatment with combined chemoradiotherapy. *Dis Col & Rec* 33:150–152, 1990.

Selected Readings

Blaustein A: *Pathology of the Female Genital Tract*. New York, Springer-Verlag, 1977.
DiSaia PG, Creasman WT: *Clinical Gynecologic Oncology*, ed. 2. St. Louis: CV Mosby, 1984.
Friedrich EG: *Vulvar Disease*. Philadelphia, WB Saunders, 1976.

80

Vaginal Hysterectomy for a Patient with Microinvasive Carcinoma of the Cervix and Symptomatic Pelvic Relaxation

George W. Morley

Case Abstract

A 35-year-old asymptomatic para I was found on recent colposcopy and conization to have a microinvasive carcinoma (3.0 mm in depth) of the uterine cervix. Margins were free of tumor. On pelvic examination, the uterus was freely movable and not enlarged, and there was some degree of cystocele and rectocele. The patient had some symptomatic but not disabling urinary stress incontinence and was not required to wear sanitary protection. The incontinence was worse when the patient was exercising or when she had an upper respiratory infection. The surgeon thought a vaginal hysterectomy could easily be accomplished on this patient and wondered whether to perform coincident anterior and posterior colporrhaphy.

DISCUSSION

A number of different issues are related to this very interesting case. This combination of problems is not an uncommon situation. First of all, in making a diagnosis, one must have a correct definition of microinvasive carcinoma (3), since serious recurrences have been reported simply because the treatment was based on an incorrect definition of this condition. The diagnosis of microinvasive or stage IA carcinoma of the cervix is defined by most gynecologic oncologists as up to 3 mm depth of invasion from the basement membrane into the underlying stroma, with no evidence of angiolymphatic invasion.

In regard to the therapy directed toward the microinvasive disease, most gynecologic oncologists recommend total hysterectomy. There is no need to favor either the transabdominal or transvaginal route for performing the hysterectomy since survival rates are the same and assessment of the regional lymph nodes is not required.

The second part of the question is the coexistence of the cystocele and rectocele with or without symptoms of stress urinary incontinence. If the patient is totally asymptomatic—that is, does not complain of apparent pelvic relaxation and does not experience urinary loss with stress—then certainly there should be no surgical "correction" of the slight variations from normalcy. All too often, an anterior colporrhaphy and posterior colpoperineorrhaphy are performed in these situations and the patient ends up with symptoms of stress urinary incontinence, dyspareunia, or other problems. There also is no evidence that a repair of either the anterior or posterior vaginal wall gives better support to the vaginal apex following a vaginal hysterectomy. Furthermore, if the vaginal repair is performed on an *asymptomatic* patient in addition to the required surgery, the cost of the entire procedure will be significantly higher, a situation that must be avoided whenever possible. The old saying "If it works, don't fix it" can be stated here as "Seldom does surgery help the asymptomatic patient."

If, however, the patient complains significantly about symptoms of stress urinary incontinence or an annoying bulge of the anterior vaginal wall, then there is no contraindication to surgery directed toward correction of the posterior urethrovesical angle and the anterior wall relaxation through an anterior colporrhaphy. If, in addition, the patient has a symptomatic rectocele, this could be corrected transvaginally with a posterior colpoperineorrhaphy (2). In general, there is no contraindication to combining surgical procedures irrespective of the presence of a malignancy since there is essentially no increased risk and no decrease in survival rates. Any risk would be related to the procedure itself, not to the fact of combination therapy. Furthermore, there are increased risks in performing these procedures separately since two anesthetics would be required. In the past it has been said that "double-headers" should be reserved for baseball and not be applied to surgery. Certainly, this may have been appropriate for a variety of reasons; however, this approach does not seem necessarily appropriate today.

If the patient has undergone an abdominal hysterectomy, the urinary stress incontinence could be treated using a retropubic approach. If the physician's preference, however, is to treat the malignancy transabdominally and the pelvic relaxation transvaginally, this too would be appropriate and would be essentially at the discretion of the surgeon. This decision would not be looked upon with disfavor even though there seems to be a less cumbersome way of handling these combined problems. Most commonly, the surgeon would probably choose either the transabdominal or the transvaginal route for the entire surgical procedure. To restate the obvious, all of the decisions related to the pelvic relaxation would have to be with the understanding and concurrence of the patient. If the symptoms of relaxation are not too bothersome, then it might be in the best interests of the patient to try medical management first and only operate for the malignancy at this time.

Finally, there is the question of when hysterectomy should be performed following the diagnostic conization. A good guideline is to perform the hysterectomy within 48 hours of the conization or to wait 6 weeks before proceeding with the more definitive therapy (1). When confronted with the treatment of a malignancy, however, most people would wait only about 4 weeks. However, others feel that it makes little or no difference when the postconization hysterectomy is performed and just depend on the liberal use of prophylactic antibiotic therapy (4). The author's bias is reflected in the first suggested approach to this question.

In summary, an appropriate decision as to the route of surgery and the extent and timing of the surgery can be met after doing a detailed history, performing appropriate diagnostic tests, and discussing thoroughly all the facets of care with the patient. There is no one answer.

References

1. Malinak LR, Jeffrey RA Jr, Dunn WJ: The conization-hysterectomy time interval: A clinical and pathologic study. *Obstet Gynecol* 23:317, 1964.
2. Thompson JD, Rock JA: *Te Linde's Operative Gynecology*, ed. 7. Philadelphia, JB Lippincott, 1992.
3. Van Nagell JR Jr, Greenwell N, Powell DF, et al: Microinvasive carcinoma of the cervix. *Am J Obstet Gynecol* 145:981, 1983.
4. Webb MJ, Symmonds RE: Radical hysterectomy: Influence of recent conization on morbidity and complications. *Obstet Gynecol* 53:290, 1979.

81

Microinvasive Cancer of the Cervix in Pregnancy

Philip J. DiSaia

Case Abstract

An 18-year-old para I, gravida II received a Papanicolaou smear as part of her initial physical examination. This was reported as abnormal with findings consistent with carcinoma in situ with possible microinvasion. A cervical conization was performed at 11 weeks gestation. Although the entire lesion appeared to be within the conization specimen and the edges were free of tumor, several nonconfluent foci of microinvasion were noted between 1 and 3 mm in depth with no vascular involvement. The gestation was now of 15 weeks duration.

DISCUSSION

Microinvasive carcinoma of the cervix is a subject that has been associated with several decades of confusion. The diagnostic issues have been confused, and some investigators have reported conflicting results on what appears to be the same subset of patients. The terminology used by various authors has varied widely. Adding a first-trimester pregnancy to this clinical dilemma seemingly "adds salt to the wound." The issues which must be addressed include abortion versus continuation of the pregnancy, treatment under either circumstance, and appropriate follow-up of the pregnancy if it is not terminated.

It is the author's belief that microinvasion should be strictly defined as invasion to a depth of no greater than 3 mm with no confluent tongues and no areas of lymphatic or vascular invasion. The volume of the invasive process is the key to predicting the aggressiveness of the disease, and the treating physician must evaluate the histologic sections personally to make a judgment on a case-by-case basis. At the author's institution, the only indication for conization in pregnancy is a colposcopically directed biopsy that suggests "possible microinvasion." The term *coin biopsy* is preferred (Fig. 81.1) to underscore the fact that the squamo-columnar junction everts during pregnancy and thus makes unnecessary what may be a dangerous excision of canal tissue.

Some authors have shown that lesions in nonpregnant patients meeting these criteria can be adequately treated with conization alone. Based on these reports and observations of 12 patients with microinvasion in pregnancy treated with conization only, the author would recommend no further therapy for this patient at this time. There is no need for termination of this pregnancy, nor for immediate definitive therapy in the form of a hysterectomy.

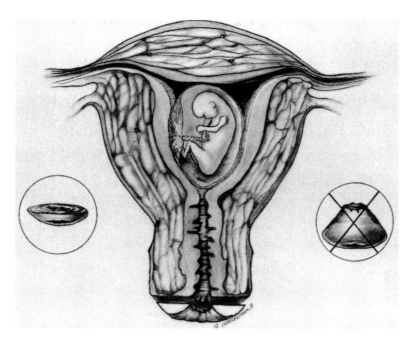

Figure 81.1.   Demonstration of shallow "coin biopsy" appropriate in pregnancy. (Reproduced with permission from DiSaia PJ, Creasman WT: *Clinical Gynecologic Oncology.* St. Louis, CV Mosby, 1993, p. 539.)

The patient should be followed with inspection of the cervix in the second trimester accompanied by repeated cytology in the third trimester when regeneration of the cervical tissue is complete. No specific route of delivery is recommended. Six weeks postpartum, the cervix should be reevaluated with cytology and colposcopy. If no further neoplastic disease is uncovered and the patient is desirous of further childbearing, it is the author's practice to withhold any further surgical therapy until such time as childbearing is complete or disease of a significant degree reappears. Whether simple hysterectomy should be recommended at the completion of childbearing in the absence of any recurrent disease is controversial. The patient undoubtedly is at some increased risk for a recurrence of cervical neoplasia. The decision for hysterectomy at this time should be made by the physician and patient, taking into consideration the probability of good patient compliance for serial cytologic evaluation, the level of cancer phobia in the patient, and other benign pathology which may coexist.

SELECTED READINGS
DiSaia PJ, Creasman WT: *Clinical Gynecologic Oncology*. St. Louis, CV Mosby, 1993.
Marcuse PM: Incipient microinvasive carcinoma of the cervix. *Obstet Gynecol* 37:360–371, 1971.
Taylor H: Early invasive cancer of the cervix. *Am J Obstet Gynecol* 85:926–939, 1963.
Wheeler CB Jr: Carcinoma of the cervix with early stromal invasion. *Am J Obstet Gynecol* 72:119, 1956.

Unexpected Uterine Malignant Tumor (Adenocarcinoma or Endometrial Sarcoma) Found When the Uterus Was Opened in the Operating Room

John J. Mikuta

Case Abstract

A vaginal hysterectomy had been performed because of perimenopausal menorrhagia in a 53-year-old patient. The uterus was of average size and there were no technical difficulties during the hysterectomy. The ovaries were grossly normal, and one appeared to contain a small follicle cyst. As a matter of departmental policy, the uterus was opened following its removal in the operating room and was found to contain a wide-based, hemorrhagic, somewhat necrotic tumor about 1 inch in diameter, located at the fundus of the uterus and grossly invading the inner third of the myometrium.

DISCUSSION

To begin with, this patient should not have had a hysterectomy without a preliminary dilatation and curettage to determine the cause of the perimenopausal menorrhagia. This could have been done as an office procedure, such as an endometrial biopsy or Vabra aspiration, or prior to the removal of the uterus by a diagnostic dilatation and curettage with a frozen section to determine whether there was any abnormality of the endometrium. There is frequently a tendency to avoid a dilatation and curettage in the absence of abnormal bleeding if there is an obvious indication for hysterectomy, particularly the presence of uterine myomas or adnexal masses. This is a mistake, and the few minutes necessary to rule out the presence of endometrial disease may obviate the kind of problem that occurred in this patient. In addition, in this patient the dilatation and curettage may have resolved the cause of the bleeding or, even without the discovery of an obvious cause, been helpful in correcting the menorrhagia.

In the situation described here, the first step should be to identify the nature of the tumor. In this case, if it turned out to be the most likely lesion, an endometrial carcinoma or a sarcoma, one should proceed appropriately with the next step, the removal of the adnexa. This might be able to be done through the vagina. However, if this is not possible, it should be done after the completion of the vaginal operation by entering the abdomen through an appropriate incision which will allow one to complete the removal of the adnexa, having first obtained washings from the peritoneal cavity using heparinized saline solution. Although peritoneal washings are routinely accepted in the management of adnexal masses and ovarian carcinomas, they must also be considered for patients who have carcinoma of the endometrium. Recent reports by Creasman et al. (1) have shown an incidence of involvement of peritoneal washings with positive cytology as high as 17% with stage I carcinoma of the endometrium. Such patients apparently also have a poor prognosis in that they tend to have recurrences in the peritoneal cavity. In addition, careful palpation of the retroperitoneal nodes and node sampling should be done as indicated by the presence of enlarged nodes.

The gynecologist must also be mindful of the way in which the prospective surgery is presented to the patient. A blanket preoperative type of permission is generally not adequate in today's medical-legal climate. It is much better to explain to the patient that at times a particular approach, such as vaginal hysterectomy or laparoscopic tubal ligation, cannot be carried out because of technical difficulties or, as in this case, unexpected findings that would alter the nature of the procedure. Prior to any surgery it is worth discussing with the patient what her wishes might be. She should have the choice of having the procedure stopped, recovering from anesthesia, and then having the possible procedure discussed with her. The advantages of using only a single anesthetic, reducing the possible spread of any malignancy that may have been discovered, and getting earlier treatment are certainly to be stressed to the patient.

REFERENCE

1. Creasman WT, DiSaia PJ, Blessing J, et al: Prognostic significance of peritoneal cytology in patients with endometrial cancer and preliminary data concerning therapy with intraperitoneal radiopharmaceuticals. *Am J Obstet Gynecol* 141:921, 1981.

SELECTED READINGS

Brown JM, Dockerty MD, Symmonds RE, et al: Vaginal recurrence of endometrial carcinoma. *Am J Obstet Gynecol* 100:544, 1968.

Butler CF, Praff JH: Vaginal hysterectomy for carcinoma of the endometrium: Forty years experience at the Mayo Clinic. In: Gray LA Sr (ed): *Endometrial Carcinoma and Its Treatment*. Springfield, IL, Charles C. Thomas, 1976.

Creasman WT, Boronow RC, Morrow CP, et al: Adenocarcinoma of the endometrium: Its metastatic lymph node potential. A preliminary report. *Gynecol Oncol* 4:239, 1976.

Jones HW III: Treatment of adenocarcinoma of the endometrium. *Obstet Gynecol Surv* 30:147, 1975.

83

Undiagnosed Invasive Squamous Cell Carcinoma in Hysterectomy Specimen

Henry C. McDuff

Case Abstract

A 47-year-old patient with uterine fibroids and menorrhagia had been examined by endometrial biopsy, and curettings reported as "cystic hyperplasia." It was the examiner's opinion that the patient had a submucous fibroid. Because of some coexisting multiparous relaxation, a vaginal hysterectomy and anterior and posterior colporrhaphy were performed. The convalescence was unremarkable, but the day before discharge, the pathology report reached the surgeon: "early invasive squamous cell carcinoma of the cervix," with invasion greater than 5 mm.

DISCUSSION

Identification of the Problem

This 47-year-old woman with known uterine fibroids and heavy menstrual bleeding was evaluated in an office setting. An endometrial biopsy was performed and the pathology report indicated "cystic hyperplasia." This is not a malignant condition, but it is a known remote precursor of "endometrial carcinoma," according to studies by Hertig (6). The patient was known to have fibroid tumors, and the physician assumed her bleeding was due to a submucous fibroid component. It would seem appropriate that a dilatation and curettage should have been done since a total evaluation of the endometrium might have identified some adenomatous or dysplastic changes to the patient's cystic hyperplasia. If that had been done, and if the D&C had been fractional, the malignancy within the endocervix would have been recognized, and appropriate treatment instituted. As the patient now presents she is at significant risk. An inappropriate operation has been performed in regard to the ultimate diagnosis. The patient also underwent a vaginal repair because of multiparous vaginal wall relaxations, and thereby tissue planes immediately adjacent to the cervix were opened and traumatized. If the invasive characteristics of the cervical lesion also identified vascular or lymphatic invasion, then a high potential for seeding of malignant cells in the areas of repair must be considered.

How Might This Problem Have Been Avoided?

The surprise diagnosis of "invasive cervical cancer" with extension greater than 5 mm poses a significant problem in regard to further study and treatment (8). The appropriate diagnosis would have been made if preoperative surveillance had been more searching. One would have to believe that a Papanicolaou (PAP) smear had been performed and that it was reported as "negative for tumor cells"; otherwise further preoperative studies would have been ordered. If a PAP smear had not been done, the physician must be held truly accountable. This must have been an occult stage IA lesion (9), not visible to the naked eye. The cervix was obviously easily visible, since there was also a significant degree of vaginal wall relaxation. The PAP smear would have included scraping of the endocervix, and this would hardly fail to identify at least a suspicion of malignancy. If the PAP smear had been reported as abnormal, office colposcopy, endocervical sampling, and biopsies would be carried out. The invasive cervical cancer would then have been identified, and appropriate treatment would have been recommended, either by radiation or radical surgery.

Historical Perspective

Total abdominal hysterectomy has been the preferred operation for benign uterine disease for the past 50 years. Prior to 1940 supracervical hysterectomy was the more popular procedure, and most clinics interested in reporting cervical cancer identified their experience with the intact uterus as well as the cervical stump, which represented 5% to 8% of any total series (9).

In 1940 total hysterectomy replaced the supracervical operation for benign surgical disease, and in the same year Papanicolaou and Traut published their hallmark article in *JAMA* (9). The advent of these changes, the PAP smear, and the total hysterectomy could conceivably write an epitaph to cervical cancer, but unfortunately the disease, though less frequent, is still an entity to be considered and respected. In this particular patient we are probably dealing with an occult lesion, and either a PAP smear was not done or it was reported negative for malignancy.

Further Study Recommended

Once the diagnosis of invasive cervical cancer has been made, additional studies should be performed to consider the type and extent of further treatment. These would include an intravenous pyelogram, cystoscopy, and sigmoidoscopy, all particularly necessary if pelvic radiation therapy is to be recommended. There is at present lingering enthusiasm for staging laparotomy for cervical cancer. This involves an abdominal incision to sample pelvic and periaortic nodes, and to thus determine if the patient is best treated by surgery or radiation.

The patient under discussion represents a stage IA occult lesion, and the potential for identifying positive nodes is remote. Lymphangiography has not lived up to expectations in evaluation of either the glandular or ductal phase, and is not recommended. The areas of greatest concern in this patient are the adjacent parametria and the upper vagina. Vigorous scrapings for cytologic study might be helpful (1).

Treatment Considerations

This patient could be satisfactorily managed by either radical surgery (3,9,7,2) or by pelvic radiation and supplemental Delclos vaginal applicator. The surgical procedure would require radical parametrectomy, upper vaginectomy, and bilateral pelvic node dissection. Ovarian preservation is a consideration which should be shared with the patient. This operation can be carried out with excellent results and minimal complications, with a 5-year survival result of 89%, about the same as for primary radical surgery for invasive cervical cancer (7,2,1).

Total pelvic irradiation plus Delclos vaginal applicator carries about the same survival figures, 85% to 90% (9,10). It is, however, also attended by certain unattractive postradiation sequelae: vaginal stenosis, dyspareunia, hormone (ovarian) dysfunction, radiation cystitis, and proctitis. These potentials should be discussed with the patient prior to further treatment.

The author's preference for treatment in light of present knowledge would involve further study that included cystoscopy and sigmoidoscopy, an intravenous pyelogram or computerized tomography scan of kidneys, and aggressive scraping of vaginal vault for cytology. Then one should wait 4 to 5 weeks, and initiate intraoperative antibiotics on the night before surgery. The author would also favor initiation of preoperative low-dose heparin therapy. Surgery would involve radical bilateral parametrectomy, upper vaginectomy, and bilateral pelvic lymphadenectomy (with possible sampling of para-aortic nodes if suspicious). If radiation therapy is suggested, the dosage schedule should be 4500 to 5000 cGy to full pelvis, followed by insertion of Delclos applicator, 4000 cGy to surface of applicator.

If residual disease is reported after review of the operative specimen, then selective and carefully tailored postoperative radiation therapy should be recommended. Careful follow-up examinations should be scheduled every 3 months for 2 years, every 6 months for 3 years, and then yearly. These examinations should include aggressive scrapings of the upper vagina, and repeat intravenous pyelograms at selected intervals for patients treated with radiation.

Prognosis

Prognosis depends upon the stage of disease, the depth of invasion, and the presence or absence of vascular or lymphatic involvement. With proper treatment, either surgery or radiation, one should expect a "cure rate" of 85% to 90% if the disease is stage I (A or B) and confined to the cervix.

Summary

Approximately 0.5% to 1.0% (4, 8) of all hysterectomies done for benign disease have reported the surprising finding of cervical cancer. Generally this is low-stage disease, stage 0 or stage I and usually occult. Biopsy of the squamo-columnar junction or endocervical curettage should identify all of these lesions preoperatively. No further treatment is suggested for in situ lesions, but radical reoperation or full pelvic irradiation with Delclos vaginal supplement is recommended for all patients with invasive disease. The outlook for cure is good; 100% for in situ lesions, and 85% to 90% for stage I disease (3,8,2,10,5).

REFERENCES

1. Bell J et al: Vaginal cancer after hysterectomy for benign disease: Value of cytologic screening. *Am J Obstet Gynecol* 65(5):699–702, 1944.
2. Chapman JA et al: Surgical treatment of unexpected invasive cervical cancer found at total hysterectomy. *Am J Obstet Gynecol* 80(6), 1992.
3. DiSaia PJ, Creasman WT: *Clinical Gynecologic Oncology*, ed 2. St. Louis, CV Mosby, 1984, pp. 122–145.
4. Finn WF: The postoperative recognition and further management of unsuspected cervical cancer. *Am J Obstet Gynecol* 63:717, 1952.
5. Heller PB et al: Cervical carcinoma found incidentally in a uterus removed for benign indications. *Am J Obstet Gynecol* 67(2):187–190, 1986.
6. Hertig AT: personal communication.
7. Lee NC, Dicker RC, Rubin GL, Ory HW: Confirmation of preoperative diagnoses for hysterectomy. *Am J Obstet Gynecol* 150:283–287, 1984.
8. Masterson JG: Discussion No. 3 by WF Finn. *Am J Obstet Gynecol* 63:717, 1952.
9. McDuff HC et al: Accidentally encountered cervical cancer. *Am J Obstet Gynecol* 71:407, 1956.
10. Orr JW Jr et al: Correlation of perioperative morbidity and conization to radical hysterectomy interval. *Am J Obstet Gynecol* 59:726, 1982.

84

Trauma to the Vena Cava During Para-Aortic Node Dissection

Jerome L. Belinson

Case Abstract

A 60-year-old woman with a grade II adenocarcinoma of the endometrium was undergoing a para-aortic dissection. Using Metzenbaum scissors, the peritoneum was dissected off of the nodal tissue and vena cava on the right side. A large amount of bleeding suddenly occurred. The nodal tissue was quickly lifted up, the bleeding markedly increased, and it was clear that the vena cava had been injured.

DISCUSSION

The inferior vena cava can be easily injured while doing a para-aortic dissection. Even if one is careful, the variability of the venous system or the adherence of a node to the vena cava may not always be predicted. However, if one is observant and precise in one's surgery, the caval injuries that occur can usually be solved without having to resort to inferior vena caval ligation.

There is a small vein that enters the inferior vena cava on its ventral surface just above the aortic bifurcation. This vein runs from the overlying nodes to the cava. Occasionally, it originates from the peritoneal surface, running through the nodes to the cava. In the author's experience, this small vein is highly predictable in its location and is also the most common cause for more serious injury to the vena cava. Generally, as one elevates the nodal tissue, the vein is either avulsed, or worse, tears a small strip in the wall of the cava. A similar injury can occur if the cava is tented slightly during dissection and cut with the scissors. It is important that one takes a calm, stepwise approach to solving the bleeding, since efforts poorly done will invariably convert simple problems to complex and dangerous ones. On a more general note, if the attachment of a variety of structures is not appreciated, the surgeon who elevates these tissues and then cuts or probes too quickly will discover that the vena cava has been tented up and a large hole has been created. This type of injury will, of course, result in massive bleeding, and is totally avoidable. First, one elevates the peritoneum or the nodes off from the cava very gently. Attachments that are identified are isolated and controlled. The author prefers the use of hemostatic clips for this purpose, although clamping and tying or the use of electrocautery will certainly work (Fig. 84.1). If cautery is used, it must not be set too high or the damage will run quickly down the vein and create a hole in the cava.

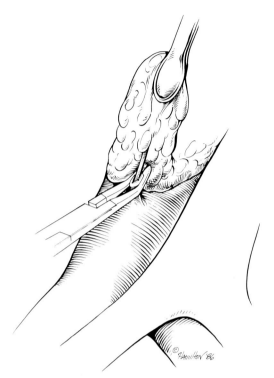

Figure 84.1. The small vein is identified and clipped as one elevates the nodal tissue off the vena cava.

In the case presented, it appears that the nature of the injury is similar to the small venous injury previously described. This, as mentioned, must be taken very seriously, since it can bleed significantly and can lead to more damage. Unless the bleeding is initially quite severe, the author prefers to try to isolate the bleeding site first. This generally means elevating the nodal tissue off the cava. Once the bleeding site is identified, direct pressure is then applied for 5 to 10 minutes, depending upon the size of the injury. If pressure alone will stop the bleeding, then one should use pressure alone. The more one has to do to stop caval bleeding, the greater the risk of further injury. If one is forced to use pressure before dissecting away surrounding tissue, one must keep in mind that as the nodes are removed the bleeding is likely to restart, although often at a much slower rate.

If the bleeding continues, the author's next choice is to try using hemostatic clips. The clips will be most effective if one can control the bleeding with a pair of vascular pick-ups. Then, while holding closed the defect with the pick-ups, one places a clip parallel to the surface of the cava just below the pick-ups (Fig. 84.2). One must be careful not to allow the tip of the hemostatic clip to cause a rent in the cava as it is being closed.

On occasion, it is fully evident that an injury to the vena cava will have to be sutured. The author prefers to control the hemorrhage first with a vascular spoon clamp. Then, using a no. 4–0 monofilament vascular suture, the defect is closed. If there is a small amount of oozing when the clamp is removed, one again uses pressure. The secret to using the spoon clamps is to include a small margin of normal caval wall around the vascular defect. The defect is then repaired within the arc of the clamp (Fig. 84.3). The

Figure 84.2.   The defect is held closed with vascular pick-ups and then a hemostatic clip is applied.

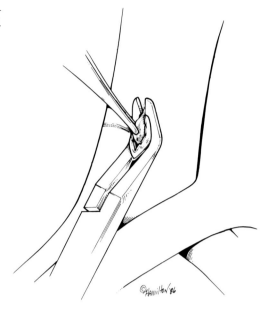

Figure 84.3.   Larger defects can be clamped and sutured using a vascular spoon clamp.

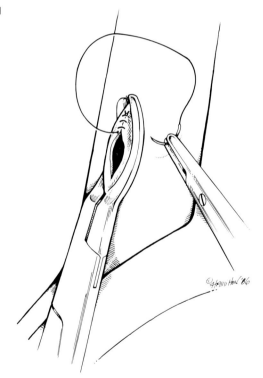

repair of the slit-type injury is also quite effectively managed using an Allis clamp, especially when the exposure is good. The Allis clamp is used to pinch the defect closed and then a no. 4–0 or 5–0 monofilament suture is placed running just beneath the clamp. In situations where one is having difficulty controlling the bleeding and exposing the injury for repair, a Fogerty catheter can also be quite useful. A no. 4 or 5 Fogerty catheter is pushed through the defect and the balloon inflated. Gentle traction on the catheter then controls the bleeding and allows one to improve the exposure.

Rarely, the inferior vena cava will be torn so severely that the anatomy is lost, alignment is impossible, and hemorrhage is overwhelming. Under these circumstances the only choice may be to ligate the vena cava above and below the injury. Fortunately, this last-resort option is available, since one is rarely working above the renal veins. However, after ligating the cava, there may still be a lumbar vein entering the injured segment that will need to be ligated. Caval ligation may be accomplished by a number of techniques. Under emergency circumstances, passing a no. 0 silk suture under the cava and tying it may be the quickest. The use of staples or caval clips can also be quite expeditious and is certainly acceptable.

SELECTED READINGS

Belinson JL, Goldberg MI, Averette HE: Paraaortic lymphadenectomy in gynecologic cancer. *Gynecol Oncol* 7:188–198, 1979.
Schwartz SI (ed): *Principles of Surgery*, ed. 4. New York, McGraw-Hill, 1984, pp. 257–259.

85

Myomectomy with Unexpected Leiomyosarcoma

Arlan B. Fuller, Jr.

Case Abstract

The uterus of a 26-year-old infertility patient with troublesome menorrhagia had multiple uterine leiomyomas, one of which was encroaching significantly on the endometrial cavity. Transabdominal multiple myomectomies were accomplished and all visible leiomyomas were removed. The patient's recovery was remarkably smooth and the pathology report was received on the morning of her planned discharge from the hospital. It reported that the largest tumor contained a leiomyosarcoma.

DISCUSSION

A 26-year-old infertility patient undergoes a procedure intended to remove her chances of childbearing and emerges with a diagnosis that threatens her fertility, her femininity, and even her life.

The diagnosis and classification of smooth muscle tumors of the female genital tract represent a challenge to the pathologist and clinician alike. Controversy surrounds the diagnostic criteria for classification of benign tumors of the uterus, borderline tumors, and leiomyosarcomas. Review of the criteria that may predict the clinical behavior of this tumor will permit a decision regarding preservation of reproductive function and prognosis for this patient. Since specific information about the histologic characteristics of the tumor is not available, discussion must be inclusive.

Leiomyomas are the most common tumors in the female pelvis and are frequent cause for hysterectomy in the United States. However, only 5% to 10% of infertility patients may have fibroids as a causative factor in their infertility, presumably a consequence of tubal obstruction (necessarily bilateral) or severe hypermenorrhea as a consequence of its submucous location.

Alternatively, myomectomy may be performed in a young woman in order to preserve fertility. If one or more fibroids are documented on successive examinations to be rapidly enlarging in a young woman not yet desirous of pregnancy, timely intervention may allow resection of the myoma(s) before it further distorts the uterine architecture and before the procedure might become technically difficult or unnecessarily morbid. Hopefully, this is an area where medical therapy with compounds such as gonadotropin-releasing hormone (GnRH) may have an increasing role in the future, particularly in the patient with multiple benign leiomyomas.

384

Meigs observed an incidence of "malignant degeneration" of 0.6%, or 9 of 1330 patients with leiomyomas. Unfortunately, this figure remains frequently quoted today; in a recent symposium on management of uterine myomas, the risk of malignant transformation was stated to be between 0.1% and 0.5%. If as many as 30% of women may have benign leiomyomas, and the incidence of leiomyosarcoma is in the range of 0.67% per 100,000 women over the age of 20 years, then the true risk of malignant change may be between 1 in 10,000 and 1 in 100,000.

The diagnosis of leiomyosarcoma on gross examination is difficult because of both the gradation of malignancy (Table 85.1) and the overlap of degenerative changes in both benign and malignant lesions. Although sarcomas typically have a necrotic or hemorrhagic center, so too may the necrotic myoma with carneous degeneration. Alternatively, the sarcoma may have merely lost the typical, whorled appearance of a benign myoma and acquired the pale gray, gelatinous appearance of a benign tumor that has outgrown its blood supply. Silverberg has examined the clinical impressions of the gynecologist and pathologist as a prognostic factor for patients with leiomyosarcomas. Significantly, when the gross impression of the tumor was that of a leiomyosarcoma, only 20% of the 10 patients studied were alive at 5 years. Conversely, when the diagnosis was not suspected clinically, 80% of the 20 patients available for follow-up were still alive.

According to Woodruff, the histologic diagnosis of leiomyosarcoma is based on the observations of hypercellularity, nuclear atypia, pleomorphism, and the number of mitoses, according to Van Dinh and Woodruff. The clinical behavior documented in any series of patients with a diagnosis of uterine sarcoma greatly depends on the criteria for inclusion of patients in the study. If one has loose criteria, including all patients with even very few mitoses, then the natural history of the disease, time to recurrence, sites of recurrence, and response to conservative therapy will differ significantly from another series in which criteria for numbers of mitoses and cellular atypia might be more strict. In his series of 43 patients, Woodruff required at least two mitoses in any high-power field to designate a tumor as a leiomyosarcoma; in some other series, the minimal criteria for inclusion are not even identified.

The intraoperative diagnosis of leiomyosarcoma would necessitate the frozen-section examination of all myomas at the time of laparotomy. Many malignant tumors can be identified by their gross appearance on cut section. Frozen-section examination can then be performed only on those tumors with necrotic centers, hemorrhage, or evidence of hyaline degeneration.

However, given the rarity of leiomyosarcomas, the uncertain reliability of frozen-section diagnosis, and the desire to employ myomectomy in young women wishing

Table 85.1 Smooth Muscle Neoplasms Diagnostic Criteria (Adapted from Kempson and Bari: *Hum Pathol* 1:331–349, 1970)

Mitoses per 10 HPF	Cytologic Atypia	Diagnosis
0–4	No	Cellular myoma
0–4	Yes	Atypical myoma
5–9	No	Borderline
5–9	Yes	Leiomyosarcoma
10 or more	Either	Leiomyosarcoma

to preserve childbearing, even if malignancy is suspected, few gynecologists would perform an abdominal hysterectomy and bilateral salpingo-oophorectomy based on frozen-section diagnosis alone. These are indeed the women who would have the most to lose with hysterectomy and would be the group who would most easily tolerate a second operation, if necessary. Moreover, the most critical case would be that of a patient with a low-grade sarcoma, where the differential diagnosis would be difficult; the high-grade sarcomas are rapidly fatal to a large population of patients, regardless of what procedure is employed.

If the diagnosis of leiomyosarcomas is to be made preoperatively (by curettage showing necrotic, atypical smooth muscle cells, or frank cancer), the appropriate procedure would involve both surgical resection of the entire tumor and precise surgical staging to determine the anatomic and pathologic extent of disease. This evaluation would involve examination of both pelvic and para-aortic nodes as well as evaluation of the extent of transcelomic spread and parenchymal organ metastases to liver and lung. Patients with disease extending beyond the uterus at the time of diagnosis have a uniformly poor prognosis in multiple series, with no survivors.

Meigs states that "if myomectomy has been done . . . immediate reoperation and total hysterectomy are necessary." The vast majority of patients cited in the literature have had at least total abdominal hysterectomy and bilateral salpingo-oophorectomy as primary treatment. Little information is available concerning the management of patients with incidental cancer found after myomectomy.

Woodruff, however, does report the outcome of nine patients treated by myomectomy alone. Three had immediate reexploration with hysterectomy and did well. Of six others treated "conservatively," five remained free of disease, and one had a local recurrence at 2 years in the uterus and abdomen and was still alive with disease at 6 years following initial therapy.

There is little evidence that postoperative pelvic radiation therapy changes the prognosis, or even the site of recurrence. The majority of recurrences are identified at extrapelvic sites in patients with anaplastic tumors.

Chemotherapy for advanced disease has produced few, if any, real successes. Reports ascribing benefit to adjuvant chemotherapy in this disease have employed historical controls and are open to criticism. Better survival in patients with stage I disease could be attributed to variations in staging of the tumor, particularly in light of the uniformly high risk of recurrence in patients with extrauterine spread of disease. Nevertheless, van Nagell and others have described fewer recurrences in stage I patients with uterine sarcomas treated with combined chemotherapy employing vincristine, actinomycin D, and cyclosphosphamide (VAC).

More than 10 mitoses per 10 high-power field (HPF) carries a poor prognosis for patients with frank leiomyosarcoma; tumors with less than 5 mitoses per 10 HPF rarely metastasize and are almost never associated with recurrence and death. These latter are the lesions that commonly occur in young women and may explain the better prognosis in premenopausal women. Van Dinh and Woodruff reported 100% 5-year survival for patients with 1 to 4 mitoses per 10 HPF, 75% survival if the mitotic count was 5 to 9 per 10 HPF, and only 20% if there were more than 10 mitoses per 10 HPF.

Silverberg and van Dinh have both reported, as have others, that tumors arising de novo in the myometrium have a much poorer prognosis than tumors arising within a leiomyoma. Survivals in the 75% range have been noted for malignant tumors in preexisting fibroids versus a 25% survival for tumors arising in the myometrium.

Silverberg noted the markedly favorable prognosis in premenopausal women; 16 of 18 premenopausal women available for follow-up were alive and well, whereas only 2 of 12 postmenopausal women enjoyed the same outcome.

It is known that leiomyomas contain high levels of estrogen and progesterone receptors relative to normal myometrium, in some cases reaching levels near that of normal endometrium. Although extensive receptor data are not available, it seems that anecdotal evidence for receptors in some uterine sarcomas does exist. One potential explanation, then, for the better prognosis in premenopausal patients may be related to the removal of both ovaries occurring at the time of hysterectomy for an estrogen-dependent tumor.

Clearly, almost all of the favorable prognostic factors are interrelated. The premenopausal patient is more likely to have a tumor with a low mitotic index, less pleomorphism and atypia, and a tumor arising in a leiomyoma. Although survival after myomectomy alone is not uniform, individualized selection of "conservative" therapy may be warranted in the properly informed patient with favorable prognostic indices.

SELECTED READINGS

Fuller AF, Patterson DC, Shimm DS: Sarcomas of the female genital tract. In: Raaf J (ed): *Management of Sarcomas* (in press).

Kempson RL, Bari W: Uterine sarcomas: Classification, diagnosis, and prognosis. *Hum Pathol* 1:331–349, 1970.

Meigs JV: *Tumors of the Female Pelvis*. New York, Macmillan, 1934.

Silverberg SG: Leiomyosarcoma of the uterus. *Obstet Gynecol* 38:613–627, 1971.

van Dinh T, Woodruff JD: Leiomyosarcomas of the uterus. *Am J Obstet Gynecol* 144:817–823, 1982.

van Nagell JR, Hanson MB, Donaldson ES, et al: Adjuvant vincristine, actinomycin D and cyclosphosphamide therapy in stage I uterine sarcomas. *Cancer* 57:1451–1454, 1986.

Wallach EE, Hammond CP, Goldfarb AF, et al: Symposium: Problems linked to uterine myomas. *Contemp Ob Gyn* 265–279, 1983.

Wilson EA, Yang F, Rees LD: Estradiol and progesterone binding in uterine leiomyomata and in normal uterine tissue. *Obstet Gynecol* 55:20–24, 1980.

86

Unexpected Carcinoma of the Ovary Reported by Pathology Five Days Following Unilateral Salpingo-Oophorectomy for Presumed Endometrial Cyst

Denis Cavanagh
Donald E. Marsden

Case Abstract

A unilateral oophorectomy for presumed endometriosis had been performed in a 23-year-old patient. At surgery, the ovary measured 12 cm in diameter, and there was no evidence of endometriosis on the opposite side nor, for that matter, elsewhere in the pelvis. Some light, filmy adhesions between the tumor and the surrounding intestine had been severed easily at the time of surgery. The tumor had been removed in its entirety, along with the tube, which was uninvolved. There was no spillage of tumor.

On the fifth, postoperative day, the pathology report indicated an adenocarcinoma of the ovary, existing in a specimen with an intact capsule, and no gross evidence of serosal penetration was described.

DISCUSSION

Identification of the Problem

The extreme seriousness of the problem must be clearly understood by all those involved in the management of this patient. A superficial assessment might lead to the conclusion that this young woman, presumably wishing to retain reproductive potential, has had a stage IA carcinoma of the ovary completely excised and has therefore been adequately treated. On the basis of the information supplied, such an assumption is completely unfounded and carries grave risks for the patient.

The prognosis and treatment of ovarian carcinoma are directly related to the clinical stage, the amount of residual tumor, and the histopathology. In this patient there is adequate information available on all of these subjects.

With respect to the clinical staging and amount of tumor possibly remaining in this patient, a number of observations relating to ovarian carcinomas actually or apparently belonging to Federation of International Gynecologists and Obstetricians (FIGO) stage I must be clearly understood.

1. Peritoneal washings will contain malignant cells in up to 36% of patients with stage I tumors with intact capsules (8), and their presence significantly affects the prognosis (3, 14) and hence the treatment.
2. The contralateral ovary, although normal to gross inspection, will harbor microscopic carcinoma in 12% to 18% of cases (9).
3. Diaphragmatic metastases have been found in over 10% of patients who, having been previously diagnosed as having stage I lesions, were subjected to surgery for restaging within a few weeks of initial diagnosis (10).
4. Para-aortic lymph node metastases have been shown to be present in approximately 10% of women with stage I ovarian carcinoma, and pelvic nodes were involved in 8% of cases (10).
5. Omental metastases were present in 3% to 5% of patients with disease that had been thought to be stage I (2, 10). Routine omentectomy in such cases may well show this estimate to be conservative.

Considering all these facts, it is not surprising that the staging of early ovarian cancer is reportedly inaccurate in 30% of cases (5). In the patient we are considering, there is no mention of any extrapelvic structures being palpated or examined for even macroscopic evidence of tumor spread. Clearly the staging was totally inadequate.

Nor is the pathology report of "adenocarcinoma . . . with an intact capsule, and no gross evidence of serosal penetration" sufficiently precise in this situation. Of particular importance here is the accurate identification of tumor type, its degree of differentiation, and microscopic evidence of serosal penetration. In a tumor of this size these judgments must be based on the examination of multiple sections from all areas of the tumor by an experienced gynecologic pathologist. Decker et al. (4) reported an 87% 5-year survival in stage I, grade I papillary cystadenocarcinomas, compared with a 54% 5-year survival in stage I, grade III papillary cystadenocarcinomas.

The seriousness of the situation for this young woman is therefore due to major inadequacies in the assessment of possible residual tumor, the staging of the disease, and the pathologic assessment of the tumor. Given these obvious deficiencies, no rational plan of therapy can be formulated.

Avoidance of This Problem

In the clinical evaluation of any female with a pelvic or adnexal mass, the possibility of ovarian malignancy must be considered. In the 20- to 30-year age group approximately 10% of ovarian tumors are malignant (13). Although only about 8% of epithelial cancers of the ovary occur in women under age 35, the proportion may be increasing (1).

With this in mind, preoperative evaluation should include, in all cases:

1. A complete history and physical examination, including cervical cytology and rectovaginal examinations.

2. Complete blood count, serology, serum electrolytes, renal and liver profiles.
3. Urinalysis and pregnancy tests.
4. Serum tumor markers CA 125, carcinoembryonic antigen (CEA), human serum beta chorionic gonadotropin, and alpha fetoprotein.
5. Chest x-ray.
6. If pregnancy has been excluded, an intravenous pyelogram should be done.

Other tests, such as barium enema, upper gastrointestinal series, liver scan, sigmoidoscopy, or colonoscopy, may be indicted by features such as dyspepsia or bowel disturbances revealed on history or by findings on physical examination. Biopsy specimens should be obtained from enlarged groin or supraclavicular nodes. If a pleural effusion is found, thoracentesis should be performed to allow cytologic examination of the effusion. On the other hand, even if ascites is present, abdominal paracentesis should be avoided because fluid will be obtained more safely at the time of laparotomy.

Sonograms, computerized axial tomography scans, and lymphangiograms are rarely helpful and are occasionally misleading (12).

The definitive investigative procedure for ovarian masses over 5 cm in diameter, or persistent masses of smaller size, or in any case where malignancy is suspected, is laparotomy. Laparoscopy may be misleading or even dangerous in the presence of ovarian carcinoma and provides inadequate information for staging.

With a mass the size that this patient had, or when there is the slightest suspicion of malignancy, a vertical incision should be used.

Immediately after the peritoneal cavity is opened the nature and volume of any ascites are noted, and samples are aspirated and sent for cytology. If ascites is not present, irrigation of the peritoneal cavity with 300 cc of saline should be performed and the fluid aspirated and sent for cytology. A soft rubber catheter and bulb syringe are used to irrigate the space between the right hemidiaphragm and the liver, which is a common site of miliary metastases.

The upper abdomen is explored first, with palpation of the retroperitoneal structures and palpation and examination of all peritoneal surfaces and intraperitoneal organs. Special attention is paid to the liver and undersurface of the diaphragm. Use of a sigmoidoscope or laparoscope may aid in obtaining sufficient illumination and better visualization of this important area. The stomach, bowel, mesentery, and omentum are all palpated and inspected. Biopsy specimens are obtained from any suspicious lesions. The para-aortic region is palpated and biopsy specimens are obtained from any palpable nodes. Even in the absence of palpable tumor deposits within it, the greater omentum should be removed if ovarian malignancy is present or strongly suspected.

When the upper abdomen has been thoroughly explored, attention is directed to the pelvis. The gross appearance of the uterus, tubes, and ovaries is noted. Adhesions, excrescences, bilaterality, and tumor rupture are suggestive of malignancy and indicate a poorer prognosis.

If at this stage there is no indication that the disease has spread beyond one ovary and the patient is young and desiring further children, consideration can be given to conservative therapy. The criteria for conservative therapy in such a case as this are:

1. Stage IA lesion (FIGO)
2. Histopathology of tumor
    a. Grade I epithelial carcinoma
    b. "Borderline tumors" ("low malignant potential")
    c. Dysgerminoma
    d. Granulosa cell tumor
    e. Arrhenoblastoma
3. Tumor encapsulated and free of adhesions
4. No invasion of the capsule, lymphatics, blood vessels, or mesovarium
5. Peritoneal washings showing no malignant cells
6. Omentectomy specimen normal
7. Sections from remaining ovary histologically negative for tumor
8. Pelvis otherwise normal

Now it is clear that not all of these criteria can be fulfilled at the initial laparotomy. If reliable frozen-section services are available, upper abdominal biopsies and omental and para-aortic nodal biopsies containing tumor on frozen section would indicate the need for the maximum surgical effort. If these are negative or reliable frozen sections are not available, decisions must be made on clinical grounds, pending permanent section results.

If conservative management still appears feasible, salpingo-oophorectomy is carefully performed to avoid rupture or leakage of the tumor. Should there still be uncertainty as to its nature, it should be cut in the operating room (away from the operating table) and checked for signs of malignancy. Again, frozen sections, if available and reliable, may be immensely useful. If malignancy appears to be or is shown on frozen section to be present, the other ovary is bivalved and wedge biopsy performed. Once more, a positive frozen section would indicate the need to abandon conservatism. The ovary should be carefully repaired using no. 5-0 polypropylene sutures, since the aim of conservatism is primarily to preserve fertility, and adhesion formation would defeat that aim.

Biopsy specimens should be obtained from any suspicious pelvic lesions or pelvic nodes.

Assuming there is still no contraindication to conservative management, the abdomen is closed, and careful and detailed operative notes are made.

The patient must be given a detailed evaluation of the situation. Should subsequent pathology or cytologic reports indicate that any of the criteria for conservative management have not been fulfilled, then reoperation with maximal surgical effort must be advised, with suitable adjunctive therapy.

If all the criteria are shown to have been fulfilled, the patient is followed carefully. When the desired family size has been achieved, total hysterectomy and removal of the remaining ovary are then carried out (1). The same careful total abdominal assessment advised for the first operation is mandatory.

Only by such a fastidious approach to this type of patient can we hope to avoid misdiagnosis, optimize treatment, and improve survival and cure rates. Nothing short of the ideal should be an accepted goal.

This Patient's Problem and Its Management

By now it will clear that the patient has received far from optimal management. Several things must be done immediately:

1. The operative specimen and slides should be seen and assessed by a competent gynecologic pathologist and, if necessary, further sections made as described above.
2. Any relevant investigations that were not done preoperatively should be performed.
3. The patient should be strongly advised to have a staging laparotomy performed, in the manner described above. Laparoscopy would not be appropriate in this situation.

Should the patient refuse repeat surgery, the dangers inherent in such a decision must be made clear to her, and monthly follow-up for 1 year with subsequent visits every 3 months advised. Appropriate serum tumor marker studies CA125 (serous tumors) and/or CEA (mucinous tumors) should be obtained bimonthly during the observation period.

If the patient agrees to reexploration, it would seem wisest to have it performed in a center where a skilled gynecologic pathologist can perform reliable frozen sections to minimize the chance of a repeat laparotomy, if sections show more advanced disease than had been suspected.

Patients with stage IA "borderline" or grade I carcinoma of the ovary appear to do equally well whether treated by unilateral salpingo-oophorectomy or total hysterectomy and bilateral salpingo-oophorectomy (7, 9). However, it has been pointed out that these reports are from older series, and survival rates were not optimal in either the conservatively or radically treated groups (11).

If the criteria for conservative management are not fulfilled, the patient should have total hysterectomy, bilateral salpingo-oophorectomy, omentectomy, and appendectomy. The aim is to reduce tumor bulk as much as possible and leave no residual tumor nodule over 1 cm in diameter ("maximal surgical effort").

Subsequently, any patient with stage I disease with poorly differentiated tumor, bilateral ovarian involvement, ascites, or positive peritoneal washings, and any patient with stage II, III, or IV disease, should receive combination chemotherapy from an experienced oncologist, using cyclophosphamide and *cis*-platinum or carboplatinum. This therapy is given once every 4 weeks for 6 to 12 courses, with careful surveillance for hematologic, cardiologic, hepatic, and renal complications. Regular gynecologic examinations, including vaginal vault cytology, and rectovaginal examinations are essential, as are appropriate serum tumor marker studies.

After 6 to 12 courses of chemotherapy, if there is no clinical evidence of recurrence, a "second look" laparotomy, performed as for the staging procedure previously described, should be done. If there is no residual tumor and peritoneal washings are negative, the patient should continue on oral cyclophosphamide, 150 mg/m^3, for 8 days per month for an additional 3 months. Thereafter the chemotherapy is discontinued, but regular gynecologic follow-up is still essential with appropriate serum tumor markers and radiologic studies.

The place of radiotherapy in the management of ovarian carcinoma is controversial at the present time, and opinions differ widely (6,15).

REFERENCES

1. Barber HRK: *Ovarian Carcinoma: Etiology, Diagnosis and Treatment*. New York, Masson, 1978.
2. Buchsbaum HJ, Keetel WC: Radioisotopes in treatment of stage IA ovarian cancer. *Natl Cancer Inst Monogr* 42:127, 1975.
3. Creasman WT, Rutledge F: The prognostic value of peritoneal cytology in gynecologic malignant disease. *Am J Obstet Gynecol* 110:773, 1971.
4. Decker DG, Malkasian GD Jr, Taylor WF: The prognostic importance of histologic grading in ovarian carcinoma. *Natl Cancer Inst Monogr* 42:9, 1975.
5. Decker DG, Webb MJ: Prophylactic therapy for stage I ovarian cancer. *Gynecol Oncol* 1:203, 1973.
6. Dembo AJ, Bush RS, Beale FA, et al: The Princess Margaret Hospital study of ovarian cancer: Stages I, II, and asymptomatic III presentations. *Cancer Treat Rep* 63:249, 1979.
7. Julian CG, Woodruff JD: The biologic behavior of low grade papillary serous carcinoma of the ovary. *Obstet Gynecol* 40:860, 1972.
8. Keetel WC, Pixley EE, Buchsbaum HJJ: Experience with peritoneal cytology in the management of gynecologic malignancies. *Am J Obstet Gynecol* 108:878, 1970.
9. Munnell EW: Is conservative therapy ever justified in stage I(IA) cancer of the ovary? *Am J Obstet Gynecol* 103:641, 1969.
10. Piver MS, Barlow JJ, Lele SB: Incidence of sub-clinical metastasis in stage I and II ovarian carcinoma. *Obstet Gynecol* 52:100, 1978.
11. Smith WG: Surgical treatment of epithelial ovarian carcinoma. *Clin Obstet Gynecol* 22:939, 1979.
12. Watring WG, Edinger DD, Anderson B: Screening and diagnosis in ovarian cancer. *Clin Obstet Gynecol* 22:745, 1979.
13. Way S: *Malignant Disease of the Female Genital Tract*. Philadelphia, Blakiston, 1951.
14. Webb MJ, Decker DG, Mussey E, et al: Factors influencing survival in stage I ovarian cancer. *Am J Obstet Gynecol* 116:222, 1973.
15. Young RC: Ovarian carcinoma: An optimistic epilogue. *Cancer Treat Rep* 63:333, 1979.

87

Nonresectable Adenocarcinoma of Ovary Which Shrinks During Chemotherapy

William T. Creasman

Case Abstract

A 15-cm fixed pelvic mass, separate from the uterus, was found in an asymptomatic 57-year-old multipara with a tentative diagnosis of ovarian carcinoma. The abdomen was opened through a midline incision. There was free peritoneal fluid from which washings were obtained, and the initial diagnosis was substantiated. There was extensive carcinomatosis. The disease was bilateral, fixed to the sidewalls of the pelvis, the broad ligament, the posterior surface of the uterus, the mesosalpinx, the descending colon, and various loops of small intestine. There were countless subserosal 1- to 2-mm nodules of metastatic tumor on the small bowel and diaphragm. Representative biopsies from the tumor were obtained. It was the opinion of the operator that the tumor was nonresectable. The abdomen was closed and the patient placed on chemotherapy involving courses of adriamycin and cis-platinum. During the course of the chemotherapy there was a good response as measured by a dramatic reduction in the size of the tumor. Upon pelvic examination it now appeared to be movable and the surgeon wondered about the propriety of reexploration and possible resection.

DISCUSSION

The situation presented by this patient was unusual when single-agent chemotherapy was standard therapy. Today, with combination chemotherapy, particularly if *cis*-platinum is included, more and more patients seem to show the clinical picture of the patient described. Yet uninhibited enthusiasm should be tempered. There is no question that patients who are optimally debulked (tumor residual equal to or less than 2 cm) have a greater chance of achieving a complete response, come for a second look more often, have a more surgical pathologically complete response, and are longer surviviors than the patient not optimally debulked. With the use of multiple-agent chemotherapy an increasing number of patients (both optimally and suboptimally debulked) seem to be experiencing a clinical response. Some preliminary data suggest that as many as 80% to 85% of patients are responding to chemotherapy. One must be extremely careful in interpreting this data, however, since two-thirds to three-quarters of the responders are only partial responders and their survivals have minimal or no increase compared with those that have no change in clinical disease.

Approximately one-third of patients with stage III or IV disease who are treated with chemotherapy will come for a second look because of a response to the treatment. If only complete responders (CRs) are included, the number is lower. Of the patients undergoing a second-look operation, only one-quarter to one-third will have surgical pathologic CRs. The rate of surgically confirmed response in two large series was 7.3% and 12.3%. Those patients with surgical CRs can expect a 20% to 40% recurrence. The overall prognosis of these patients with current modalities is therefore very dismal.

Since there is such a poor overall survival in this group of patients, approaches are now being evaluated which were once considered radical. The first question this patient poses is whether she could have been optimally debulked by a more experienced surgeon. Apparently only a biopsy was obtained. It is recognized that there are some situations in which no surgeon can adequately debulk a patient. Preliminary data do suggest that a significant number of patients said to be unresectable were reexplored and optimally debulked. Some required removal of part of the gastrointestinal tract with reanastomosis. The amount of tumor remaining behind after the surgical procedure continues to be an extremely important (if not the most important) prognostic criteria for prolonged survival. Even in "unresectable" cases the adnexal masses can be removed and partial omentectomy can be performed in essentially every situation. Approaching the pelvic mass(es) retroperitoneally always facilitates removal, and also decreases blood loss considerably. The decision to reexplore the patient immediately after the initial exploration is often difficult. Clinical judgment, reports from the primary surgeon, and political consideration are all taken into the decision-making process. Sometimes the patient is not reexplored immediately even though it is felt that optimal debulking may be achieved. The patient is given three courses of chemotherapy, and if there is a clinical response, reexploration at that time is performed. In several instances, optimal debulking, even down to "no gross remaining disease," has been accomplished. The number of cases are few and definitive statements concerning what, if any, role this protocol will accomplish cannot be made.

The role of secondary surgery in ovarian cancer continues to be debated. For many years a second look at laparotomy has been considered standard therapy in the United States. At one time almost all patients who had completed a prescribed number of chemotherapy courses would undergo a surgical exploration (second-look laparotomy) to determine if the patient was tumor-free, and if so, therapy could be stopped. In those in whom gross disease was identified, attempts at secondary debulking were done in hopes of improving long-term survival. Today a true second-look laparotomy is done only if a patient has had a complete clinical response and there is no laboratory evidence of persistent disease, including a normal Ca 125. Even under those circumstances as many as one-half of those undergoing a second-look laparotomy will have persistent disease. In those who have a surgical complete response, experience has indicated that up to one-half may recur. Because of these dismal results, most investigators outside of the United States really question whether a second-look laparotomy should be part of standard therapy and, in fact, have discontinued doing this procedure.

Previous anecdotal experience indicated that secondary surgical debulking results were bleak. More recently it has been suggested that debulking surgery at the time of the second-look laparotomy or attempts at debulking in a patient with known persistent disease after a prescribed number of courses of chemotherapy may be of benefit. If a patient can be debulked to essentially no gross disease at the time of the secondary surgery, her prognosis increases considerably. In a collected series of 600 patients who had disease present at the time of the second-look laparotomy, only about 20% at the completion of the debulking had microscopic disease present. Of those with microscopic disease, only about a third survived. This latter figure represents only 6% of those undergoing the second-look laparotomy. The cost-benefit ratio obviously has to be taken into consideration. Nevertheless, in the small subset of patients who can be optimally debulked, survival does appear to be improved. If these individuals could be determined preoperatively, obviously the morbidity of doing a large number of patients without apparent benefit would help in the overall management of these individuals.

A recently reported abstract from the European Cooperative Group noted in a prospective randomized study that interventional debulking surgery did appear to improve survival in patients with advanced epithelial ovarian carcinoma. Several hundred patients with suboptimal stage III and IV ovarian cancer were evaluated. After the initial debulking surgery, all had significant disease remaining. They then received three courses of cytoxan cisplatin and if no progression was noted were randomized to receive an interval debulking or continue the chemotherapy. Those who did undergo the interval debulking had an exploratory laparotomy with the surgical intent to optimally debulk the patient's tumor. After surgery that group of patients continued the chemotherapy and received the same amount of drugs as the group of non-interval-debulking patients. Although the study is ongoing, the preliminary data suggest that those who underwent the interval debulking had a longer progression-free interval that was statistically significant. Probably of more importance is that the mean survival of those patients undergoing the interval debulking was 27 months versus 19 months for the patients who did not have the interval surgery. Again this difference is highly significant. For the first time this prospective randomized study suggests that there may very well be a place for interval debulking. Prior data were anecdotal or nonrandomized. Although this is only a preliminary report, the results are encouraging. The Gynecologic Oncology Group in the United States is planning to evaluate interval debulking in a similar group of patients in an attempt to confirm these encouraging results.

Even with newer chemotherapeutic agents (most recently Taxol) patients with advanced ovarian cancer have a dismal prognosis. It has been appreciated for many years that surgical debulking, particularly if optimal debulking can be performed, is extremely important in the overall prognosis of patients with ovarian cancer. It is important that we continue to evaluate the possible role of surgery after the initial debulking to see if it may be an important adjunct in the overall management of ovarian cancer patients.

Selected Readings

Creasman WT: Evaluation of debulking surgery at second-look laparotomy. In: Sharp F, Mason WP, Creasman WT (eds): *Ovarian Cancer.* London, Chapman & Hall, 1992, p. 375.

van der Burg MEL, van Lent M, Loborska A, Colombo N, et al: Intervention debulking surgery does improve survival in advanced epithelial ovarian cancer. *ASCO* 12:818, 1993.

Section IX

Problems of Minor Gynecologic Surgery

88

Perforation of Uterus at Dilatation and Curettage

John C. Lathrop

Case Abstract

A fractional D&C was recommended for a 65-year-old patient with a 1-year history of watery vaginal discharge which had recently become bloody. Menopause had been at age 50 years, and supplemental estrogen administration of 2 years duration had been given immediately after the menopause. The patient was a moderately obese multipara, but was neither diabetic nor hypertensive.

The endocervical portion of the fractional curettage proceeded easily enough, producing scant, grossly benign curettings. However, when the uterine sound was introduced to measure uterine depth, its passage appeared to encounter little resistance. A curette was introduced, and the tip proceeded with ease well beyond the estimated depth of the cavum, suggesting perforation of the wall of the uterus.

DISCUSSION

Given the history of a watery, bloody discharge and her age, this patient must be considered a likely candidate for endometrial carcinoma. In order to establish the diagnosis and institute appropriate therapy, sampling of the endometrium is essential. Since it is probable that the sound and the curette have both perforated the uterus, the surgeon is understandably reluctant to persist in further attempts to complete the procedure in the usual fashion. Nevertheless, efforts to obtain endometrial tissue must be pursued in spite of the recognized perforation.

Uterine perforation at the time of curettage may occur for a variety of reasons. In a 65-year-old woman, the endometrium has become atrophied and the myometrium is thinner. If malignancy is present in the uterine wall, the likelihood of perforation is even greater (6). Marked degrees of unrecognized anteversion or retroversion of the fundus allow perforation to occur more readily by permitting misdirection of the sound or curette (Fig. 88.1). In keeping with the principles of performing a D&C as outlined by Word et al. (8), it is imperative that the position of the uterus be determined by bimanual examination before any instruments are inserted. Adherence to this guideline will reduce the incidence of perforation to a minimum. When instruments are inserted, care must be taken to avoid the overzealous use of force in their manipulation.

Upon recognition of the perforation of the uterus, subsequent management is considered in two phases: (a) treatment of the perforation; (b) establishment of the

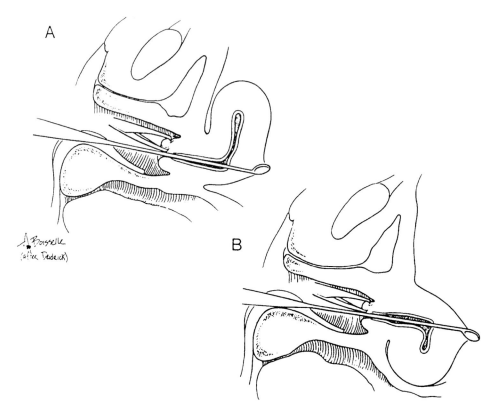

Figure 88.1.   **A.** Perforation of the posterior wall of an anteflexed uterus. **B.** Perforation of the anterior wall of a retroflexed uterus.

histologic diagnosis. Most uterine perforations occurring during diagnostic D&C in post-menopausal patients cause no significant clinical problems. A simple, noninvasive test, real-time ultrasonography, may be employed to scan the cul-de-sac for accumulation of blood. A negative scan in the presence of a clinically stable patient would permit management by simple observation over a period of 1 or 2 days for signs of bleeding, infection, or adjacent organ injury (7). If intraperitoneal bleeding to a significant degree is suspected, clinically or by real-time ultrasonography, a culdocentesis may be readily carried out for confirmation. Should gross blood be aspirated or if there is a serious concern regarding adjacent organ injury, laparoscopy would be advisable to evaluate the necessity of a formal celiotomy. If the perforation site can be visualized and is found to be actively bleeding, electrocoagulation of the area under direct vision can be attempted. Should cautery fail to stop the bleeding or be contraindicated for any reason, the translaparoscopic application of microfibrillar collagen (Avitene) may be tried (4). If these methods fail to sufficiently control bleeding or if serious trauma to an adjacent organ, requiring repair, is observed, laparotomy would be indicated. If infection occurred, antibiotics could be utilized and colpotomy performed later if an abscess presented in the cul-de-sac.

The management of a perforation produced by a uterine sound does not differ significantly from management of an injury produced by a curette in the atrophic postmenopausal uterus. One might anticipate a somewhat lower incidence of complications following perforation with a sound because of its size, shape, and lack of sharp edges.

Hysteroscopy, utilizing either gas or liquid as a distention system, is contraindicated in the presence of a uterine perforation since it would not be possible to distend the uterus (5). Contact hysteroscopy might be of some value in identifying the perforation site, although there has not been wide experience with this method at this time. It would be more useful in assessing the nature and anatomic location of intrauterine pathology. It has no value in determining the extent of extrauterine injury.

Perforations occurring in the presence of cervical carcinoma are managed according to the principles applying to any other type of uterine perforation at curettage. In this instance, however, it would be prudent to make no further attempts at endometrial sampling since the primary diagnosis is already established and the histologic evaluation of the endometrium will have little or no influence on the determination of treatment of the primary disease.

The question of dissemination of endometrial carcinoma to an intraperitoneal location is often considered in discussions of uterine wall perforation at the tumor site. Assuming that the primary diagnosis of malignancy is established, the initiation of therapy in the form of external radiation or surgery is usually undertaken promptly according to the appropriate clinical findings. Studies have shown that there is no significant survival difference for these patients as a result of the perforation. For this reason, the principles of management of the incident would be similar to those described for the nonmalignant state.

In younger patients having curettage performed during pregnancy, such as an incomplete or therapeutic abortion or a hydatidiform mole, the anatomic location of the perforation would have greater significance. Midline perforations in the anterior or posterior wall could be treated conservatively with observation for complications. Lateral perforations, with their greater likelihood of injury to the uterine vessels dilated in the gravid state, would indicate laparoscopic examination if there was any indication of broad ligament hematoma formation, or laparotomy if significant intraperitoneal hemorrhage appeared to have occurred (3).

In the patient in question, diagnosis of the primary disease process must be promptly established by obtaining for study tissue samples of the endometrium. This could be done by first carefully reassessing the position of the fundus with a repeat bimanual examination.

If the operator is an experienced hysteroscopist, the contact hysteroscope may be gently inserted into the endometrial cavity to accurately identify the geographic location of the tumor (1). This would facilitate and minimize the amount of curetting necessary to obtain an adequate specimen and reduce the risk of reperforation of the uterus. It would also identify any bowel or omentum previously drawn into the uterine cavity by the curette at the time of perforation. Very cautious passage of the sound could then be executed in the appropriate axis of the uterus, trying consciously to avoid the site of prior perforation. If this is successful, the cervix could then be dilated and the curette carefully passed into the endometrial cavity, and thorough curetting of the fundus should then be accomplished. An alternative possibility would be to perform a laparoscopic examination and then, with the laparoscope in place, execute the D&C under direct intra-abdominal vision (2). Evaluation of possible dissemination of a malignant process represents an added benefit of prelaparotomy laparoscopy but by itself is insufficient justification to warrant this procedure following simple perforation of the uterus.

In the absence of indications for emergency intervention, the standard order of diagnostic procedure should be carried out with the aim of establishing an accurate histologic diagnosis. Gross evaluation of the endocervical curettings is of no significance in this patient since their benign appearance does not eliminate the possibility of uterine malignancy. Should cancer prove to be present in the uterus, other forms of therapy, such as radiation or chemotherapy, might be more appropriate to consider as the first step in the optimal treatment plan. The interests of the patient are best served when laparotomy, if indicated, can be deferred to fit into a thoughtful and well-conceived plan of treatment.

REFERENCES

1. Barbot J, Parent B, Dubuisson J: Contact hysteroscopy: Another method of endoscopic examination of the uterine cavity. *Am J Obstet Gynecol* 136:721, 1980.
2. Ben-Baruch G, Menczer J, Shaley J, et al: Uterine perforation during curettage: Perforation rates and postperforation management. *Isr J Med Sci* 16:821, 1980.
3. Berek JS, Stubblefield PG: Anatomic and clinical correlates of uterine perforation. *Am J Obstet Gynecol* 135:181, 1979.
4. Borten M, Friedman EA: Translaparoscopic hemostasis with microfibrillar collagen in lieu of laparotomy. *J Reprod Med* 28:804, 1983.
5. Neuwirth RS: *Hysteroscopy*. Philadelphia, WB Saunders, 1975, p. 40.
6. Rutledge F, Ehrlich C: *Adenocarcinoma of the endometrium*. In: Gray LA (ed): *Endometrial Carcinoma and Its Treatment*. Springfield, IL, Charles C. Thomas, 1977, Chap. 12, p. 128.
7. Shaley E, Ben-Ami M, Zuckerman H: Real-time ultrasound diagnosis of bleeding uterine perforation during therapeutic abortion. *J Clin Ultrasound* 14:66, 1986.
8. Word B, Graylee LC, Wideman GL: The fallacy of simple uterine curettage. *Obstet Gynecol* 12:642, 1958.

Pelvic Mass Following Conization

Barrie Anderson

Case Abstract

Cold-knife conization of the cervix using a no. 11 pointed scalpel blade had been performed on a 52-year-old multipara to better evaluate and treat a severe cervical dysplasia which had extended into the endocervical canal. Deep hemostatic stitches of chromic catgut had been placed at the 3 and 9 o'clock positions lateral to the cervix. After conization, the vaginal edge was caught in a running-lock hemostatic suture of chromic catgut.

Postoperatively the patient felt weak and developed a persistent low-grade fever and troublesome backache, the latter thought to have been due to her position in the stirrups on the operating table at the time of the conization.

The symptoms persisted and the patient was examined in the doctor's office 2 weeks postoperatively, disclosing a marked tenderness around the cervix at the vault of the vagina, and a raw purulent site of the recent conization. There was a hemoglobin of 10 gm. A local cellulitis was diagnosed and the patient placed on a broad-spectrum antibiotic. The symptoms of weakness, backache, and fever worsened progressively and the patient was readmitted 5 weeks after surgery. The hemoglobin was now 8.5 gm. An intravenous pyelogram (IVP) demonstrated compression and lateral displacement of the right ureter and a computerized axial tomography (CAT) scan revealed a 6- to 8-cm cystic mass posterior to the cervix on the patient's right. This was confirmed by pelvic examination under anesthesia.

DISCUSSION

The origin of the hematoma in the right broad ligament and retroperitoneal area in this patient resulted from lack of hemostasis in either the descending cervical branch of the uterine artery or the uterosacral ligament branch of the vaginal artery. This can occur during conization when the dissection of the cervical canal is identified incorrectly so that the incision perforates the cervix high in the endocervical canal, in this case on the right and posteriorly. Bleeding in this area may not be expressed vaginally and can be difficult to identify and to control. Constant checking of the direction of the canal and its relationship to the incision during the procedure can prevent such perforations. This can be facilitated by placing a sound in the endocervical canal and aiming the point of the blade toward it at all times. In such a maneuver the handle of the knife will describe a very large circle with the point remaining essentially stationary.

Another cause for bleeding in this area may be inadequate ligation of the descending cervical branch of the uterine artery. In the postmenopausal woman, cervical atrophy and obliteration of the vaginal fornices may make it difficult to place a lateral suture high enough along the cervix to ligate this artery satisfactorily. Reflecting the vaginal mucosa away from the cervix, as at the beginning of a vaginal hysterectomy, can allow for better access to the descending cervical branch, which should be ligated at the level of the internal os. Also, care must be taken to place the suture perpendicular to the endocervical canal. If the needle is angled too much, the cervical artery may be perforated or missed entirely, with subsequent bleeding upon removal of the cone specimen.

In addition, better hemostasis may be obtained from the lateral sutures if they are not tied until after the removal of the cone specimen. After decrease in cervix bulk following removal of the specimen, it is not uncommon for sutures to become less snug and therefore less hemostatic. This is particularly true in a small or atrophic cervix. To prevent this, lateral sutures can be placed and held with hemostats until completion of the surgical excision, when they can be tied.

Finally, suturing of only the portio vaginalis may not be sufficient to control hemorrhage from deeper branches of the cervical artery but may place sufficient pressure to prevent vaginal exit of the blood, thus forcing it into a retroperitoneal location and delaying diagnosis. An alternate closure that allows better hemostasis and control of deeper vessels is the Sturmdorf closure, which has both a deep and a superficial component and approximates portio epithelium with endocervical epithelium (3,4). Other methods of hemostasis include electrocautery or injection of the cervix with Pitressin. Any postoperative bleeding from the latter two methods would be immediately evident vaginally.

Differential diagnosis in this patient would have to include ureteral obstruction, retroperitoneal hematoma, and pelvic inflammatory disease. The presence of backache should direct attention to the retroperitoneal area and to the kidneys, especially in the presence of fever. Ureteral obstruction could have resulted from a poorly placed lateral hemostatic suture at either 3 or 9 o'clock as the ureters pass from a lateral position near the cervix medially down the anterior vaginal wall to the trigone at a point about 3 to 4 cm below the anterior vaginal fornix. Atrophy in the postmenopausal cervix blurs landmarks and increases the risk of accidental ureteral compromise. Unilateral ureteral obstruction would be expected to give localized costovertebral angle tenderness, with fever arising from infection beyond a partially or completely obstructed ureter. An IVP early in the course of the process should be diagnostic.

Serial hemoglobin and hematocrit measurements would direct attention to possible occult blood loss. Again, back pain should direct attention to the retroperitoneum, and pelvic examination and IVP can help identify the location of the hematoma.

Retroperitoneal drainage of this hematoma through a lower quadrant abdominal incision, extended vertically into the flank, is ideal because tissue planes are easily developed from this approach (1). Blood vessels can be more easily traced and bleeding points identified. Other vulnerable structures such as the ureter can be avoided. Ureteral repair in the event of damage is also more easily accomplished. Finally, longterm negative suction drainage is more practical and comfortable through such an incision rather than through a vaginal approach.

Assuming that the cervical neoplasia has been completely removed, the patient should do well. The Jackson-Pratt drain should be left in place until total drainage in 24 hours is 10 to 15 cc or less. Broad-spectrum antibiotic coverage tailored to bacterial cultures and sensitivities should be continued for a full therapeutic course. Should hysterectomy be necessary in the near future, consideration should be given to prophylactic antibiotics, which appear to eliminate the increased morbidity of hysterectomy performed soon after cervical conization (2,5,6).

In the patient described above, because of the distance of the mass from the vault of the vagina, a tentative diagnosis of infected hematoma in this area was made, and through a flank incision a retroperitoneal exposure of this hematoma was accomplished with ease. The ureter was traced for its length, and found to be uninvolved. The hematoma was evacuated as well as possible, and a Jackson-Pratt drain placed in the cavity of the hematoma. The patient's postoperative course was uneventful and she was discharged on her fifth postoperative day.

REFERENCES

1. Byron RL, Yonemoto RH, Riihimaki DU, et al: Retroperitoneal ligation of the hypogastric arteries for pelvic hemorrhage. *Am Surg* 33:25–28, 1967.
2. Forney JP, Morrow CP, Townsend DE, et al: Impact of cephalosporin prophylaxis on conization-vaginal hysterectomy morbidity. *Am J Obstet Gynecol* 125:100–103, 1976.
3. Krebs HB: Outpatient cervical conization. *Obstet Gynecol* 63:420–424, 1984.
4. Stafl A: Cervical intraepithelial neoplasia. In: Thompson JD, Rock JA (eds): *Te Linde's Operative Gynecology*, ed. 7. Philadelphia, JB Lippincott, 1992.
5. Van Nagell JR, Roddick JW, Cooper RM, et al: Vaginal hysterectomy following conization in the treatment of carcinoma-in-situ of the cervix. *Am J Obstet Gynecol* 113:948–951, 1972.
6. Orr JW, Shingleton HM, Hatch KD, Mann WJ, Austin JM, Soong S-J: Correlation of perioperative morbidity and conization to radical hysterectomy interval. *Obstet Gynecol* 59:726–731, 1982.

SECTION X

OBSTETRIC SURGERY

Disruption of a Fourth-Degree Laceration

John O. L. DeLancey

Case Abstract

A 26-year-old gravida I, para 0 had labor induced at 42 weeks of pregnancy. After a second stage of 3 hours, forceps were used to deliver a 4800-gram fetus. A midline episiotomy was used and extended into the rectum with considerable collateral laceration. This was repaired in the delivery room. On the fourth day postpartum the patient had a fever to 101.8°F and purulent discharge was found from the wound. During pelvic examination the wound opened spontaneously throughout its entire length. Initial debridement removed several pieces of necrotic external anal sphincter muscle. The patient defervessed and on the day after the episiotomy opened she asked why this had happened and when the episiotomy could be closed.

DISCUSSION

Management of episiotomy breakdown centers around a choice between early repair and delayed repair. It should, however, include analysis of how this situation might have been prevented. A prolonged gestation, oxytocin augmentation, instrumental delivery, and prolonged second stage of labor are all factors that predispose to fourth-degree laceration. Consideration might have been given to performing a mediolateral episiotomy, which would have dramatically decreased the likelihood of an extension into the rectum from occurring. The idea that rectal extension is inevitable is not supported by data, and performance of mediolateral episiotomy is associated with fewer extensions into the rectum than midline episiotomy. Not only is rupture of the perineum associated with occasional breakdown, as evidenced by the present case, but it also causes damage to continence even when the incision heals uneventfully (3). In addition, prolonged second stage of labor, in an attempt to avoid episiotomy, may increase the neurologic injury that is associated with prolonged second stages of labor (1).

Repair of a fourth-degree laceration at the time of delivery should receive the same care that repair of a chronic fourth-degree laceration does. Good lighting, proper exposure, adequate assistance, and an individual sufficiently experienced to repair these lesions are essential. Cleansing the fecal material from the field and using atraumatic technique are important. The rectal submucosa, internal anal sphincter, external anal sphincter, and perineal body must all be carefully identified and repaired.

In the event that a properly repaired fourth-degree laceration comes apart, it is *possible* to repair it at any time. The *best* time for repair has not been universally agreed upon. The likelihood that the repair will heal without another disruption, however, depends on several factors. The cause of the initial breakdown, the state of the tissues, any associated diseases, and the clinical condition of the patient will all influence the choice and timing of repair. If the repair came apart because it was repaired improperly so that the sutures were insecurely anchored in the tissue or the knots insecurely tied, immediate repair makes sense. Once any necrotic tissue has been removed and the possibility of infection cleared, primary suturing is acceptable.

Early Repair

An episiotomy that has been infected should not be repaired until the tissues are no longer septic and all necrotic tissue has been removed. Once disruption has occurred, patients understandably wish to have the situation corrected quickly, and the physician whose repair has failed has a similar desire for an expeditious resolution to an unhappy situation. Early repair is possible, and when carefully performed has an acceptable failure rate, but it is critical to examine what measures were required prior to repair to prevent infection and breakdown (5,6). Before one attempts to suture the laceration, uncompromising preoperative preparation is needed, often requiring several days of inpatient care prior to reapproximation. Thrice daily physician debridement and intravenous antibiotics are often necessary. Repairing an infected episiotomy immediately without this type of rigorous preparation will result in recurrence of the defect and further damage to the tissues. Therefore, this type of early repair should not be performed casually with inadequate tissue preparation.

Many surgeons with extensive experience in this area prefer to wait until the laceration has had a chance to clean itself, and for the edema and friability of the tissue to resolve. With a mildly constipating diet, antidiarrheal medications when needed, daily sitz baths, and normal function of the levator ani muscles, continence is surprisingly good, and this allows a woman to be at home with her family and newborn infant while the body resolves the infection and sloughs the necrotic tissue. In most situations, there are surprisingly few problems with continence when awaiting repair, since the intact puborectalis maintains closure to solid stool even without the external sphincter. There are tremendous pressures to repair these lacerations early, but this should not be done unless the tissues are remarkably clean and demonstrably free of infection. It is not a decision between early repair and delayed repair of an infected episiotomy, but between daily debridement and intravenous antibiotics followed by repair, and recovery at home followed by repair.

Other Considerations

In addition to considering possible infection as an etiologic agent in the breakdown of episiotomy, other factors should be excluded as well. Inflammatory bowel disease, extensive condylomas, severe insulin-dependent diabetes mellitus, and malnutrition may play a role in impaired healing. When these conditions have resulted in wound breakdown, they should be corrected or controlled to the extent possible before attempting another repair. In these instances a labial fat pad graft (4) placed at the site of the closure may help to improve the blood supply in the area and increase the likelihood that healing will occur without breakdown.

Preoperative Preparation

Authors vary in their opinions concerning the technical details of preoperative preparation for repair of a disrupted episiotomy, but they agree on the basic principles. Healthy tissues, an empty bowel, preoperative antibiotic therapy, and anatomic repair are all critically important. Two to 3 days of clear liquid diet with two bisacodyl (Dulcolax) tablets given the morning before surgery and two Fleet enemas on the evening before the operation clear the colon unless long-standing constipation has been present. In the latter event, cathartics and enemas should be started 2 days before surgery. Alternatively, 4 liters of chilled GoLYTELY may be ingested the day prior to the operation. In any event, the author has found that cathartics given the evening before the operation or enemas on the morning of the surgery may result in continuous drainage during the operation with increased possibility of infection.

Surgical Repair

Understanding the anatomy of the anal continence mechanism is a key to understanding repair of chronic fourth-degree laceration. Restoration of both the internal and external anal sphincters must be accomplished. These sphincters occur over a length of about 4 cm (2) and are more than the single band of striated muscle often depicted in surgical illustrations. Digital examination of the healthy nullipara reveals a long sphincter zone, and restoration of this length of sphincter should be the goal of a repair.

Repair begins with identification of the anatomic defect. The scar is examined to identify the available tissues. Most commonly, the vaginal mucosa heals directly to the rectal mucosa so that the sphincter and perineal body are separated. The end of the muscle should be identified by watching for the retraction of the dimple in the perineal skin when the sphincter contracts. In addition, the bulk of the muscle may be palpated with a finger in the rectum and thumb on the perineum. If the muscle does not contract, concomitant nerve injury should be suspended. The results of repair in these instances are less than perfect because the restored sphincter still does not have its normal contractility (8). Nevertheless, reapproximation is appropriate because it allows whatever sphincter is still functional to contribute to continence. After the incision has healed, pelvic muscle strengthening either with or without biofeedback can help the remaining muscle hypertrophy to try to compensate for the lost muscle.

The goal of the operation is to restore the vaginal and rectal tubes to their individual positions and to bring the separated sphincters and connective tissue of the perineal body together in the midline between these two viscera. Repair is accomplished by separating the vaginal wall from the rectum along the line of scarring. If considerable scarring is present from infection and granulation, this may be excised. Careful closure of the submucosa of the rectum begins the repair. The author prefers a running suture begun above the apex of the defect because this lessens tissue strangulation and eliminates the bulk of suture knots in the area of healing. Next, the internal anal sphincter (often thought of as a fascial layer) is similarly approximated followed by 4 to 6 interrupted sutures approximating the external anal sphincter. The perineal body is then reconstructed and the vaginal mucosa and perineal skin closed.

In instances where infection has been present, some of the muscle may have become necrotic and been lost, either because of necrosis and liquefaction, or because of necessary removal during debridement. This is especially true when there was a ragged, irregular tear associated with the laceration. In these instances, the length of the remaining muscle and the tension on the muscle that would result from reapproximation must be assessed. If unusual tension exists on the suture line after the sphincter has been brought together, a relaxing or "paradoxical" incision, as described by Miller (7), would be made. This is accomplished by a single stab incision at the 5 o'clock position with subsequent suturing of the skin defect. Since the sphincter muscle is constantly contracting, the suture line is under constant tension in normal repairs. When tension caused by a tight sphincter is added, this can cause separation of the suture line during the healing process. The paradoxical incision seems to "paralyze" the muscle temporarily by interrupting its continuity during the initial healing process and allows the suture line to heal. Probably, because the connective tissue surrounding the sphincter in the area of the relaxing incision remains intact, the ends of the severed muscle are gradually bridged by firm scar tissue. This second injury to the sphincter does not defeat the success of the repair, and results with the incision are actually better than without.

With care and attention to detail, the results of these repairs should be excellent.

REFERENCES

1. Allen RE, Hosker GL, Smith ARB, Warrell DW: Pelvic floor damage and childbirth: A neurophysiological study. *Br J Obstet Gynaecol* 97:770–779, 1990.
2. Aronson MP, Lee RA, Berquist TH: Anatomy of anal sphincters and related structures in continent women studied with magnetic resonance imaging. *Obstet Gynecol* 76:846–851, 1990.
3. Crawford LA, Quint EH, Pearl ML, DeLancey JOL: Incontinence following rupture of the anal sphincter during delivery. *Obstet Gynecol* 82:527–531, 1993.
4. Elkins TE, DeLancey JOL, McGuire EJ: The use of modified Martius graft as an adjunctive technique in vesicovaginal and rectovaginal fistula repair. *Obstet Gynecol* 75:727, 1990.
5. Hankins GDV, Hauth JVC, Gilstrap LC, et al: Early repair of episiotomy dehiscence. *Obstet Gynecol* 75:48, 1990.
6. Hauth JC, Gilstrap LC, Ward SC, Hankins GDV: Early repair of an external sphincter ani muscle and rectal mucosal dehiscence. *Obstet Gynecol* 67:806, 1986.
7. Miller NF, Brown W: The surgical treatment of complete perineal tears in the female. *Am J Obstet Gynecol* 34:196, 1937.
8. Snooks SJ, Henry MM, Swash M: Faecal incontinence due to external sphincter division in childbirth is associated with damage to the innervation of the pelvic floor musculature: A double pathology. *Br J Obstet Gynaecol* 92:824–828, 1985.

Postpartum Rectovaginal Fistula — When to Repair? Future Delivery — Vaginal or Cesarean?

Bruce H. Drukker

Case Abstract

A 24-year-old primigravida was delivered by spontaneous vaginal delivery of a 3280-gram female infant following labor of 16 hours duration. At the time of delivery, which was complicated by shoulder dystocia, the patient sustained a fourth-degree laceration of the perineum, which was repaired at the time of delivery. By the third postpartum day, the patient began passing small amounts of fecal material and flatus through the vagina. Pelvic and vaginal examination showed a 2-cm laceration of the anterior rectal wall communicating with a defect in the lower posterior wall of the vagina. The perineum and perineal body appeared to be intact. The patient requested immediate correction of the condition.

DISCUSSION

Development of signs such as passing flatus or stool per vagina during the immediate or late postpartum period is a disturbing and unpleasant surprise for the patient and her physician. Postpartum rectovaginal fistulas are not a common problem, and most are preventable. Most commonly, these fistulas occur following unsuspected fourth-degree perineal lacerations following vaginal or forceps delivery. The next most frequent cause is a median episiotomy with or without fourth-degree extension. This type of extension has been reported to occur between 3% and 11% of the time during median episiotomy (10). Brantley and Burwell, as well as Legino et al., note rectovaginal fistula in less than 1% and 1.5%, respectively, in patients who have had fourth-degree tears at the time of delivery (1,6). Goldaber et al. note shoulder dystocia associated with 17% of women with perineal wound dehiscence following fourth-degree laceration, compared with only 4% of women without dehiscence (3). The changing trend toward noninterventional obstetrics favors spontaneous vaginal delivery, infrequent episiotomy, and alternative delivery positions. These changes may lead to an increase in rectovaginal fistula. This increase also may be related to attempted repair of perineal lacerations or episiotomies in positions permitting less than adequate exposure and visualization. Every effort must be made to avoid repair of an episiotomy or spontaneous perineal laceration in a compromised situation without proper lighting, instruments, position, and assistance when needed.

The clinical situation presented of an early postpartum rectovaginal fistula can be classified as type III rectovaginal fistula (8). This occurrence can be attributed to delivery through an introitus and perineum not sufficiently "stretchable" to permit passage of the head and shoulders without damage. How could this be prevented? Judgment of perineal and introital capacity is the discerning factor. If following perineal distention there is not adequate "give" of the tissue, a precise midline episiotomy is preferable to the situation which developed in the patient described in this chapter, that is, a spontaneous perineal tear. When making the episiotomy, one must recall the position of the anterior rectal wall, which can be tightly applied to the perineum. The instrument for episiotomy incision, either scissors or scalpel, must be carefully placed. The author prefers a sharp scalpel blade with a wooden tongue depressor placed against the posterior vaginal wall, distending the perineal body and protecting the fetal scalp. An episiotomy, although common, should be regarded with caution.

Repair of spontaneous laceration or episiotomy must be done with the patient in a location and position that provide adequate exposure and light to permit careful inspection and surgical repair. Often a birthing bed or birthing chair does not permit appropriate exposure. Small, separate, or contiguous anterior rectal wall openings can often be visualized during repair by inserting a gloved index finger into the rectum, separating the perineal tissue, vulva, and posterior vaginal wall, and exploring for an opening. If a separate opening is found, the rectum should be incised distal to the opening and a surgical fourth-degree episiotomy completed. Following complete delineation and opening of the rectum to the point of the aperture, closure should begin, inverting the edges with no. 3-0 polygalactin interrupted suture using a fine-taper needle. Sutures should be placed at 0.5-cm intervals, inverting the rectal mucosal edge. A second inverting layer of similar suture is advisable, placed through the perirectal fascia. Thereafter, the episiotomy or laceration can be repaired in a routine fashion with no. 2-0 interrupted polyglycolic acid sutures through the fascial covering of the sphincter muscle. These basic steps should significantly reduce the potential for fistula.

When a fistula appears within 24 hours after delivery, assessment for closure is necessary. Although tradition mitigates against primary closure proximate to the diagnosis of the fistula, this narrow time frame coupled with precise surgical technique offers an opportunity for successful closure with sufficient success to permit attempting the procedure (4,5,7). It must be done quickly, however, to remain within the time frame. If closure is attempted at this time, the patient must have a rapid bowel preparation with an oral purgative such as polyethylene glycol and electrolyte oral solution and mechanical cleansing of the lower colon as necessary. At the time of transvaginal surgery, immaculate perineal and vaginal cleansing with povidone iodine solution is mandatory. A minimally moistened, tightly rolled laparotomy pad can be placed in the recently distended vagina against the cervix to prevent uterine contamination during vaginal preparation. The packing can remain in place during the surgical procedure if it does not compromise exposure. The pad should be removed, of course, immediately following surgery.

The basic principles of surgery to effect closure at this time include development of healthy vascular, nonnecrotic tissue planes, absence of contamination, and absence of tissue tension. Since bacterial contamination is a major deterrent to success, a prophylactic intravenous antibiotic such as an ampicillin/sublactum drug should be started prior to any repair to ensure satisfactory peak serum levels at the time of operation. Because of the potential for contamination despite adequate preparation and initial antibiotic prophylaxis, an appropriate intravenous short-term antibiotic regimen should follow the initial operative dosing. At surgery, the recently repaired episiotomy or primary perineal and vaginal laceration incisions should be opened, all remaining sutures removed, necrotic tissue resected, and edges freshened to obtain healthy tissue. The rectal sphincter should be opened at the sight of previous repair and the rectum opened as well, slightly above the area of the fistula. The fistula tract then should be removed and the entire area copiously irrigated with saline to ensure significant reduction in bacterial tissue contamination. These maneuvers essentially convert the perineum, vagina, and fistula into a new fourth-degree laceration with good vascularity and healthy tissue. Repair should begin using a no. 3–0 polygalactin-type suture on the rectal wall, inverting the freshened mucosal edge. Sutures should be interrupted and placed at 0.5-cm intervals. The perirectal fascia should be closed in a similar fashion after the mucosa has been completely closed from the apex of the fistula to the anal opening. The rectal sphincter should be approximated by placing interrupted polygalactin no. 2–0 suture through the muscular fascia, thus bringing into apposition the fresh edges of the sphincter muscle located within the fascial ring. Often five or six sutures are necessary, with care taken to place these sutures in both cephalad and caudad positions of the fascial ring. One must not rely on one or two sutures to maintain the fascial integrity. No sutures are required in the muscle per se. The remaining portion of the perineal defect can be repaired as in an episiotomy, using absorbable suture and closing the perineum with a subcuticular no. 3–0 polygalatic acid suture. A very small, closed, low-pressure suction drain placed just below the vaginal wall can be used but is rarely necessary. If it is used, it should be left in place for only 24 hours. Postoperatively, a low-residue, high-fiber, nonconstipating diet with a stool softener (9) should be used for 14 days. Sphincterotomy by scalpel at the 5 to 6 o'clock position can be considered if the rectal mucosal defect is of significant length— that is, greater than 4 cm—or if there is any suggestion that there will be increased pressure on the anterior rectal wall due to a tight sphincter. This type of sphincterotomy heals spontaneously without fecal incontinence. If a fistula redevelops following this closure, another repair should be delayed until all infection and induration have subsided and complete scarification has occurred. Delay of 8 to 12 weeks is usual. Prior to surgery, colon cleansing, as previously described, is necessary. Surgical repair can take a number of approaches. Isolation loop colostomy is not routinely necessary for closure at this time.

If the fistula is located proximate to the introitus and external to the hymenal tags, it can be repaired by recreating a fourth-degree midline episiotomy, excising the fistula tract, reapproximating the rectal mucosa, and repairing the sphincter as previously described. The remaining closure is similar to an episiotomy. For a fistula located higher in the vagina, the so-called type III, a transvaginal approach without creation of an episiotomy is appropriate. In this situation, a circumferential incision through the vaginal mucosa around the fistula opening is dissected and the fistula tract identified, including its attachment to the rectum. With meticulous care, the entire fistula tract is removed, thus creating an opening to the anterior rectal wall somewhat larger than the fistula tract. Meticulous closure of the rectal wall is necessary using interrupted no. 3–0 polyglycolic acid sutures on a small-taper needle. Suture placement should be 0.5 cm apart, or closure can be effected by a purse-string suture that does not crimp the anterior rectal wall too tightly. The perirectal fascia is closed in a linear fashion, and the vaginal mucosa can be closed with interrupted no. 2–0 polyglycolic acid sutures. If additional reinforcement of the repair is necessary, a bulbocavernosus fat pad flap can be created from either labium and sutured over the perirectal fascia closure. A transperineal repair has also been described which may give more mobilization of tissue proximate to the fistula, improve visualization of the rectal orifice of the fistula, and decrease the occasional tendency for vaginal constriction. This approach should be considered seriously if a very large fistula is present (11). Repair of fistulas close to the introitus will, in some situations, result in a thin perineal body. In these situations, initial development of cruciate incisions across the perineal body with advancement of skin flaps following levator plication and sphincter apposition will recreate normal distance between the anus and introitus (2). It is important to restore as much muscular integrity of the perineum as possible if the area is shortened or defective.

Unfortunately, rectovaginal fistula repair will fail on rare occasion, despite meticulous preparation and careful technique. Should a fistula repair fail following a second attempt, isolation loop colostomy should be considered before embarking on a third repair. The colostomy should be fashioned to prevent seepage of colonic contents from one stoma to another, which can occur with proximate stoma locations often created by loop colostomies. If colonic contamination is prevented, spontaneous fistula closure will, in some situations, occur following diversion. If spontaneous closure does not occur, surgical correction in a clean field will yield excellent results following basic surgical principles for fistula repair. After the fistula has healed completely and there has been documented evidence of integrity of the anterior rectal wall and posterior vaginal wall, colon reanastomosis can be accomplished at a convenient time, usually 3 to 4 months later.

Should a patient become pregnant following repair of a rectovaginal fistula, the characteristics of the vagina during pregnancy, with its increased vascularity and mobility of the tissue, do not preclude vaginal delivery. The patient should be made aware of the potential of possible fistula recurrence, particularly if a subsequent fourth-degree laceration occurs, and be given the opportunity to opt for cesarean section. However, since the chance of recurrence is very minimal, vaginal delivery should be considered the prime mode for parturition in these situations.

REFERENCES

1. Brantley JT, Burwell JC: A study of fourth degree perineal lacerations and their sequelae. *Am J Obstet Gynecol* 80:711–714, 1960.
2. Corman ML: Anal incontinence following obstetrical injury. *Dis Colon Rectum* 28:86, 1985.
3. Goldaber KG, Wendel PJ, McIntire DD, Wendel GD: Postpartum perineal morbidity after fourth-degree perineal repair. *Am J Obstet Gynecol* 168:489–493, 1993.
4. Hankins GD, Hauth JC, Gilstrap LC, Hammond TL, Yeomans ER, Snyder RR: Early repair of episiotomy dehiscence. *Obstet Gynecol* 75:48–51, 1990.
5. Hauth JC, Gilstrap LC, Ward SC, Hankins GD: Early repair of an external sphincter ani muscle and rectal mucosal dehiscence. *Obstet Gynecol* 67:806–809, 1986.
6. Legino LJ, Woods MP, Rayburn WF, McGoogan LS: Third-and-fourth-degree perineal tears: 50 years' experience at a university hospital. *J Reprod Med* 33:423–426, 1988.
7. Owen J, Hauth JC: Episiotomy infection and dehiscence. In: Gilstrap LC, Faro S (eds): *Infections in Pregnancy*. New York, Alan R. Liss, 1990, pp. 61–74.
8. Rosenshein NB, Genadry RR, Woodruff JD: An anatomic classification of rectovaginal septal defects. *Am J Obstet Gynecol* 137:439, 1980.
9. Rothenberger DA, Goldberg SM: The management of rectovaginal fistulae. *Surg Clin North Am* 63:61, 1983.
10. Shieh CJ, Gennaro AR: Rectovaginal fistula: A review of 11 years experience. *Int Surg* 69:69, 1984.
11. Thompson JD, Masterson BJ: Transperineal repair of rectovaginal fistula. *Ob/Gyn Illustrated*, The UpJohn Company, 1985.

Section XI

Medical, Endocrine, and Miscellaneous Problems

92

The HIV-Positive Patient's Right of Confidentiality in Surgery

Thomas E. Elkins
Douglas Brown

Case Abstract

A 30-year-old hospital employee was admitted with acute pelvic inflammatory disease and a large tubo-ovarian abscess. Despite 72 hours of intensive antibiotic therapy, her condition worsened. As preparation for surgery was being made, the patient explained to her physician that she was tested as HIV-positive several months before at the local public health clinic (where testing is anonymous). She requested that this fact be kept a secret, especially from others on the hospital staff. The physician was concerned about the risks of exposure to others on the operating team and asked the patient to let her tell them. She adamantly refused to do so.

DISCUSSION

In some hospitals today, including the one in which this case occurred, this situation represents an ethical dilemma for physicians. The principles involved are important ones to examine: patient confidentiality and privacy versus protection of uninformed third parties. This conflict has most often involved sexual partner notification. However, many of the same concerns are noted in cases such as this one.

Commitment to a patient's privacy and confidentiality is an essential feature of a doctor-patient relationship. As worded in the Hippocratic Oath: "What I may see or hear in the course of treatment . . . I will keep to myself, holding such things shameful to be spoken about" (3). Modern codes of ethics, such as the International Code of Medical Ethics in 1949, have spoken of confidentiality as an absolute (7). More recently, the American Medical Association, the American Psychiatric Association, the American College of Physicians, the Infectious Diseases Society of America (11), and the American College of Obstetricians and Gynecologists (1) have all specifically reaffirmed the need for confidentiality for HIV patients.

The primary reasons for maintaining confidentiality without exceptions are at least two. (1) The potential harm a breach of confidentiality can bring upon a HIV-positive patient is well known. Discrimination, isolation, labeling, anger, and even abuse have occurred to those whose HIV status has become known (2). As stated by the Centers for Disease Control, the voluntary testing, screening, and participation of HIV-positive patients are essential for gaining control of this epidemic. Cooperation from those who are HIV-positive is certainly increased if patient anonymity can be preserved (5).

Some do not see patient confidentiality as beyond exception. Instead, they view specific confidentiality as one of several competing ethical principles the physician should bring into cases (4,8). For many years, appealing to concern for public health, the state has demanded reporting and contact notification for such diseases as tuberculosis, cholera, and certain venereal diseases. However, from the onset of HIV recognition, there has been an "HIV exceptionalism" in this regard (13). Reasons for this approach include the severe discrimination against HIV-positive persons, the stigmatization of those in the homosexual and/or drug abuse communities, and the strong advocacy of gay and lesbian groups (2). In fact, as the HIV epidemic has spread, this "exceptionalism" has waned. Twenty-six states have now enacted laws mandating named reporting of HIV-positive patients. This has led to a much larger identification of other HIV-positive persons, and earlier treatment programs for all those identified (6).

Court cases are often cited to justify giving greater weight to public safety concerns than to individual autonomy and privacy. One such case is the Tarasoff case in which a psychiatrist was told of an intended murder and failed to notify the victim (12). The court stated that "the protective privilege ends where the public peril begins" (12). More recently a Louisiana man was imprisoned for continuing to have sexual intercourse knowing he was HIV-positive, without telling his partner or using safer sex methods (the partner became HIV-positive as a result) (9).

However, these situations hold little resemblance to the case under discussion. In the issue of contact notification, the risk of harm is direct and sufficiently possible. Efforts to control a growing epidemic depend on notification. In the case presented, appropriate surgical technique, including strict attention to universal precautions, sufficiently prevents exposure to patients' bodily fluids. If a direct needle stick occurs from an HIV-positive patient, the risk remains small. The Center for Disease Control has reported that 1963 persons have had 2008 needle sticks from HIV-positive patients, and only 6 seroconversions have occurred (an infection rate of 0.31%) (9). In the 1990s, any surgical procedure should invoke universal precautions. This is especially true for cases resulting from severe pelvic inflammatory disease, for reasons even beyond that of HIV fears. Nine years into the HIV epidemic, only 27 health care workers had become infected. From September 1986, until August 1987, between 167 and 202 health care workers died from hepatitis B (also a sexually transmitted disease), whereas none died from AIDS (10). In the case presented for this discussion, therefore, notifying the operating room team about this particular patient's HIV status is unnecessary, although reminders about universal precautions should be constant in such a setting. In 1994, breaching the patient's confidence and trust in order to remind professionals to do their job well seems unwarranted and even harmful.

What will it be like in the year 2000? Those in our urban inner cities where HIV rates are already high can begin to tell us. Patients with any form of sexually transmitted disease presentation will likely be under universal HIV testing with mandatory partner or contact notification. Universal precautions will be constant concerns for those accustomed to performing surgery, since any patient can be HIV-positive. Negative attitudes toward persons who are HIV-positive will be replaced by compassion as the epidemic moves closer to us all. The discussion in this case will probably be far from anyone's mind.

REFERENCES

1. ACOG Ethics Committee. Patients who are HIV-positive and physician responsibilities. No. 130. American College of Obstetricians and Gynecologists. Washington, DC.
2. Bayer R: Sounding board: Public health policy and the AIDS epidemic. *NEJM* 324:1500–1503, 1991.
3. Beauchamp TL, Childress JF: *Principles of Biomedical Ethics*. New York, Oxford University Press, 1983.
4. Bok S: The limits of confidentiality. *Hasting Center Report* 13:24–31, 1983.
5. Centers for Disease Control. Additional recommendations to reduce sexual and drug-related transmission of [HIV]. *Morbidity and Mortality Weekly Report* 35:152–155, 1986.
6. Centers for Disease Control. Public health uses HIV-infection reports—South Carolina 1986–1991. *Morbidity and Mortality Weekly Report* 41:245, 1992.
7. Code of Ethics, 1949 World Medical Association, in *Encyclopedia of Bioethics*. New York, The Free Press, 1978.
8. Emson HE: Confidentiality: A modified value. *J Med Ethics* 14:87–90, 1988.
9. Gerbering JL, Henderson DK: Management of occupational exposures to blood borne pathogens: Hepatitis B virus, hepatitis C virus, and human immunodeficiency virus. *Clin Infect Dis* 14:1179–1185, 1992.
10. Protection against viral hepatitis: Recommended actions of the Immunization Practiced Advisory Committee. *Morbidity and Mortality Weekly Report* 39(PR-2):1–26, 1990.
11. Smith ML, Martin KP: Confidentiality in the age of AIDS: A case study in clinical ethics. *J Clin Ethics* 236–241, 1993.
12. Tarasoff v. Regents of the University of California, 17 Cal. 3d 425, 551, p. 2d 334 (1976).
13. Wachter RM: Sounding board: AIDS activism and the politics of health. *NEJM* 326:128–129, 1992.

Procidentia in an Elderly Multipara

J. George Moore

Case Abstract

A chronically hypertensive 88-year-old multipara, no longer able to wear a supportive pessary, developed a total procidentia. The patient was moderately hypertensive, 190/110, though she had been taking hydrochlorothiazide and methyldopa daily for a number of years. She lived alone, managing her own affairs, and seemed alert and in otherwise good health.

DISCUSSION

It is generally agreed that age alone is not a contraindication to indicated surgical procedure. Medical complications certainly influence the choice of procedures that will correct the clinical problem. In this instance, one must ensure that blood electrolytes are in proper balance and that maximal cardiovascular stability has been attained.

In a patient on hydrochlorothiazide and methyldopa, plasma potassium must be maintained between 3.5 and 4.5 mg/dl. Electrocardiography should ensure that cardiac irregularities are minimized, and a lidocaine intravenous infusion should be used to maintain stability of cardiac rhythm postoperatively. Hypertension must also be controlled postoperatively, especially during periods of pain. An arterial line should be placed intraoperatively and maintained postoperatively. If hypertension exceeds 200 mmHg systolic or 125 mmHg diastolic, vasodepressive medication should be employed, using hydralazine or even nitroprusside if necessary.

The surgical procedure chosen to correct the procidentia depends on the condition of the patient. Ideally a vaginal hysterectomy, correction of the enterocele, and a complete colpectomy (total colpocleisis) is the procedure of choice for a complete procidentia. Adding the colpectomy to the procedure generally secures a lasting correction of the prolapse. If the patient will not consent to vaginal obliteration and if a total colpectomy is not elected, a careful repair of the endopelvic supports to create a narrow, deep vagina with a well-supported, high perineum is indicated to preclude a subsequent prolapse of the vagina. If a functional vagina must be maintained, a sacrospinous colpopexy (with enterocele repair) is likely to give the best functional result. An abdominal hysterectomy or uterine suspension will *not* correct the procidentia.

In a debilitated patient, a LeFort procedure (1,2) (partial colpocleisis) under local anesthesia might be considered. This latter procedure can be done quickly with minimal blood loss, and it maintains reasonable uterine support with a very low recurrence rate. The partial colpocleisis does have drawbacks. Recurrence is likely if an enterocele is left unrepaired, and stress incontinence will ensue unless a urethral plication is done and unless the perineum is built up close to the urethra. In the LeFort procedure, the relatively strong posterior vaginal wall, when sutured to the anterior wall, has a tendency to pull the urethra down, resulting in incontinence with minimal increase in intra-abdominal pressure. Modification of the LeFort procedure to provide a functional vagina is generally not indicated because of poor satisfaction and the increased chance of recurrence. Another undesirable feature of the LeFort procedure is the difficulty in investigating subsequent uterine bleeding, in that a D&C is virtually impossible.

Total procidentia implies that the entire uterus (including the corpus) is outside the vagina. In most cases, the complete uterine prolapse is accompanied by a cystocele, rectocele, and enterocele, and correction of each of these defects is required. This entails correction of the enterocele (high ligation of the enterocele sac, preferably with nonabsorbable suture material and careful approximation of the uterosacral ligaments) along with an anterior and posterior colporrhaphy. If a vaginal hysterectomy is carried out (and it should be), a total colpectomy (complete colpocleisis) almost certainly precludes recurrence. Even with a complete colpocleisis, repair of the enterocele and reconstruction of the pelvic support are essential. If the enterocele is not corrected, a vaginal evisceration can occur in the late postoperative course.

REFERENCES

1. LeFort L: *Bull Gen de Therap* 92:337, 1877.
2. Spiegelberg O: Colporraphia mediana. *Berl Klin Woch* 9:249, 1872.

94

Surgical Patient with History of Previous Thrombophlebitis

Robert E. Rogers

Case Abstract

Vaginal hysterectomy with colporrhaphy was recommended for a 350-lb, 62-year-old, multiparous, normotensive patient with a progressive and symptomatic genital prolapse, including a second-degree prolapse of the uterus, a large cystocele, enterocele, rectocele, and perineal defect. The patient had been unable to retain a pessary. Following a cholecystectomy 12 years previously, the patient developed a pulmonary embolus on the fifth postoperative day, which was treated by 3 months of anticoagulant therapy. There was no history of previous phlebitis or of varicose veins.

DISCUSSION

The patient with an increased risk for thromboembolism is becoming a more common problem today because surgeons are operating on older patients, frequently with medical and surgical problems that would have been absolute contraindications for surgery in earlier years.

The incidence of thromboembolism is variable and depends on the age and medical condition of the patient and on the operative procedure performed. The incidence of thromboembolism in a large series of gynecologic patients is approximately 1 in 1000 operations. A number of factors contribute to this incidence: surgical or nonsurgical trauma, obesity, age over 40 years, varicose veins, previous thromboembolic disease, estrogen use, atherosclerotic cardiovascular disease, cardiac failure, and immobilization. It is important to realize that 95% of pulmonary emboli arise from thrombi in the deep venous system of the pelvis and lower extremities. The gynecologic surgeon must be alert to the fact that every patient is a possible candidate for thrombosis and thromboembolism.

The patient presented here has at least three of the risk factors mentioned above; therefore, she must be considered at high risk for a repeat thromboembolic event. The only risk factor under either the patient's or the physician's control is the patient's obesity. The possibility of the patient making any meaningful reduction in weight is doubtful. All patients with this risk factor should be counseled and helped to reduce obesity. The success in this area has been limited.

Two approaches to this problem must be considered, mechanical and medical. The mechanical approaches include ambulation, compression of superficial veins with fitted elastic hose, stimulation of the calf muscles to act as a blood pump, intermittent compression of the leg, and proper protection of the legs at the time of surgery.

Three mechanical approaches are recommended in the patient presented. The first of these is fitted elastic hose. In the morbidly obese patient an adequate fit of these garments is difficult and requires prior planning. Most often the garment is not available "off the shelf" and must be ordered. The hose should be available at the time that the patient is admitted to the hospital, and the patient should wear them at the point that her usual activity is limited, generally the day of admission.

A second mechanical factor is the placement of the patient in stirrups. The greatest care must be given to avoiding point compression of the lower extremities in stirrups. For this reason the orthopedic stirrup or the "hanging stirrup" should be chosen. The leg should be arranged in the stirrup so as not to compress any portion of the extremity. The antiembolism hose must be in place, elevated on the thigh and unwrinkled throughout the procedure.

The third mechanical consideration is early ambulation, within hours of surgery. The patient may start by simply standing at the bedside and breathing deeply. Early and frequent ambulation must be encouraged. Meticulous attention must be given to the elastic hose to make certain that they are properly pulled up on the thighs. Occasionally in the morbidly obese patient it may be necessary to tape the hose to the upper thigh.

Medical measures involve the alteration of the patient's blood coagulability. Several approaches are available: low- and full-dose heparin, low-dose heparin with dihydroergotamine, oral anticoagulation, intravenous Dextran, and preoperative aspirin therapy.

In the patient presented, one might consider operating using the mechanical methods and not altering coagulability. Most surgeons weighing the risk of altering coagulability against the risk of operating without anticoagulants will choose to alter the patient's clotting function.

Operating under full anticoagulation is possible, but in most surgical situations, particularly when the vaginal route is chosen, it is not recommended. The best solution would be limited alteration of clotting ability during the surgery and immediate postoperative period.

Dextran 70 or Dextran 40 has occasionally been used for prophylaxis. It is generally given in volumes of at least 500 ml over a 4- to 6-hour period starting at the time of the operation and then repeated daily for 2 to 5 days. Dextran may be associated with a slight increase in bleeding. In elderly patients it carries a danger of fluid overload.

Low-dose aspirin is said to reduce the incidence of thrombophlebitis and thromboembolism. There is no documentation of its usefulness in pelvic surgery.

Subcutaneous low-dose heparin given in a dose of 5000 units 2 hours preoperatively and then every 8 to 12 hours postoperatively has been shown to be an effective prophylaxis in many studies. When this agent is used, there is an increase in intraoperative and postoperative bleeding, and wound hematomas prove to be significantly increased.

A combination of heparin sodium, 5000 units, and dihydroergotamine mesylate, 0.5 mg, has become available for prevention of deep vein thrombosis. This combination appears to inhibit at least two of the factors which lead to phlebitis; hypercoagulability and stasis. Dihydroergotamine has been shown to exert a selective constrictive effect on the veins and venules and to some degree a constricted effect on the arterioles and arteries. Venous return appears to be accelerated and venous stasis prevented. The combination of heparin sodium and dihydroergotamine mesylate is available as Embolex® (Sandoz).

At the time of the planned vaginal hysterectomy and colporrhaphy the patient should be carefully positioned with particular attention to the support of the legs. The planned operation should be carried out in a routine fashion, but particular attention must be given to hemostasis. In this situation an electrocautery is useful to coagulate small vessels that one might ignore in the course of most vaginal operations. A vaginal pack is advisable after the operation is complete, even if the surgeon does not customarily use one. Pressure on small bleeding vessels will control bleeding and prevent vaginal hematomas. The surgeon must be aware that delayed bleeding and wound hematomas are most common, even with low-dose heparin.

SELECTED READINGS

Hirsch J, Genton E, Hull R: A practical approach to the prophylaxis of venous thrombosis. In: *Venous Thromboembolism*. New York, Grune & Stratton, 1981, pp. 108–121.

Mosier K: Pulmonary thromboembolism. In: *Harrison's Principles of Internal Medicine*. New York, McGraw-Hill, 1983, pp. 1561–1567.

95

Hysterectomy in Morbidly Obese Patients

Donald G. Gallup

Case Abstract

A 48-year-old parous woman was scheduled for a hysterectomy and removal of the ovaries because of a rapidly growing 16-week suspected leiomyomatous uterus. Pre- and postprogestin treatment endometrial biopsies showed adenomatous hyperplasia. In addition to having an enlarged uterus, the patient was 62 inches tall and weighed 250 pounds. Minidose heparin was initiated preoperatively. After the large redundant panniculus was grasped with towel clips, it was pulled cephalad with tape and removed from the operating field by the attachment of light weights. A Pfannenstiel incision was made in the subpannicular fold to create the "shortest distance" to the female pelvic organs. Despite limited exposure, the scheduled procedure was performed with minimal blood loss (320 ml) and the histopathology eventually revealed only mild adenomatous hyperplasia. The patient was on postoperative antibiotics for 3 doses every 6 hours, and on I.M. Demerol and Phenergan for pain.

About 18 hours postoperatively, the patient was noted to be unresponsive. Arterial blood gases revealed a PO_2 of 50 and a PCO_2 of 49. She was transferred to the intensive care unit and intubated. After 4 days she was extubated and returned to the surgical floor. On the fifth postoperative day, the patient's temperature registered 39°C. The wound examination revealed weeping of purulent material, and it was opened to the level of the intact fascia. The patient spent an additional 4 days in the hospital undergoing wound care. She was discharged to home health care, and the wound eventually healed by secondary intention as was noted 5 weeks postoperatively.

DISCUSSION

This complicated case might have had a more favorable outcome with careful attention to preoperative management, incision choice, and postoperative care. Because of their physical size, obese patients have unique perioperative problems. Most complications are related to ventilation disorders, circulation problems, thromboembolic phenomena, and wound dehiscence. Additionally, these patients are difficult to operate on from a purely technical standpoint. The obese patient is defined by the Metropolitan Insurance Company tables as weighing 30% more than desirable body weight. Morbid obesity is defined as exceeding desirable weight by either 100% or 100 kg.

427

Preoperative Evaluation of Associated Medical Problems and Postoperative Care

One-third of moderately to severely obese patients have impaired pulmonary function. The spectrum ranges from the patient who has minimal problems perioperatively to the patient with sleep apnea syndrome. All obese patients have ventilatory and perfusion abnormalities. Ventilation/perfusion mismatch may be tolerated well by the patient less than 50 years of age, but may overwhelm an older patient.

Because chest wall (muscular) movement is compromised by weight, the work of breathing and subsequent oxygen consumption are higher in the obese patient. Cardiac perfusion is reduced because of increased preload (the pressures found in the pulmonary vasculature which have to be overcome for blood flow through the pulmonary tree) and afterload (systemic blood pressure), which further compromises oxygen delivery and saturation. Hypoxia is common in these patients, and combined with respiratory depression from anesthesia and analgesics, may render the elderly obese patient obtund. Blood gases and pulmonary function tests (PFTs) should be considered. Preoperative instruction in incentive spirometry and early ambulation may minimize atelectasis. In the short-necked patient, a preoperative anesthesia consultation should be obtained. The use of patient control analgesia (PCA), which decreases respiratory depression by limiting the quantity of narcotic necessary, is beneficial. This presented patient might have been identified as high risk by more careful preoperative workup.

The sleep apnea syndrome should be identified preoperatively. Patients with this syndrome are usually severely obese. Clinically, they have large, floppy uvulas (resulting in snoring), morning headaches, and sleep disturbances. The patient who has sleep apnea will have a history of sleeping during the day and problems staying awake. These patients should be recognized preoperatively, because the use of narcotics may cause significant problems in the postoperative period, including hypoxia leading to a respiratory arrest and death. If a patient is suspected of having sleep apnea syndrome, she should be referred to a pulmonologist for a sleep study.

Because of the difficulties with ventilation, narcotics should be administered with caution in obese patients. PCA pumps are especially desirable for pain control in these patients. Intramuscular narcotics have varying peaks and troughs of drug levels temporally related to dosage interval. Because the pump allows for a more constant infusion, the peak drug level is decreased. In a 24-hour period, less narcotic is used, better pain management is achieved, and, most importantly, less respiratory depression occurs.

The relationship between obesity and thromboembolic phenomena is well recognized. Multiple studies have shown an increase in pulmonary embolism in obese versus nonobese patients. Surgical series have proven that heparin prophylaxis can decrease the incidence of thromboembolic phenomena to levels found in normal individuals. Two prophylactic methodologies are available to prevent deep venous thrombophlebitis (DVT). The most commonly used is 5000 to 7500 units of heparin given subcutaneously every 12 hours. A dose response curve exists, and if a patient weighs more than 100 kg, a higher dose is probably indicated.

The use of pneumatic stockings is becoming more popular as a means of preventing DVT. In the author's institution, if a surgery will take longer than 2 hours, these stockings are used in conjunction with heparin prophylaxis. After the induction of anesthesia, the stockings are not removed until 24 hours postoperatively, or until the patient can ambulate.

Incision Choice in the Obese Patient

In general, incisions for obese patients can be transverse or vertical. For *major* gynecologic procedures, the traditional transverse incision is inappropriate for most obese patients because of limited exposure. Wound complication rates in obese women undergoing abdominal hysterectomy have been reported in as many as 30% of the patients. Krebs and Helmkamp have reported a wound infection rate of 24% in massively obese patients when a periumbilical transverse incision is used (4). Because muscle cutting may be needed for this incision, entry time can be lengthy and the incisions relatively bloody. If *any* transverse incision is chosen for obese patients, it should be far removed from the anaerobic, moist environment of the subpannicular fold.

The author has used a technique to operate obese patients which has resulted in a wound complication rate of only 3%. This technique is outlined below.

A. Careful cleansing of the umbilicus and preoperative showers.
B. Clip preparation of abdominal hair.
C. Use of a midline incision after retracting the panniculus caudad, below the superior margins of the symphysis (Fig. 95.1).
D. Use of a wound protector to improve exposure in the pelvis. Special long-bladed fixed retractors help. A Bookwalter retractor is an option.
E. Closure of pelvic peritoneum is unnecessary after hysterectomy.

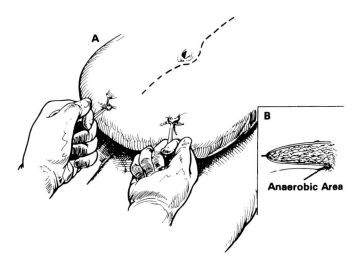

Figure 95.1.   Towel clips are used to retract the panniculus caudad. A midline incision can be extended cephalad to the umbilicus. The anaerobic area posterior to the subpannicular fold is avoided. (Reprinted with permission from Gallup DG: Opening and closing the abdomen. In: Phelan JP, Clark SL (eds): *Cesarean Delivery.* Elsevier Science Publishing [Chapman & Hall], 1988, p. 178.)

Figure 95.2. One no. 1 or no. 2 polypropylene suture is started from each end and tied in the middle. This mass closure technique incorporates all layers. A hemoclip is placed in the short end to prevent untying of the six throws of the knot. With Maxon, a clip is not used. (Reprinted with permission from Gallup DG: Opening and closing the abdomen. In: Phelan JP, Clark SL (eds): *Cesarean Delivery.* Elsevier Science Publishing [Chapman & Hall], 1988, p. 179.)

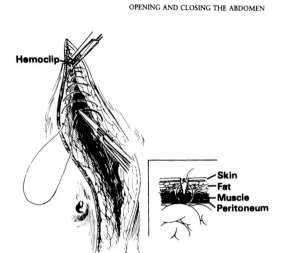

OPENING AND CLOSING THE ABDOMEN

Hemoclip

Skin
Fat
Muscle
Peritoneum

F. Fascial closure with either:
    1. Smead-Jones internal retention suture with polypropylene or polyglyconate.
    2. Running, mass closure with no. 2 polypropylene or no. 1 polyglyconate. (These bites should be closely spaced, about 1 to 1.5 cm apart and about 2 cm lateral to the cut edge of the fascia.) The running technique distributes tension equally over a continuous line. With polypropylene, a clip is placed on the short end of the knots to prevent unraveling (Fig. 95.2). With polyglyconate (Maxon) six throws are used for each knot, and the knots are buried.
G. Subcutaneous sutures should not be used, but a closed drainage system is placed anterior to the fascia and left in about 72 hours, depending upon drainage. (Although several studies [2,3,6] suggest a benefit from subcutaneous drains, randomized prospective trials have not been done). One retrospective study of massively obese patients suggests they are not helpful (7).
H. The skin is closed with staples, which are not removed for 2 weeks.

Other Options

Some investigators suggest a beneficial effect from prophylactic antibiotics, but these are not used in the author's institution. Panniculectomy at the time of hysterectomy has been advocated, but the small number of patients reported in the recent literature have a wound infection rate of 20% to 30%. If the panniculectomy is done first, exposure in the pelvis is improved. Increased blood loss and increased operating time are other disadvantages of these combined procedures.

Delayed closure of incisions is also advocated. In this technique, no. 3-0 nonfilament interrupted skin sutures are placed and loosely tied, but the wound is packed open with dressing sponges layered posterior to the suture. These are changed with sterile saline moistened dressings three times a day. Around postoperative day 5, if the wound appears clean, the sutures are simply tied and the incision reinforced with steri-strips.

Finally, the patient reported in this case could have been managed by secondary closure rather than by secondary intention healing. These closures can be done under local anesthesia (1). After an infected wound is opened, it is initially debrided under local anesthesia. Saline-soaked gauzes are changed as noted above, and most wounds are ready for closure in 4 to 5 days, when they appear beefy-red and are free of necrotic tissue. After local anesthesia, no. 1 polypropylene sutures, 3 to 4 cm from the skin edge, are used to approximate the wound and reinforced with steri-strips.

REFERENCES

1. Dodson MK, Magann EF, Meeks GR: A randomized comparison of secondary closure and secondary intention in patients with superficial wound dehiscence. *Obstet Gynecol* 80:321, 1992.
2. Gallup DG: Modification of celiotomy techniques to decrease morbidity in the obese gynecologic patient. *Am J Obstet Gynecol* 150:171, 1984.
3. Gallup DG, Nolan TE, Smith RP: Primary mass closure of midline incisions with a continuous polyglyconate monofilament absorbable suture. *Obstet Gynecol* 76:389, 1990.
4. Krebs HB, Helmkamp F: Transverse periumbilical incision in the massively obese patient. *Obstet Gynecol* 63:241, 1984.
5. Menendez MA: The contaminated closure. In: O'Leary JP, Woltering EA (eds): *Techniques for Surgeons.* New York, John Wiley, 1985, pp. 36–37.
6. Morrow CP, Hernandez WL, Townsend DE, et al: Pelvic celiotomy in obese patients. *Am J Obstet Gynecol* 127:335, 1977.
7. Scott HW, Law HD, Sandstead HH, et al: Jejunoileal shunt in surgical treatment of morbid obesity. *Ann Surg* 171:770, 1977.

96

Compartment Syndrome

David H. Nichols

Case Abstract

A patient's legs had been elevated for 3½ hours in candy cane stirrups placed beneath the calves. Within a few postoperative hours the patient complained of considerable pain in the right leg, and examination of the right calf demonstrated diffuse swelling. The right dorsalis pedis artery pulsations were readily apparent, however, and appeared comparable in intensity to those of the opposite leg.

DISCUSSION

Compartment Syndrome

Prolonged stirrup pressure beneath the calf of more than 3 hours duration, while leaving arterial circulation intact, may obstruct arteriolar flow within one or more fascial compartments of the leg. Ischemia promotes edema, and since tissue expansion is limited within a fascial compartment, compression of nerves as well as of circulation may compromise function. This condition, although rare, is called the compartment syndrome (1). It may be suspected by the combination of leg pain and visible swelling postoperatively, despite palpations of a normal dorsalis pedis pulse. The pain is accentuated by passive stretching of the muscles within the compartment and may progress rapidly to numbness, burning, and difficulty in moving the leg.

The compartment syndrome should be apparent to the astute observer in the recovery room following surgery, and prompt consultation should be obtained from a vascular or orthopedic surgeon. If muscle pressure measurements are elevated in a diagnosis established within the first 12 postoperative hours, emergency surgical fasciotomy should be performed to relieve excess pressure within the affected compartment and thus reverse the pathologic process (2).

If the diagnosis is made at a time beyond the first 12 postoperative hours, the affected tissues are probably in an early stage of necrosis. In this case the trauma of surgical decompression would introduce a significant risk of surgical infection to these already partly necrotic tissues and should not be performed. To aid circulation during the recovery phase, the patient's legs should be positioned at the level of her heart.

If permanent damage has not occurred, the prognosis for full recovery is good, although often slow and over a period of many weeks. Foot drop and decreased sensation over the feet herald progression of the disease process, with permanent nerve and muscular damage.

Prevention of the syndrome requires padding the stirrups supporting the legs and paying special attention to avoid passive dorsiflexion of the ankle. Passive repositioning of the legs during a long surgical procedure will provide some prophylaxis.

If Allen universal stirrups have been used, it is important to properly position the feet within the stirrups so that the heel of the foot will bear some measure of support.

REFERENCES

1. Adler LM et al: Bilateral compartment syndrome after a long gynecologic operation in the lithotomy position. *Am J Obstet Gynecol* 162:1271, 1990.
2. Whitesides TE et al: A simple method for tissue pressure determination. *Arch Surg* 110:1311, 1975.

Adnexal Abscess
After Vaginal Hysterectomy

David H. Nichols

Case Abstract

Vaginal hysterectomy without repair was performed shortly following menstruation upon a 42-year-old multipara with chronic menorrhagia. No "preventive" antibiotic was given because of a history of allergy to penicillin. A low-grade afternoon fever was noted on the third day, which responded within 48 hours to gentamicin and clindamycin therapy. Hospitalization was otherwise uneventful, and the patient was discharged the morning of the sixth postoperative day. Because of fever and left lower abdominal pain, the patient was readmitted on the eighth postoperative day, and a vaginal cuff abscess diagnosed, incised, and drained of 10 cc of purulent material which grew a culture of antibiotic-resistant Enterococci *and* Bacteroides fragilis. *The patient was discharged 2 days later and the Penrose drain removed from the vagina a week later. On day 20 after the original surgery, the patient was rehospitalized because of severe left-sided lower abdominal pain. An ill-defined, tender, 5-cm cystic left adnexal mass was palpated and its presence confirmed by sonography.*

DISCUSSION

Because the ovaries often are brought closer to the vaginal cuff with peritonealization following vaginal hysterectomy than with peritonealization following total abdominal hysterectomy, they are perhaps more vulnerable to postoperative infection in the premenopausal patient, particularly in the presence of a vaginal cuff infection (1). This might be related to their vulnerability around the time of ovulation, or to the presence of a culture medium within the ovary from a postovulatory corpus hemorrhagicum (Fig. 97.1). This patient must be considered to have an adnexal abscess or oophoritis until proven otherwise, as, for example, by laparoscopic examination. Although certain antibiotics (clindamycin, cefamandol, cefoxitin, and metronidazole) are believed to have superior qualities of abscess penetration, ovarian abscess may be resistant to such therapy. Because the ovary is higher within the pelvis than the tubes, it may be inaccessible to safe transvaginal postoperative drainage, and may require a transabdominal oophorectomy or salpingo-oophorectomy for resolution. This may be in contrast to the clinical resolution of salpingitis during conservative or nonsurgical treatment by rest and appropriate antibiotic administration. Posthysterectomy ovarian abscess, occasionally subsequent to ovulation, characteristically becomes clinically evident a week or two following

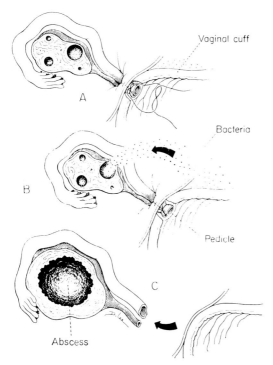

Vaginal cuff

Bacteria

Pedicle

Abscess

Figure 97.1. Possible mechanism for the development of an adnexal abscess after vaginal hysterectomy is shown diagrammatically. **A.** The close proximity of the adnexal structures to the vaginal cuff after vaginal hysterectomy is depicted. **B.** Postoperative ovulation exposes the stroma of the ovary to bacterial invasion from the infected vaginal cuff. **C.** Disintegration of suture holding the pedicle to the vaginal cuff permits retraction of adnexal abscess high into the pelvis. (Reproduced with permission from Ledger WJ et al: Adnexal abscess as late complication of pelvic operations. *Surg Gynecol Obstet* 129:973–978, 1969.)

the patient's discharge from an apparently uneventful posthysterectomy hospital course. The patient may call and describe an onset of fever with a severe noncramping, often unilateral, pelvic pain. If an adnexal abscess is identified, the presence or absence of hydronephrosis or retroperitoneal hematoma may be studied by sonography. If ovarian abscess cannot be excluded, a diagnostic laparoscopy should be performed. If the diagnosis is confirmed, the ovary and usually the tube should be excised by transabdominal laparotomy.

This problem is prevented by practicing meticulous hemostasis during surgery, by using an appropriate preoperative antibiotic or antibacterial, and possibly by burying the adnexal stump beneath the vaginal wall during the operative procedure, leaving a finger-tip-size opening in the posterior portion of the vaginal vault for drainage.

In the patient described, laparoscopy confirmed the diagnosis, and a transabdominal left salpingo-oophorectomy was performed. Recovery was uneventful.

REFERENCE

1. Ledger WJ, Campbell C, Taylor D, Willson JR: Adnexal abscess as late complication of pelvic operations. *Surg Gynecol Obstet* 129:973–978, 1969.

98

Psychiatric Consequences
of Gynecologic Surgery

Andrew E. Slaby

Case Abstract

Total abdominal hysterectomy with elective bilateral salpingo-oophorectomy was performed upon an unmarried 29-year-old schoolteacher to relieve discomfort associated with a large fibroid uterus. Surgery was uncomplicated and convalescence smooth. An incidental finding at surgery was superficial ovarian endometriosis.

Following discharge from hospital, the patient gradually became despondent and depressed over her lost reproductive capacity and progressively withdrawn and resentful. She was brought to the hospital emergency room some 6 months after surgery, unconscious following an alleged overdose of sleeping tablets.

DISCUSSION

Hysterectomy is second only to cesarean section as the most commonly performed surgical procedure in the United States. Until 1981, it was the most common (12). Reactions to hysterectomy vary, but are as diverse and multidetermined as those reported in the puerperium, which have long been recognized as a time of increased risk for psychiatric disorder (3,5,8). Although the intensity and character of response may differ, reactions are present to a greater or lesser degree in all cases. Response would be anticipated to be greatest among those who are younger and have not yet borne a child and most severe when hysterectomy occurs concomitantly with the loss of a child as a complication of pregnancy.

The most frequent responses to hysterectomy and loss of reproductive capacity in the premenopausal years are depression, anger, anxiety, and psychosomatic complaints (6,11,12). In fact, it has been reported that there is a greater than average prevalence of gynecologic problems in anxious women (12). Loss of the uterus, even by women with several children or by women who do not posit any immediate desire to have a child—such as nuns, individuals vowing never to marry and have children, and lesbians not desiring children or marriage to man—is difficult. Reactions to hysterectomy, as to elective sterilization (1,2,9,10,13), are dependent on age, marital status, religion, ethnic background, social class, previous psychiatric status, number of children borne, reason for surgery (e.g., cancer), social support, husband or partner's response, and plans for divorce or remarriage (unpredictable events in many cases). An exaggerated response is expected if a woman's self-esteem is predicated on successfully bearing children and heirs and on rearing them, as in some fundamentalistic religious groups. The true prevalence of regret after sterilization is reported to be 3.6% to 20% (13).

Both premenopausal and postmenopausal women perceive hysterectomy as mutilation of their bodies. The organ historically defining their roles as potential mothers and women has been removed. Prior to menopause, loss of the uterus surgically represents forfeiting the ability to have children. It is the end of an era, the end of the reproductive era. The younger the woman, the greater the possibility of such a reaction. If a hysterectomy takes place near the anticipated time of menopause, there may be a less dramatic response. The range of response in such instances would be expected to resemble that in menopause. Since capacity to bear a child no longer exists after menopause, the primary issue is loss of an organ that in part defines a woman's body as different from a man's. In addition, the fear exists that organs are removed unnecessarily or because of medical indications (e.g., cancer) not revealed to the patient. In the former instance, a woman may feel that she is one of many people she reads about in the popular press who have undergone unnecessary surgery. Patients have become medically sophisticated. Many feel that the decision to undergo surgery should be one of both surgeon and patient, with the patient educated as to the consequences both of having and not having surgery. When an alliance is formed between the woman and her surgeon allowing full informed participation by the patient in any decision, and this alliance is documented in the patient's chart, future litigation pursuant to unexpected complications is minimized. If a malignancy is suspected, what is the possibility that a clinical laboratory test such as a PAP smear of a biopsy may be in error? Frank discussions with patients and their significant others prior to an operation regarding the indications and contraindications of surgery, and the limitations of tests, and projected outcomes with and without surgery can serve to reduce anxiety prior to surgery and anger and depression afterward.

Depression is a normal response to the loss of the uterus, much as it is to menopause and loss of a breast by surgery or loss of testes from orchiectomy. Patients with a family or past personal history of affective illness are at higher risk to develop the signs and symptoms of a depression at such times (11). In one study of 102 women who underwent hysterectomy, the incidence of depression was higher before surgery than afterward (6). Risk factors for posthysterectomy depression included prior history of affective illness, lower socioeconomic status, and high preoperative scores on anxiety. Fears of cancer and of adverse sexual effects were the main sources of anxiety. Divorced women, regardless of surgery, are at eight times the risk for psychiatric problems requiring hospitalization (10). Divorce, in fact, is rated nearly as stressful as death of spouse on Rahe and Holmes's Life Events Scale. Psychologic consequences of gynecologic procedures are reduced when women learn more about their problems and are supported by their families and others with similar problems.

The first step in management of depression as a complication of hysterectomy is to anticipate it and discuss the possibility with the patient, spouse (or spouse equivalent), and family if she so desires. Women referred to gynecologists, when compared to controls, report more psychiatric problems (12), especially if divorced, separated, widowed, or complaining of pelvic pain (4). Included in the discussion should be a description of early symptoms of depression. In the case summarized at the beginning of this chapter, it was apparent that the patient was slipping into depression. She was portrayed as "despondent and depressed" and becoming more withdrawn and resentful. These symptoms and signs suggest to a clinician or family that expected depression has become greater than anticipated and that psychiatric consultation is necessary to commence treatment and to evaluate the risk of self-destructive behavior. The patient was a young single woman living alone. In such instances, follow-up visits must be scheduled so that a depression may be identified sufficiently early to prevent the morose mood from causing a patient to cancel appointments and slip unrecognized into a suicidal state. The rate of completed suicide among those with untreated major depression is 15% (11).

Prior to surgery, the full meaning of a hysterectomy and loss of reproductive capacity, if in the premenopausal years, should be discussed and the patient allowed to participate in the decision to pursue surgery, given the reality of the psychologic and medical consequences of having surgery. An alternate surgical approach to hysterectomy, such as myomectomy, may be elected. Loss of a uterus also ironically allows a greater equality with a man. A woman is no longer burdened with the vicissitudes of the menstrual cycle and has, without fear of the medical complications of birth control, the freedom to have sexual liaisons without fear of pregnancy. Some women may focus more on this, especially if professional and more androgynous in their orientation than women who feel that their uniqueness is lost or that some men may reject them because they cannot give them children. The fear of being barren is particularly great if a woman is young and unmarried at the time of hysterectomy and would like to bear children or feels a potential husband will reject her because she cannot have children. A comparable response may occur with women who are married to men who determine their virility by fathering children to validate their heterosexual orientation and manhood. Finally, a young woman in an unhappy marriage considering a divorce and a remarriage to a more suitable partner may feel her chances are compromised if she is not able to offer a man the possibility of fathering a child (10).

Sexual satisfaction is reported as improved by women undergoing elective sterilization. When difficulty arises, it is usually anticipated by disturbances at initial assessment (9). Tubal ligation is not analogous to the mutilation and irreversible impact of hysterectomy, and the assumption of sterility can be reversed by microsurgical corrective techniques.

Most women have strong emotional bonds to their gynecologists because of the intimacy of discussing gynecologic problems and sexual life and because of the physical examination. This is so even if a gynecologist is a woman, appears aloof, or is not consciously "liked" by the patient. Intimacy alone serves to bond, and choices may be made out of fear or a feeling of vulnerability in a bonded relationship rather than rationally. It is, therefore, all the more imperative that all aspects of an anticipated procedure be presented as objectively as possible and a patient allowed to participate to the greatest degree possible in decisions made.

Early signs of depression that should be discussed with a patient are significant sleep disturbance (difficulty falling asleep, awakening in the middle of the night, and early morning awakening, or the antipode, hypersomnia), appetite and weight disturbance, decreased libido, increased "blues," diurnal variation in mood with feeling worse in the morning, tearfulness, feelings of worthlessness, pessimism about the future, and suicidal thoughts. If a patient does not know if she has lost weight because of failure to have weighed herself, one should ask if her clothes are fitting loosely. A family history of depression, suicide, alcoholism, mania, and bankruptcy (as an indication of mania) suggest vulnerability to affective illness in the face of stress, even if the patient herself has not yet had a depressive episode.

The incidence of depression increases with each decade of life (1). Hysterectomy performed prior to menopause is not at greatest risk for depression under usual circumstances, and a history of depression would be less likely in a premenopausal woman undergoing hysterectomy than in a postmenopausal woman, who may have experienced her first depression at menopause. Women who experience depression at menopause or following the birth of a child would be anticipated to experience another at the time of hysterectomy. This would obviously not be due to loss of opportunity to have children in a postmenopausal woman, since that has already occurred, but rather because of another mutilation of the image of womanhood and because of fear of cancer if the hysterectomy was performed because of the presence of malignancy.

Evaluation of suicidal potential is an integral part of the evaluation of a depression by a physician. Suicide risk is increased in women who have a personal or family history of suicide, are currently depressed, or are divorced, separated, or widowed. Suicide risk is greatest among those with major depression or manic depressive illness, schizoaffective disorder, dysthymic disorder, and borderline personality disorders (11). Other factors increasing suicide risk are a lack of social supports and predominant homosexual orientation (2,4,7).

Loss of a uterus is always ambivalent. As stated earlier, it represents both the end of an era and the ultimate in sexual freedom. A man seldom experiences what a woman does prior to menopause when she becomes aware that she can never again produce a child. Men, even in their 80s and 90s, may father a child with a woman in their reproductive period if they so wish, although the risk of problems increases with age at the time of fatherhood, as it does with women. But a woman after menopause or hysterectomy cannot bear a child—that option has forever perished into time. There is both the feeling of rage at not being able to do so and, in this era of androgyny, some potential for happiness. There is the feeling of freedom, the ability to compete with men without the hindrance of menstruation, and the reality that pregnancy can be avoided without the artificial means of birth control. Some equality with men is ironically achieved at a core level when a woman may elect to have a sexual liaison for pleasure without the fear of pregnancy or the need to avoid it by artificial means. Thus what may appear to be a solely or predominantly negative event is ambivalent, and in this ambivalence exists tension that enhances conflict and anxiety.

The use of groups for women who have undergone hysterectomy, either self-help or more formalized groups, allows women to explore the many facets of such surgery together and to provide support to each other at a time of stress. Women in posthysterectomy groups discuss the issues around hysterectomy, such as their identity as women, fear of occult cancer, and fear—sometimes real—that men may see them as barren and therefore not wish to pursue them as marital partners or wish to divorce them because of their inability to have children. They also discuss the ambivalence. Nothing helps one to understand as much as being understood.

If consequences of surgery do not meet expectations, sensitivity to the possibility of postoperative litigation is particularly required when confronting patients with a past or current history of psychiatric illness or with a family history of affective illness, anxiety disorders, or schizophrenia. Even when indications for surgery and technical skill comport with the highest standards of care, the cost in terms of time and money to establish that fact affects patient, family, and surgeon. Adverse legal consequences are minimized by clear documentation that risks, benefits, and alternatives to surgery were discussed with the patient and family and that the option for consultation with another gynecologist for a second opinion was provided. If a patient is actively psychiatrically ill, concurrent management with a psychiatrist is useful.

In summary, hysterectomy is a complicated procedure, both surgically and psychologically, and responses to it are complex and not always easily predictable. Problems are minimized, however, by exploring preoperatively the risks and benefits of such surgery with women and by allowing them to participate, as they should, in decisions about what is happening to their bodies. Early identification of possible areas of conflict and ambivalence allows patient and gynecologist to develop plans of management that obviate more destructive consequences. All gynecologists should be aware of early signs of depression and know how to evaluate self-destructive potential. Whenever there is doubt as to whether a depression is present or whether suicidal potential is severe, a psychiatrist should be consulted to help manage the case. Management includes both psychotherapy and sociotherapy, in addition to the use of antidepressants when endogenous signs of a depression (e.g., sleep and appetite disturbance) accompany the affective change.

REFERENCES

1. Baker M, Quinkert K: Women's reactions to reproductive problems. *Psychol Reports* 53:159–166, 1983.
2. Blendin KD, Cooper JE: Letter to editor re: The regrets of sterilized women. *Lancet* 2:578–579, 1984.
3. Brokington IF, Martin C, Brown GW, Goldberg D, Margison F: Stress and puerperal psychosis. *Br J Psychiat* 157:331–334, 1990.
4. Byrne P: Psychiatric morbidity in a gynecology clinic: An epidemiologic surgery. *Br J Psychol* 144:28–34, 1984.
5. Klompenhouwer JL, van Hylst AM: Classification of postpartum psychosis: A study of 250 mother and baby admissions in the Netherlands. *Acta Psychiat Scand* 84:255–261, 1991.
6. Lalinec-Michaud M, Engelmann F: Depression and hysterectomy: A prospective study. *Psychosomatics* 7:550–558, 1984.
7. Lieb J, Lipsitch II, Slaby AE: *The Crisis Team*. New York, Harper & Row, 1974.
8. Miller WH, Bloom JD, Resnick MP: Chronic mental illness and perinatal outcome. *Gen Hosp Psychiat* 14:171–176, 1992.
9. Psychological sequelae of female sterilization. *Lancet* 2:144–145, 1984.
10. Renshaw D: Divorce. *Ob Gyn Ann* 13:313–330, 1984.
11. Slaby AE: *Handbook of Psychiatric Emergencies*, ed. 4. Norwalk, CT, Appleton-Lange, 1993.
12. Swales PJ, Shiekh JI: Hysterectomy in patients with panic disorder (Letter to the Editor). *Am J Psychiat* 149:846–847, 1992.
13. Wright AF: letter to editor re: The regrets of sterilized women. *Lancet* 2:578, 1984.

99

Genital Injuries Following Sexual Assault

David Muram

Case Abstract

A 12-year-old girl was brought to the emergency department with complaints of vaginal bleeding, nausea, and vomiting. The patient confided to her physician that she had been sexually assaulted on her way to school that morning, some 12 hours prior to her admission. She had been sexually active for the past 6 months, and was not using any contraceptive method.

The patient was noted to be febrile. The abdomen was diffusely tender, and bowel sounds were diminished. Pelvic examination revealed an attenuated hymen and a small hymenal laceration, which extended onto the perineal skin. A small amount of old blood was noted in the vagina. Inspection of the vagina showed a large vaginal laceration in the posterior fornix, creating a fenestration into the peritoneal cavity. Bowel loops were seen through this opening.

DISCUSSION

The physician treating victims of sexual assault must be versed in counseling and demonstrate empathy for the victim. The patient often feels alienated and unprotected. Whereas family and friends support patients at the time of illness, following rape the patient is often isolated and lonely. This places an extra burden on the staff, since they may be the only people on whom the victim can depend. The patient should be provided with an opportunity to ask questions, and these questions must be answered candidly.

A complete medical history is required for the proper management of the patient. In addition, the examiner should solicit a description of the assault. Although the evaluator should not attempt to assume the role of a police investigator, it is important to obtain a detailed history from the victim. An account of the incident is extremely valuable. It may reveal an unusual area of injury and thus uncommon sites for evidence collection, and in some states an account of the incident found in the medical record may be used in court as evidence.

The primary objective of the physical examination is to attend to the medical needs of the victim. In addition to the specimens collected for the proper medical management of the patient, such as a pregnancy test, the examiner must collect samples to be used by the forensic laboratory. Although collection of evidence is done simultaneously with the examination, it is discussed separately in the last section of this chapter.

The external genitalia and anus should be inspected, and all abnormalities should be noted and diagrammed in the record. The use of a colposcope or other magnifying tools, such as surgical loops, may help detect minor injuries (10,11). The use of

441

toluidine blue has been useful in delineating minor trauma to the vagina as well as minor lacerations in the fossa navicularis and the posterior fourchette (2,4,5). Speculum examination for the thorough inspection of the vagina is necessary in all patients exhibiting signs of penetrating injury. Bimanual abdominopelvic examination then follows to determine the presence or absence of preexisting pelvic pathology, such as gravid uterus or adnexal mass.

Repair of injuries

Many victims do not sustain serious physical injury as a result of the assault, particularly if they have been sexually active prior to the assault. Superficial injuries (bruises, edema, local irritation) resolve within a few days and require no special treatment. Meticulous perineal hygiene is important in the prevention of secondary infections. Sitz baths should be utilized to remove secretions and contaminants. In some patients with extensive skin abrasions, broad-spectrum antibiotics should be given as prophylaxis. Vulvar hematomas often require no treatment. Small hematomas can usually be controlled by pressure with an ice pack, and even massive swelling of the vulva usually subsides promptly when cold packs and external pressure are applied. Occasionally, large hematomas will continue to increase in size and should be incised with the clots removed and bleeding points identified and ligated. Large vulvar tears require suturing. This is best done under anesthesia, using fine absorbable suture material (7,8).

Bite wounds should be irrigated copiously, and necrotic tissue cautiously debrided. A noninfected fresh wound can often be closed primarily, but most bite wounds should be left open. Closure is completed when granulation tissue is formed. After 3 to 5 days, secondary debridement may be required to remove necrotic tissues. Antitetanus immunization should be given if the child is not already immunized. Broad-spectrum antibiotics should be utilized in a therapeutic rather than a prophylactic manner (7,8).

Vulvar and vaginal lacerations often require surgical repair to control bleeding and to approximate the tissues. These can be done using either local or regional anesthetics. Many vaginal lacerations are superficial, limited to the mucosal and submucosal tissues. Such lacerations, if not bleeding, may be left to heal spontaneously. When bleeding is present, hemostasis can be accomplished using fine suture material. Vaginal wall hematomas form when bleeding persists underneath the repaired vaginal mucosa. The internal pressure created by the blood clot often controls the bleeding. If the bleeding continues, the overlying mucosa is incised, the blood clot evacuated, and the bleeding points identified and ligated.

If the laceration extends to the vaginal vault, surgical exploration of the pelvic cavity is necessary to rule out extension into the broad ligament or peritoneal cavity and injuries to intraperitoneal organs. Bladder and bowel integrity must be confirmed by inspection, catheterization, and rectal palpation (8).

In the case described above, the patient was taken to the operating room and the vaginal laceration was repaired. At laparotomy, acute salpingitis was noted. No other intraperitoneal injuries were seen. The postoperative course was unremarkable. However, cervical cultures, which were obtained at the time of surgery, grew *Chlamydia trachomatis*. The patient was treated with doxycyclin, and reported to be well following her discharge.

Collection of Evidence

Although the primary objective of the physical examination is to attend to the medical needs of the victim, the examination has a secondary purpose as well—to collect samples that can later be used as evidence. Whereas specimens collected for the proper medical management of the patient should be collected on all victims, samples for the forensic laboratory should be collected only if the assault occurred within 72 hours from the examination. All specimens collected for forensic purposes must be noted in the record with a description of the location from which they were obtained and any associated findings, such as saliva collected from the patient's neck near a bite mark. All items collected must be individually packaged and clearly labeled, and the containers and envelopes sealed and signed by the examiner. Each label must include the following:

1. Patient identification
2. Specimen
3. Site from which it was collected
4. Date and time collected
5. Examiner's initials

All the specimens must be placed in a container and sealed with a special evidence tape properly labeled, with a routing slip attached. The physician may wish to use commercially available kits specially designed for this purpose. The kit is then given to the police investigator, who signs for it in the record and on the routing slip. All persons handling the materials must sign for it. Such a system is necessary to maintain the chain of evidence; otherwise these specimens may not be admissible in court. If the kit needs to be stored in the physician's office, it must be placed in an inaccessible area, preferably locked, until it can be given to the police investigator or to the forensic laboratory (6,9).

The clothing worn by the patient during the assault is collected and placed in a bag. A description and condition of the clothes should be attached. During the general inspection, all foreign material such as sand, grass, and so on should be removed and placed in clearly labeled envelopes. Scrapings from underneath the fingernails and loose hairs on the skin are collected. A Wood's lamp can be used to detect the presence of seminal fluid on the patient's body because the ultraviolet light causes semen to fluoresce. The stain may be lifted off the skin with moistened cotton swabs for further analysis (1,3).

The specimens required include the following:

1. **General**
Outer and underclothing if worn during or immediately following the assault.
Fingernail scraping.
Dried and moist secretions and foreign material observed on the patient's body. Use Wood's lamp to detect semen.
Oral Cavity
Swabs for semen (11) if within 6 hours of assault.
Culture for gonorrhea (GC) and other sexually transmitted diseases (STDs).
Saliva—for reference.

Genital Area
Dried and moist secretions and foreign material.
Comb public hair. Collect all loose hair and foreign material.
Vaginal swabs (2).
Wet mount.
Dry mount slides (11).
Culture for GC and other STDs.
Anus
Dried and moist secretions and foreign material.
Rectal swabs (11).
Dry mount slides (11).
Culture for GC and other STDs.
Blood
Blood type.
RPR.
Pregnancy test (blood or urine).
Alcohol/toxicology (blood or urine).
Urine
Urinalysis.
Pregnancy test (blood or urine).
Alcohol/toxicology (blood or urine).
Other
Saliva. Use clean gauze or filter paper.
Head hair. Cut and remove.
Pubic hair. Cut and remove.

REFERENCES

1. Aiken MM, Muram D, Keene PR, Mamelli JA: Evidence collection in cases of child abuse: The detection of seminal fluid. *Adolesc Pediatr Gynecol* 6:86–90, 1993.
2. Bays J, Lewman LV: Toluidine blue in the detection at autopsy of perineal and anal lacerations in victims of sexual abuse. *Arch Pathol and Lab Med* 116:620–621, 1992.
3. Gabby T, Winkleby MA, Boyce T, Fisher DL, Lancaster A, Sensabaugh GF, Crim D: Sexual abuse of children: The detection of semen on skin. *AJDC* 146:700–703, 1992.
4. Lauber A, Souma G: The use of toluidine blue for documentation of traumatic intercourse. *Obstet Gynecol* 60:644–648, 1982.
5. McCauley J, Gorman RL, Guzinski G: Toluidine blue in the detection of perineal lacerations in pediatric and adolescent sexual abuse victims. *Pediatrics* 78:1039–1043, 1986.
6. Muram D: Child sexual abuse. *Obstet Gynecol Clin North Am* 19:193–207, 1992.
7. Muram D: Child sexual abuse. In: Sanfilippo J, Muram D, Lee P, Dewhurst JC (eds): *Pediatric and Adolescent Gynecology*. Philadelphia, WB Saunders, 1994, Chap. 23, pp. 365–382.
8. Muram D: Genital tract trauma in pre-pubertal children. *Pediatr Ann.* 15:616–620, 1986.
9. Muram D, Hostetler BR, Jones CE: Adolescent assault. *The Female Patient* 18:54–59, 1993.
10. Norvell MK, Benrubi GI, Thompson RJ: Investigation of microtrauma after sexual intercourse. *J Reprod Med* 29:269–271, 1984.
11. Slaughter L, Brown C: Colposcopic findings in victims of sexual assault. *Am J Obstet Gynecol* 166:83–86, 1992.

Medicolegal Complications Consequent to Unauthorized Surgery

David Landel Nichols
John W. Caldwell

Case Abstract

A 28-year-old nullipara with a history of unilateral salpingectomy 4 years previously for ectopic pregnancy was hospitalized because of moderately severe, crampy, lower abdominal pain and tenderness, accentuated by motion of the cervix. A pregnancy test was positive, and another ectopic pregnancy was suspected. Written operative consent was obtained for "laparoscopy and possible laparotomy," and the patient was taken to surgery the day following admission, where laparoscopy confirmed the presence of an unruptured pregnancy in the remaining tube. Laparotomy was performed, and the tube and uterus were removed, followed by an "incidental" appendectomy.

The postoperative abdomen was distended, but bowel sounds were initially present. By the third postoperative day, the patient was febrile, the abdomen was diffusely painful and tender, and bowel sounds were absent. A diagnosis of peritonitis was established, and at repeat laparotomy it was found that the tie around the appendiceal stump had slipped, and there was full communication between the cecal lumen and the abdominal cavity, with spillage of intestinal contents.

Following appropriate treatment and a long stormy postoperative course, the patient brought suit against her surgeon some months later, alleging grave damages and complaining that no consent had been given for either the hysterectomy or appendectomy.

DISCUSSION

The lion's share of medical malpractice litigation is sparked by a patient complaint familiar to plaintiffs' lawyers: "I would not have let the doctor operate on me had I only known what the risks were!" Though the law of *contracts* is the foundation of the doctor-patient relationship (wherein the doctor agrees to treat the patient, and the patient agrees to pay the doctor for these services), in recent years it has become the law of *torts* that governs informed consent in the United States. A tort is a civil wrong or injury usually done by one person owing a legal duty to another, a breach of that duty, and some type of injury resulting from the breach. Although lack of informed consent has been characterized in some jurisdictions as assault and battery, many states now frame lack of informed consent as medical or professional negligence, actionable as a tort, with no reference to assault and battery.

The doctor-patient relationship has substantially changed over the last 25 years. Whereas once patients deferred to the judgment of their doctors, they now seek a greater role in determining how and by whom they will be treated. As the current national debate on health care continues, it is unlikely that this trend of increased patient involvement in their own medical care will abate.

In its landmark decision in an informed consent case, the District of Columbia Court of Appeals, quoting from an earlier case, stated: "The root premise is the concept, fundamental in American jurisprudence, that "every human being of adult years and sound mind has a right to determine what shall be done with his own body . . ." (1).

In the above abstract, after examination of the patient and review of the laboratory tests, the doctor informed the patient that the probable cause of her abdominal pain and tenderness was an ectopic pregnancy. The patient consented to an exploratory laparoscopy and possible laparotomy to treat the probable ectopic pregnancy. The law of torts came into play when the surgeon removed the appendix and uterus.

Some patients may not have strong feelings about an incidental appendectomy, especially when there are no postoperative complications. It is, however, very unlikely in this day of in vitro fertilization that this nullipara would agree with her surgeon's decision to remove the uterus. If the surgeon had contemplated either of these procedures before the operation, he or she should have disclosed this to the patient with all the other information a valid informed consent requires. Courts have found against doctors in cases like this even when the patient was postmenopause. In a Louisiana case, the patient had complaints of side and stomach pain. Her doctors recommended exploratory abdominal surgery and a colonoscopy. At surgery, three conditions were found, one of which was adhesions of the left fallopian tube and ovary. The surgeon decided to remove both the tube and ovary. The court found that the surgeon exceeded the consent given by the patient, and since the adhesed tube and ovary were not life-threatening, the court ordered the surgeon to pay damages of $1,000 (2).

All surgeons know that the law, with very limited exceptions, requires the informed consent of their patients before they may operate. States are divided into two main groups in developing standards for what doctors are required to tell their patients in order to obtain a valid consent. Some states have statutes which indicate the disclosure standard. In most states, however, it has been the courts which have determined the controlling disclosure standard.

The older standard, often called the professional community standard, requires a doctor to disclose to the patient that information which a reasonable medical practitioner would disclose under the same or similar circumstances. In other words, a doctor's duty to disclose information adequate for informed consent is determined by other health care professionals. Nearly half of the states follow some variation of this standard. For a patient to prevail in a lawsuit for failure to obtain informed consent under this standard, the patient would have to provide the court with testimony from a medical expert that the treating doctor had failed to disclose sufficient information to the patient.

The newer standard, adopted by more than twenty states, is patient-based. Here a doctor must disclose any information which a reasonable patient would want to know before deciding to submit to the proposed treatment. In a lawsuit, this standard generally relieves the patient of producing the testimony of a medical expert on the issue of informed consent. Many of the "reasonable patient" states, however, require that the patient prove not only that the doctor provided insufficient information for informed consent, but also that she would have withheld her consent if the undisclosed information had been provided.

In 1977, Texas, a state that has adopted the reasonable patient standard, established a medical disclosure panel consisting of six physicians and three lawyers. The panel's statutory duty is to identify procedures that require the disclosure of risks and those that do not. The panel reviews the two lists annually. Failure to comply with the disclosure requirements of the published lists creates a rebuttable presumption that the doctor negligently failed to comply with disclosure standards. Compliance with the lists creates a rebuttable presumption that sufficient information was disclosed to the patient. In cases where the panel has not determined a duty of disclosure, the Texas statute appears to invoke the reasonable patient standard (4).

Although the law may vary from state to state, informed consent generally requires that a surgeon disclose to the patient the following information before surgery:

1. Diagnosis
2. Proposed treatment, including its risks and probable results
3. Alternative treatments, including their risks
4. Prognosis if treatment is not accepted

The information should also include the names of the physicians who will perform the proposed procedure. Risks include more than undesired results but also known consequences. For example, sterility is a known consequence, not a hazard, of a hysterectomy.

In his scholarly analysis of disclosure standards, McCallum suggests that risk disclosure is advisable when the probability of maloccurrence exceeds 1%. He goes on to say that "even more remote contingencies should be disclosed if the result is extreme in comparison to the elective nature of the surgery" (3).

When a patient claims that the physician performed some procedure without the patient's consent, the burden generally shifts to the physician to show that a valid consent was obtained or not needed. A witnessed, written consent form is the best evidence of informed consent. The form should indicate that the witness not only saw the signing of the consent form but also heard the physician provide the listed information to the patient. In an effort to avoid litigation over the issue of informed consent, some physicians have tried to use blanket consent forms in which the patient defers to the judgment and skills of the physician. Courts have been reluctant to validate the use of "carte blanche" consent forms. Courts will view with more favorable inferences a consent form that is specific and tailored to an individual patient and the proposed treatment.

The law recognizes a limited number of exceptions to the disclosure requirements cited above. Though an extensive discussion of them would exceed the scope of this chapter, the two exceptions most commonly utilized are worth mentioning: emergencies and therapeutic treatment. An emergency is generally when the patient's life or serious impairment is at risk. Even in emergency cases, the physician should try to obtain consent from the patient or someone who is authorized to consent on behalf of the patient. When consent is impossible and a true emergency exists, the law generally presumes consent. It does not, however, authorize the physician to go beyond that treatment which is necessary to avoid the life-threatening situation or threat of serious impairment; and irrespective of the treatment, the patient must be fully informed later of what transpired.

The therapeutic exception recognizes that some patients may become so emotionally ill when medical information is disclosed that disclosure forecloses rational thought or poses serious psychological harm to the patient. In these situations, the physician may choose not to volunteer to disclose, although he or she may not lie to a direct question; nor may the physician withhold information just because the patient may choose not to follow his or her advice.

The use of specially tailored, written consent forms accomplishes two purposes. These forms record exactly what the physician told the patient before the treatment. Of course, this may be a two-edged sword in those cases where the physician provided inadequate information to the patient. The form also serves as a checklist to remind the physician what information needs to be provided. Physicians, like lawyers, often speak a language which is foreign to their patients. It is of great importance that the physician explain everything in language which a layperson can understand. Good medical practice makes no allowance for misunderstandings.

Although the law differs from state to state, the general principles discussed above serve as an overview and starting point. The recommended practice is to disclose, in addition to any information required by a state's statute or medical board, any information which may affect a reasonable person's decision to undergo treatment.

Recommended Surgical Resolution of Factual Hypothetical

The *surgical* problem in this case relates to peritonitis resulting from fecal leakage from the cecum after slippage of an appendiceal tie. This might have been prevented by double ligature of the appendiceal stump. Similar leakage can develop from intestinal perforation by necrosis following spillage from phenol used to "cauterize" the appendiceal or tubal stump. For this reason, the editors long ago abandoned the routine use of phenol and alcohol for this purpose, substituting local swabbing with povidone-iodine (Betadine). Once the catastrophe was recognized in the patient described above, the proper treatment was laparotomy with religation of the stump, drainage, and the general intensive supportive treatment of peritonitis. (Ed.)

REFERENCES

1. Canterbury v. Spence, 464 F.2d 772 (D.C. Cir. 1972).
2. Guin v. Sison, 552 So.2d 60 (La. Ct. App. 1989).
3. McCallum RD: Gynecological errors and medical malpractice. In: JH Ridley (ed): *Gynecologic Surgery*, ed. 2. Baltimore, Williams & Wilkins, 1981.
4. Tex. Rev. Civ. Stat. Ann. art 4590i §§ 6.01–6.07 (Vernon 1993).

INDEX